RC280.B8 H878 2018eb
08006341
HER2-Positive Breast Cancer

HER2-Positive
Breast Cancer

HER2-Positive Breast Cancer

SARA HURVITZ, MD
Division of Hematology/Oncology
David Geffen School of Medicine
University of California, Los Angeles

KELLY MCCANN, MD, PHD
Division of Hematology/Oncology
David Geffen School of Medicine
University of California, Los Angeles

ELSEVIER

ELSEVIER

3251 Riverport Lane
St. Louis, Missouri 63043

HER2-POSITIVE BREAST CANCER ISBN: 978-0-323-58122-6

Content Strategist: Robin Carter
Content Development Manager: Christine McElvenny
Content Development Specialist: Jennifer Horigan
Publishing Services Manager: Deepthi Unni
Project Manager: Janish Ashwin Paul
Designer: Gopalakrishnan Venkatraman

Printed in United States of America

Last digit is the print number: 9 8 7 6 5 4 3 2 1

I dedicate this book to my mother, Beth, whose optimism and humor in the face of her own battle with breast cancer is an inspiration to me and my patients.

List of Contributors

Dennis J. Slamon, MD, PhD
Professor of Medicine
Department of Medicine
Division of Hematology and Oncology
David Geffen School of Medicine
Jonsson Comprehensive Cancer Center
University of California Los Angeles
Los Angeles, CA, USA

Kelly E. McCann, MD, PhD
Health Sciences Clinical Instructor
Department of Medicine
Division of Hematology and Oncology
David Geffen School of Medicine
Jonsson Comprehensive Cancer Center
University of California Los Angeles
Los Angeles, CA, USA

Yanling Ma, MD, MS
Associate Professor of Pathology
Department of Surgical Pathology
Keck School of Medicine
University of Southern California
Los Angeles County and USC Medical Center
Los Angeles, CA, USA

Michael F. Press, MD, PhD
Harold E. Lee Chair in Cancer Research
Professor of Pathology
Department of Surgical Pathology
Keck School of Medicine
Norris Comprehensive Cancer Center
University of Southern California
Los Angeles, CA, USA

Mahdi Khoshchehreh, MD, MS
Resident Physician in Anatomic and Clinical Pathology
Department of Surgical Pathology
Keck School of Medicine
University of Southern California
Los Angeles, CA, USA

Grace Namjung Kim, MD
Assistant Professor of Pathology
Department of Surgical Pathology
Keck School of Medicine
University of Southern California
Los Angeles, CA, USA

Melody Cobleigh, MD
Associate Professor of Medicine
Department of Internal Medicine
Division of Hematology
Oncology and Cell Therapy
Rush University Medical Center
Chicago, IL, USA

Ruta Rao, MD
Associate Professor of Medicine
Department of Internal Medicine
Division of Hematology, Oncology and Cell Therapy
Rush University Medical Center
Chicago, IL, USA

Sarah Sammons, MD
Department of Medicine
Division of Hematology/Oncology
Duke Cancer Institute
Duke University
Durham, NC, USA

Kimberly Blackwell, MD
Professor of Medicine
Department of Medicine
Division of Hematology/Oncology
Duke Cancer Institute
Duke University
Durham, NC, USA

Nancy U. Lin, MD
Associate Professor of Medicine
Medical Oncology
Dana-Farber Cancer Institute
Boston, MA, USA

José Pablo Leone, MD
Instructor in Medicine
Department of Medicine
Division of Medical Oncology
Harvard Medical School
Dana-Farber Cancer Institute
Boston, MA, USA

Ayal A. Aizer, MD, MHS
Instructor in Radiation Oncology
Radiation Oncology
Dana-Farber Cancer Institute
Boston, MA, USA

Peter A. Fasching, MD
Professor
Comprehensive Cancer Center Erlangen-EMN
University Hospital Erlangen
Department of Gynecology and Obstetrics
Erlangen, Bavaria, Germany

Michael Untch, MD, PhD
Prof Dr Gynecology and Obstetrics
Helios Klinikum Berlin Buch
Berlin, Germany

Mohammad Jahanzeb, MD, FACP
Professor of Clinical Medicine
Hematology-Oncology
Medical Director
U Sylvester Deerfield Campus
Associate Center Director for Community Outreach
    Sylvester Comprehensive Cancer Center University
    of Miami
Miller School of Medicine
FL, USA

Reshma Mahtani, DO
Assistant Professor of Medicine
Sylvester Cancer Center
University of Miami
Deerfield Beach, FL, USA

Ana Cristina Sandoval-Leon, MD
Breast Oncology Fellow
Department of Medicine
Division of Medical Oncology
Sylvester Comprehensive Cancer Center
University of Miami
Miami, FL, USA

Javier Cortes, MD, PhD
Dr. Medical Oncology
Ramon y Cajal University Hospital
Madrid, Spain

Vall d'Hebron Institute of Oncology (VHIO)
Barcelona, Spain

IOB Institute of Oncology, Quironsalud Group
Madrid & Barcelona, Spain

Debora de Melo Gagliato, MD
Assistant Physician
Clinical Oncology
Hospital Sirio Libanes
Sao Paulo, Brazil

Sara M. Tolaney, MD, MPH
Associate Director
Clinical Research
Breast Oncology
Susan F. Smith Center for Women's Cancers
Dana-Farber Cancer Institute
Boston, MA, USA
Assistant Professor of Medicine
Department of Medicine
Division of Medical Oncology
Harvard Medical School
Boston, MA, USA

Romualdo Barroso-Sousa, MD, PhD
Clinical Fellow
Department of Medicine
Division of Hematology/Oncology
Dana-Farber Cancer Institute
Boston, MA, USA

Eric H. Yang, MD
Assistant Clinical Professor of Medicine
Department of Medicine
Division of Cardiology
David Geffen School of Medicine
University of California Los Angeles
Los Angeles, CA, USA

Aashini Master, DO
Assistant Professor of Medicine
Department of Medicine
Division of Hematology and Oncology
David Geffen School of Medicine
Jonsson Comprehensive Cancer Center
University of California Los Angeles
Los Angeles, CA, USA

Ruth M. O'Regan, MD
Chief
Division of Hematology Oncology
Medicine
University of Wisconsin
Madison, WI, USA

Marina N. Sharifi, MD, PhD
Oncology Fellow
Department of Medicine, Division of Hematology and
    Oncology
University of Wisconsin Madison
Madison, WI, USA

Mary L. (Nora) Disis, MD

William R. Gwin, III, MD
Acting Instructor
Medicine
University of Washington
Seattle, WA, USA

Hope S. Rugo, MD
Professor of Medicine
Director, Breast Oncology and Clinical Trials Education
Medicine
University of California San Francisco Comprehensive
    Cancer Center
San Francisco, CA, USA

Mirela Tuzovic, MD
Cardiovascular Fellow
UCLA Cardio-Oncology Program
Division of Cardiology
Department of Medicine
University of California at Los Angeles
Los Angeles, CA, USA

Megha Agarwal, MD
Assistant Clinical Professor of Medicine
UCLA Cardio-Oncology Program
Division of Cardiology
Department of Medicine
University of California at Los Angeles
Los Angeles, CA, USA

Nidhi Thareja, MD
Assistant Clinical Professor of Medicine
UCLA Cardio-Oncology Program
Division of Cardiology
Department of Medicine
University of California at Los Angeles
Los Angeles, CA, USA

Preface

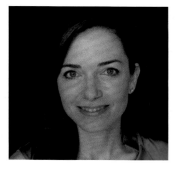

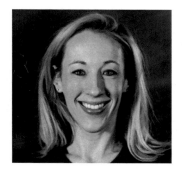

Sara A. Hurvitz, MD

Associate Professor of Medicine, Department of Medicine, Division of Hematology/Oncology, David Geffen School of Medicine at the University of California Los Angeles, Los Angeles, CA.

Kelly E. McCann, MD, PhD

Health Sciences Clinical Instructor, Department of Medicine, Division of Hematology/Oncology, David Geffen School of Medicine at the University of California Los Angeles, Los Angeles, CA.

In the span of a few decades, HER2+ breast cancer has been transformed from a disease with a terrible prognosis to one with a wealth of treatment options and an outcome that is now similar to or better than that associated with HER2-negative breast cancer. Although HER2+ breast cancer is still considered an aggressive cancer, it is a targetable one thanks to the development of HER2-directed therapies and optimized combination strategies. We open this text with discussions of HER2 biology, an understanding of which is essential for drug development, followed by controversies in HER2 testing of tumor tissue. Next we discuss treatments for inoperable and metastatic HER2+ disease, including optimal first-line treatments, options for second-line therapy and beyond, and management of metastatic disease in the central nervous system, an increasingly common problem in our patient population as we have made gains in long-term control of systemic disease. Naturally, significant advances in drug therapies in the metastatic setting

move on to evaluation in the curative setting, but here the strategies differ widely based on drug approvals, stage, hormone receptor status, and the preferences of patients and healthcare providers. Neoadjuvant (preoperative) approaches utilizing pathologic complete response as a surrogate marker for longer-term outcomes has allowed more rapid advances in HER2-targeted approaches for early-stage disease. In the curative setting, it is crucial to consider the consequences of our therapies; in Section 4, we give consideration to cardiac and noncardiac toxicities of HER2-targeted therapies. De-escalation strategies for patients with early-stage and hormone-receptor positive HER2+ cancers are an attempt to optimize the risks and benefits of cytotoxic and HER2-targeted medications. Finally, we explore therapies on the horizon, including kinase inhibitors, antibody-drug conjugates, immunotherapies, and trastuzumab biosimilars.

Acknowledgements

We would like to acknowledge the women whose courageous participation in clinical trials has advanced the treatment of HER2-positive breast cancer for future generations.

Contents

CHAPTER 1

The Molecular Biology of HER2 and HER2-Targeted Therapies

KELLY E. MCCANN, MD, PHD • DENNIS J. SLAMON, MD, PHD

DISCOVERY OF THE ONCOGENE *erbB*

Our current understanding of the molecular biology of cancer began with the idea that cancer might be an infectious disease. As Louis Pasteur and Robert Koch uncovered the agents responsible for cholera, tuberculosis, cholera, and anthrax in the late 19th century, cancer was also thought by some to be a transmissible disease based on experiments in which tumors were explanted from one animal and successfully implanted in another of the same species.[1,2] Peyton Rous discovered that finely filtered, cell-free tumor extracts from Plymouth Rock chicken sarcomas were capable of inducing sarcomas in hens of the same breed and correctly determined that the agent responsible must be viral in nature.[3,4] The virus, eventually named the Rous Sarcoma Virus (RSV), is a single-stranded RNA retrovirus that is reverse-transcribed into DNA, integrates into the host genome, and replicates using the host's transcription and translation machinery to create new RNA viruses in capsid packages.[5] Decades after Peyton Rous's publications, RSV was found to be capable of transforming chicken embryo fibroblasts in petri dishes into cells with characteristics of sarcoma tumor samples: change in morphology from spindle-shaped to round, rapid growth, loss of contact inhibition, and immortality.[6] Of the four genes in RSV's genome, the transforming agent was found to be the one gene not involved in viral replication and was given the name *src*.[7]

Although DNA was shown to be the carrier molecule for the transforming information underlying the malignant phenotype in 1944, genetic analysis was limited to simple viral genomes until the middle of the 1970s. By the late 1970s, advances in molecular biology as well as gene cloning and sequencing made it feasible to study more complex genomes. Using a radio-labelled *src* DNA probe, Michael Bishop and Harold Varmus were surprised to discover that the *src* gene was native to the normal chicken genome.[8] In its accidental development as a cancer-causing virus, RSV had randomly integrated into the chicken genome near *src* and incorporated the *src* coding RNA into its virus particles.[9] Given that *src* is known to be a critical signaling tyrosine kinase that promotes cell growth and differentiation, inappropriate expression of *src* carried into cells by RSV was capable of transforming normal cells into potentially tumorigenic ones.[10]

This work inspired additional searches for retroviruses with co-opted host oncogenes and the discovery of genes such as *myc*, *abl*, *ras*, and *raf*. *Kit* was found in the Hardy-Zuckerman feline sarcoma virus in a cat with sarcoma. *Abl* was found in the Abelson murine leukemia virus causing pre-B-cell lymphoma in a mouse. *ErbB* was found in a chicken with erythroleukemia caused by the avian erythroblastosis ES4 retrovirus, and related gene *neu* was found in the neuroblastomas and glioblastomas of rats treated with the mutagen ethylnitrosourea.[11, 12] As with *src*, expression of these genes can be oncogenic under circumstances of constitutive protein activation, but they otherwise fulfill roles in normal cellular proliferation, differentiation, and survival functions.

ErbB2/HER2/NEU GENE AMPLIFICATION IN HUMAN BREAST CANCER

Interestingly, almost all of the proto-oncogenes co-opted by retroviruses were found to be highly conserved among invertebrate and vertebrate species, including *Homo sapiens*. Four slightly different versions of the *erbB* gene were eventually discovered in humans in the 1980s and 1990s, and *erbB2* and *neu* were found to be the same gene. *ErbB2* was found to be increased in copy number in some human gastric and breast cancers. In 1987, we published the initial finding that 20%–25% of breast cancer patients had tumors with amplification of the *erbB2* oncogene (now known more commonly as *HER2* for human epidermal growth factor receptor 2) and that these malignancies had a dramatically poorer prognosis than those without *HER2* amplification (Fig. 1.1). Patients with *HER2* amplification had a median survival of 3 years compared with 6–7 years if *HER2* was not amplified.[13]

The *HER2* gene is located on the long arm of chromosome 17 (17q), and its genetic amplification is a consequence of aberrant replication of a segment of 17q encompassing multiple genes.[14] The molecular mechanisms underlying *HER2* gene amplification remain an active area of research. It has been hypothesized that unusually large areas of DNA sequence repeats on either side of *HER2* may form secondary structures during DNA replication, resulting in collapse of the replication fork with formation of DNA double-strand breaks, thus resulting in DNA repair processes that duplicate the HER2 gene.[15] Interestingly, having multiple copies of chromosome 17 (polysomy 17) as a result of aneuploidy in cancer cells does not seem to result in overexpression of *HER2* by mRNA or protein analysis.[16] The pathologic overexpression of the gene product seems to be restricted to those tumors containing HER2 amplification.[17]

HER2 IS A TYROSINE KINASE RECEPTOR

As stated earlier, HER2 is one of four transmembrane type I tyrosine kinase receptors in the ErbB family, which also includes EGFR (HER1), HER3, and HER4.[18] HER2 shares homology with other ErbB members in having four extracellular domains, a helical transmembrane domain, an intracellular tyrosine kinase catalytic domain, and conserved phosphotyrosine residues at the C-terminus (Fig. 1.2), but HER2's baseline protein conformation is fundamentally different.[19] EGFR, HER3, and HER4 are receptors anchored within the cell membrane in an inactive monomeric form with extracellular subdomains II and IV tethered together (Fig. 1.3).[20–22] On ligand binding, each of these three types of receptors undergoes a conformational change to an open state that exposes binding sites for dimerization with a second ErbB receptor protein. ErbB homo- and heterodimerization result in phosphorylation of C-terminal tyrosine residues. These sites serve as docking sites for adapter proteins mediating downstream intracellular signaling through the MAP kinase RAS/RAF/MEK/ERK, JAK/STAT, and PI3K/AKT/mTOR pathways (Fig. 1.4).[23,24]

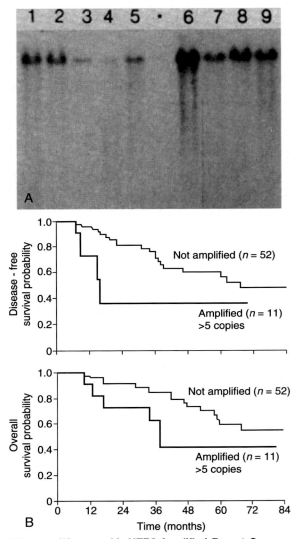

FIG. 1.1 **Women with *HER2*-Amplified Breast Cancers Were Found to Have a Poorer Prognosis than Those Without *HER2* Gene Amplification.** **(A).** Using Southern blot analysis with a radiolabeled HER2 DNA probe, HER2 gene copy number was determined in 189 breast tumor samples. In this representative Southern blot, samples 3 and 4 have a single copy of HER2, samples 1, 2, 5, 7, and 9 have 2–5 copies, and tumors 6 and 8 have 5–20 copies. **(B).** Node-positive patients with >5 copies of the HER2 gene were found to have poorer disease-free survival and overall survival on Kaplan-Meier analysis. (Adapted from Figs. 1 and 3 in Slamon DJ, et al. Human breast cancer: correlation with relapse and survival with amplification of the HER-2/*neu* oncogene. *Science* 1987;235 (4785):177–182 by permission.)

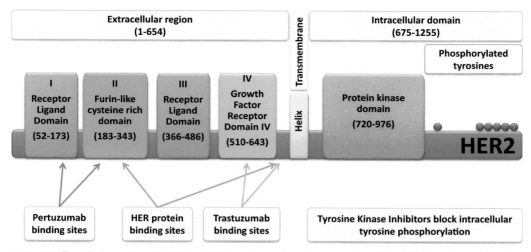

FIG. 1.2 **Protein Domains of HER2.** HER2 has four extracellular domains. Other ErbB family proteins bind to extracellular domain II and a region near extracellular domain IV, the antibody pertuzumab binds to extracellular domains I and II, and the antigen for trastuzumab is located in and C-terminal to domain IV.[18,37] Tyrosine kinase inhibitors such as lapatinib and neratinib interfere with intracellular protein kinase activity.[60]

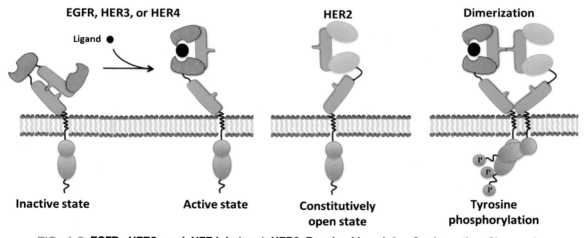

FIG. 1.3 **EGFR, HER3, and HER4 but not HER2 Require Ligand for Conformation Change for Dimerization.** EGFR, HER3, and HER4 undergo a ligand-activated conformational change to adopt an open conformation for dimerization. HER2 rests in the open conformation independently of ligand, thus being immediately available for dimerization with other ErbB family members. (Adapted from Marchini C, et al., under creative commons 3.0 license.[60])

More than 10 soluble protein ligands have been identified for the ErbB family of receptors, but HER2 itself neither needs a ligand for activation nor has it been shown to bind one. Unlike the other three family members, HER2 rests in the open conformation at baseline.[25,26] This has important implications for normal cell function and for oncogenic transformation. HER2 is the preferred binding partner for other ErbB proteins due to a constitutively open protein state that facilitates homodimerization with other HER2 proteins or heterodimerization with ligand-activated EGFR, HER3, or HER4 (Fig. 1.3).[27–29]

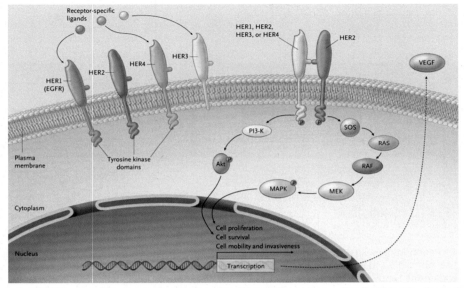

FIG. 1.4 **ErbB Family of Transmembrane Tyrosine Kinase Receptors.**   The ErbB family of proteins are tyrosine kinase receptors. HER2 does not have a known ligand, and HER3 lacks an intracellular tyrosine kinase domain. Dimerization of HER2 with EGFR (HER1), a second HER2 protein, HER3, or HER4 results in activating autophosphorylation of the tyrosine residues on the intracellular kinase domains of the receptors. The activation signal is carried downstream via the PI3K/AKT and Ras/Raf/MEK pathways. *Akt*, Ak strain transforming; *MAPK*, mitogen-activated protein kinase; *MEK*, MAPK/ERK kinase; *PI3-K*, phosphatidylinositol-3 kinase; *Raf*, rapidly accelerated fibrosarcoma; *Ras*, rat sarcoma; *VEGF*, vascular endothelial growth factor. (Used with permission from Hudis CA. N Engl J Med 2007; 357:39–51.[61,67])

Because intracellular pathways downstream of ErbB receptors culminate in the expression of proteins involved in cell growth, proliferation, survival, and migration, they are indispensable for normal cellular functions but can also play a direct role in oncogenesis if inappropriately or constitutively activated. HER2 is involved in epithelial cell differentiation and migration during embryogenesis and breast development during puberty and may play a role in cardiac development based on HER2 knockout mouse models.[30–32] Overexpression of HER2 on the cell surface can result in spontaneous homodimerization and thus activation of the ErbB intracellular tyrosine kinase signaling pathway without the necessity of a ligand.[33]

DRUGS TARGETING PATHOLOGIC HER2 SIGNALING

HER2 gene amplification has been described in numerous cancers, including gastric, esophageal, ovarian, endometrial, lung, and bladder malignancies and is estimated to be amplified in 20%–25% of breast cancers, making HER2 an attractive target for antineoplastic therapies.[34,35] The five Food and Drug Administration (FDA)-approved HER2-targeted therapies and their FDA-approved indications are presented in Table 1.1, and a timeline for their approval is presented in Fig. 1.5.

Trastuzumab and pertuzumab are IgG1 monoclonal antibodies directed against the extracellular domain of HER2. Trastuzumab binds to extracellular subdomain IV, and pertuzumab binds to the ligand-binding extracellular subdomain I and dimerization domain II (Fig. 1.2).[19] Trastuzumab was developed in the 1990s and was initially FDA-approved in 1998 in combination with chemotherapy or as a monotherapy depending on the clinical scenario.[36] Pertuzumab's first FDA-approved indication was attained in 2012; thus far, pertuzumab has only been FDA-approved to be used in combination with trastuzumab and a taxane-based chemotherapy regimen.[37] Because clinical trials have shown that the addition of pertuzumab to trastuzumab-based therapy further improves clinical efficacy, the mechanisms underlying this synergy are an active area of basic science research in an effort to understand HER2 biology.[38] In addition to interfering

TABLE 1.1
FDA-Approved HER2 Inhibitors

HER2 Inhibitor	Target	Mechanism of Action	FDA-Approved Indications for HER2+ Breast Cancer	Toxicities	Resistance
Trastuzumab (Herceptin)	Recombinant humanized IgG1 monoclonal antibody to the extracellular domain (subdomain IV) of HER2	<ul><li>Downregulation of HER2 receptor expression</li><li>Inhibition of HER2 dimerization</li><li>Inhibition of cleavage of the extracellular domain</li><li>Inhibition of HER2-mediated intracellular signaling pathways</li><li>Induction of cell apoptosis through undetermined mechanisms</li><li>Immunologic mechanisms via ADCC and complement-mediated cell lysis</li></ul>	**Early stage**<ul><li>Neoadjuvant or adjuvant therapy in combination with chemotherapy +/− pertuzumab</li></ul>**Metastatic**<ul><li>1st line in combination with paclitaxel +/− pertuzumab</li><li>2nd or 3rd line as a single agent</li></ul>	<ul><li>**Cardiotoxicity** (subclinical and clinical decrease in LV EF, arrhythmia, HTN)<ul><li>Must monitor LV EF prior to and during treatment. Withhold if >16% absolute decrease from baseline LV EF.</li></ul></li><li>**Infusion reactions** (discontinue if anaphylaxis, angioedema, interstitial pneumonitis, ARDS)</li><li>**Embryo-fetal toxicity** (oligohydramnios, pulmonary hypoplasia, neonatal death)</li><li>**Pulmonary toxicity** (increased cough, dyspnea, rhinitis, sinusitis)</li><li>**GI toxicity**, including nausea, vomiting, and diarrhea</li></ul>	<ul><li>Mutations in extracellular HER2 domain causing decreased binding affinity to trastuzumab</li><li>Decreased expression of HER2</li><li>Expression of p95HER2, a truncated form of the receptor with loss of extracellular domain</li><li>Activation of alternative growth factor receptor pathways, such as IGFR1, estrogen receptor, and MET receptor</li><li>Activating mutations in intracellular signaling proteins, such as PI3K</li></ul>

Continued

TABLE 1.1
FDA-Approved HER2 Inhibitors

HER2 Inhibitor	Target	Mechanism of Action	FDA-Approved Indications for HER2+ Breast Cancer	Toxicities	Resistance
Pertuzumab (Perjeta)	Recombinant humanized IgG1 monoclonal antibody against the extracellular dimerization domain (subdomain II) of HER2	• Inhibits heterodimerization of HER2 with other ErbB family members (EGFR, HER3, HER4) • Immunologic mechanisms such as ADCC	**Early stage** • Neoadjuvant or adjuvant therapy in combination with trastuzumab and chemotherapy **Metastatic** • In combination with trastuzumab + docetaxel in the first-line metastatic setting	• **Cardiotoxicity** (subclinical and clinical decrease in LV EF, arrhythmia, HTN) ○ Must hold if drop in LV EF <40% or LV EF 40%−45% with a 10% or more absolute reduction from baseline • **Infusion reactions** (discontinue if anaphylaxis, angioedema, interstitial pneumonitis, ARDS) • **GI toxicities** (nausea, vomiting, diarrhea) • **Embryo-fetal toxicity** (birth defects, neonatal death)	• Mutations in extracellular HER2 leading to decreased binding affinity to pertuzumab • Decreased expression of HER2 • Increased expression of ErbB family members (EGFR, HER3) • Activation of alternative growth factor receptor signaling pathways
Ado-trastuzumab emtansine (Kadcyla)	ADC with trastuzumab chemically conjugated to emtansine (DM1)	• ADC is internalized by HER2+ cancer cells by receptor-mediated endocytosis with release of the potent antimicrotubule agent emtansine in the lysosomal compartment • Inhibition of HER2-mediated intracellular signaling • Immunologic mechanisms such as ADCC	**Metastatic** • 1st line if disease recurrence within 6 months of completing adjuvant HER2-directed therapy • 2nd line after prior trastuzumab and/or taxane-based chemotherapy	• **Cardiotoxicity** (subclinical and clinical decrease in LV EF, arrhythmia, HTN) ○ Must hold if drop in LV EF <40% or LV EF 40%−45% with a 10% or more absolute reduction from baseline • **Infusion reactions** • **Hepatotoxicity** with LFT elevation (transient) • **Pulmonary toxicity** (increased cough, dyspnea, rhinitis, sinusitis) • **Neurotoxicity** (peripheral sensory neuropathy) • **Fatigue**	• Mutations in extracellular HER2 domain causing decreased binding affinity to trastuzumab • Decreased expression of HER2

Drug	Mechanism	Indication	Toxicities / Warnings	Resistance
Lapatinib (Tyverb)	Small molecule inhibitor of EGFR and HER2 tyrosine kinase activity; reversible ATP competitor	**Metastatic** • In combination with capecitabine	• **Contraindicated in patients with liver failure** • **Drug-drug interactions** ◦ Metabolized by CYP3A4 and CYP3A5; use with caution in patients on warfarin • **Cardiac toxicity** secondary to mitochondrial dysfunction in cardiomyocytes (decrease in LV EF, arrhythmia) ◦ Cardiac function monitoring with echo for LV EF ◦ EKG monitoring for QTc prolongation • **Myelosuppression** • **Dermatological toxicity** (rash, hand-foot syndrome) • **GI toxicity** (diarrhea common) • **Loss of appetite** • **Fatigue**	• Genetic mutations that decrease binding • Activation of alternative growth factor signaling pathway, such as estrogen-receptor signaling
Neratinib (Nerlynx)	Small molecule inhibitor of EGFR, HER2, HER3, HER4 tyrosine kinase activity; covalently binds to the intracellular domain; irreversible	**Early stage** • Adjuvant therapy after completion of HER2-directed chemo-therapy and trastuzumab ×1 year	• **GI toxicity** (diarrhea in 95%, nausea, vomiting) ◦ Loperamide prophylaxis advised per package insert • **Loss of appetite** • **Fatigue** • **Hepatotoxicity** ◦ Dose adjustment required in severe liver failure	• Genetic mutations abrogating binding of neratinib to the intracellular domain

Standard dosing of therapies is as follows:

• Trastuzumab loading dose of 4 mg/kg IV followed by maintenance dose 2 mg/kg IV weekly or 8 mg/kg IV loading dose with maintenance dose 6 mg/kg every 3 weeks

• Pertuzumab loading dose 840 mg IV followed by maintenance dose of 420 IV every 3 weeks.

• Ado-trastuzumab emtansine 3.6 mg/kg IV every 3 weeks

• Lapatinib 1250 mg by mouth daily (absorption increased with food) in combination with capecitabine or lapatinib 1500 mg by mouth daily in combination with letrozole

• Neratinib 240 mg by mouth daily with food

ADC, antibody-drug conjugate; *ADCC*, antibody-dependent cellular cytotoxicity; *EKG*, electrocardiogram; *IGFR1*, insulin-like growth factor receptor I; *LV EF*, left ventricular ejection fraction.

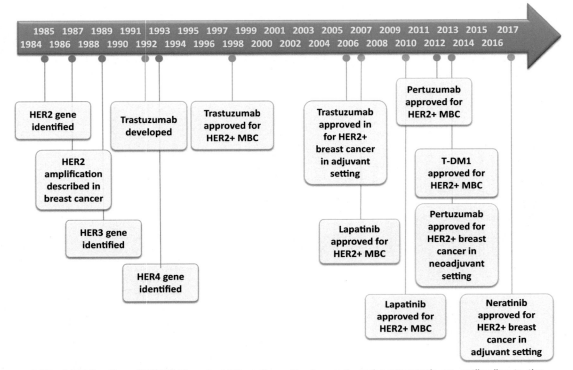

FIG. 1.5 **Timeline of HER2-Targeted Therapies.** Trastuzumab and pertuzumab are antibodies to the extracellular domain of HER2. Lapatinib and neratinib are small molecule tyrosine kinase inhibitors. T-DM1 is an antibody-drug conjugate of trastuzumab linked to microtubule inhibitor emtansine. *MBC,* metastatic breast cancer.

with homo- and heterodimerization and thus intracellular signaling pathways, the HER2-targeted antibodies have also been shown to engage the immune system in vitro and in murine models.[39–41] The mechanism by which antibody binds to the cell surface and recruits immune cells is called antibody-dependent cell cytotoxicity (ADCC).

Ado-trastuzumab emtansine (T-DM1) is an antibody drug conjugate resulting from trastuzumab attached to a potent microtubule inhibitor by a chemical linker.[42] T-DM1 is internalized by HER2+ cancer cells by endocytosis. After internalization, the chemical linker is cleaved in the lysosome, and emtansine is released into the cell to impede replication by binding to tubulin. T-DM1 is approved in the HER2+ metastatic breast cancer as monotherapy.[43]

Small molecule tyrosine HER2 receptor kinase inhibitors (TKIs) act on the intracellular kinase domain to disrupt autophosphorylation. Most TKIs inhibit multiple tyrosine kinases rather than being specific for one TKI. The first FDA-approved TKI was imatinib for CML

in 2001.[44] In addition to inhibition of the BCR-ABL fusion protein in CML, imatinib inhibits the c-KIT kinase in gastrointestinal stromal tumors (GISTs) and platelet-derived growth factor receptor (against which it was first developed).[45] The efficacy of an EGFR-inhibiting TKI, gefitinib, was described in a subset of non–small cell lung cancer patients in 2003 and later found to be those with mutations conferring a constitutive activation of EGFR in 2004, namely L858R and exon 19 deletion mutations of HER1.[46-49]

Two tyrosine kinase inhibitors have been approved for HER2+ breast cancer. Lapatinib is a tyrosine kinase inhibitor that disrupts the activity of EGFR and HER2 by competitively binding at the ATP-binding pocket in the catalytic kinase domain.[50] Neratinib is a pan-HER inhibitor that covalently binds the intracellular domain and is thus irreversible.[51] Lapatinib was FDA-approved in 2007 in the metastatic setting in combination with capecitabine and in 2010 in combination with letrozole for HER2+, hormone receptor–positive breast cancer patients.[50] Tucatinib is a more recent kinase inhibitor in late-stage clinical development that specifically targets the HER2 kinase.[52]

Interestingly, with the advent of whole exome sequencing for oncogenic driver mutations in tumor samples, HER2 activating mutations have also been found in *HER2*'s tyrosine kinase domain and the extracellular domain, although it is *HER2* gene amplification that drives the majority of HER2+ breast cancers. Activating point mutations, small insertions, and deletions result in increased protein signaling but not in increased expression and thus cannot be identified using fluorescent in situ hybridization or immunohistochemistry. Activating mutations are cautiously estimated to be present in 1%–2% of breast cancer patients, but because the breast cancer population is so large, this is not an inconsequential number of breast cancer patients.[53] Extrapolating from experience with activating *EGFR* (also known as *HER1*) mutations in lung adenocarcinomas, treatments with tyrosine kinase inhibitors such as neratinib are being tested, but to date there is no convincing evidence that cancers with activating mutations in the HER2 kinase or its extracellular domain responds to HER2-targeted therapies.

MECHANISMS OF RESISTANCE TO HER2-TARGETED THERAPIES

Trastuzumab revolutionized the treatment of women with HER2+ breast cancers, but it was quickly discovered that a significant number of patients with metastatic HER2+ breast cancer who initially respond to trastuzumab developed progression within 12 months.[54] Resistance mechanisms to trastuzumab and pertuzumab can be quite different from resistance mechanisms that develop in response to lapatinib and neratinib due to the inherent dissimilarities in antibody-mediated therapeutic approaches versus that of small molecule inhibitors (summarized in Table 1.1), and so HER2+ tumors may respond to HER2-targeted TKIs after progression on trastuzumab +/− pertuzumab.[42,55,56] To illustrate this point, a truncated, active form of HER2 lacking the extracellular domain called p95ErbB2 has been described; trastuzumab is unable to bind to p95, but lapatinib inhibits kinase activity of p95HER2 by acting intracellularly.[57] So far, the findings with p95HER2 have been largely restricted to preclinical models rather than actual patient tumors. As a second example, trastuzumab is thought to be unable to cross the blood-brain barrier at standard doses administered peripherally, but lapatinib has been shown to have efficacy in brain metastases that developed during trastuzumab therapy.[58] Because the HER2-targeted antibodies and TKIs work by different mechanisms, it follows that the

combination of dual HER2-targeting therapies with an antibody and a TKI may be more efficacious than either alone. In fact, the combination of trastuzumab and lapatinib has been successfully tested in the metastatic setting and is an option for trastuzumab-exposed HER2+ disease per NCCN guidelines.[59, 60]

It has been 31 years since the HER2 alteration and its association with disease outcomes in human breast cancer was first described.[13] This observation introduced a new subtype of the disease beyond the prior classification based solely on the status of the estrogen/progesterone receptor pathway. Subsequent studies regarding why HER2 gene amplification and resulting pathologic overexpression of the gene product leads to a more aggressive clinical phenotype made the alteration a logical therapeutic target.[13,17,61−63] Preclinical research led to translation into clinical studies that ultimately resulted in the regulatory approval of trastuzumab in 1998 as the initial therapeutic for HER2+ breast cancer.[64−66] Despite the 31 years since the initial description of this alteration, the 20 years since the approval of trastuzumab, and an abundance of published research on the HER2+ subtype, methods of HER2 testing, mechanisms of action of trastuzumab and other HER2-targeting agents, and mechanisms of resistance to these drugs, multiple questions and controversies surrounding HER2+ breast cancer and its treatment remain. This volume reviews and addresses a number of these critical issues in an attempt to bring the reader up to date on the status of HER2+ breast cancer and its treatment.

REFERENCES

1. Brock TD. *Robert Koch: A Life in Medicine and Bacteriology.* Washington, DC: American Society for Microbiology; 1999.
2. Feinstein S. *Louis Pasteur: The Father of Microbiology.* New York, NY: Enslow Publishing; 2008.
3. Rous P. A transmissible avian neoplasm. (sarcoma of the common fowl). *J Exp Med.* 1910;12(5):696−705.
4. Rous P. A sarcoma of the fowl transmissible by an agent separable from the tumor cells. *J Exp Med.* 1911;13(4):397−411.
5. Smith B. Principles of virology. *Vet Rec.* 2017;180(10):254.
6. Temin HM. Mechanism of cell transformation by RNA tumor viruses. *Annu Rev Microbiol.* 1971;25(1):609−648.
7. Avery OT. Studies on the chemical nature of the substance inducing transformation of pneumococcal types: induction of transformation by a desoxyribonucleic acid fraction isolated from pneumococcus type III. *J Exp Med.* 1944;79(2):137−158.
8. Stehelin D, Varmus HE, Bishop JM, Vogt PK. DNA related to the transforming gene(s) of avian sarcoma viruses is

present in normal avian DNA. *Nature.* 1976;260(5547): 170–173.

9. Stehelin D, Guntaka RV, Varmus HE, Bishop JM. Purification of DNA complementary to nucleotide sequences required for neoplastic transformation of fibroblasts by avian sarcoma viruses. *J Mol Biol.* 1976;101(3):349–365.

10. Thomas SM, Brugge JS. Cellular functions regulated by src family kinases. *Annu Rev Cell Dev Biol.* 1997;13(1): 513–609.

11. Cooper GM. *Oncogenes.* 2nd ed. Boston: Jones and Bartlett Publishers; 1995.

12. Flint SJ. *Principles of Virology: Molecular Biology, Pathogenesis, and Control.* Washington, D.C.: ASM Press; 2000.

13. Slamon D, Clark G, Wong S, Levin W, Ullrich A, McGuire W. Human breast cancer: correlation of relapse and survival with amplification of the HER-2/neu oncogene. *Science.* 1987;235(4785):177–182.

14. Sahlberg KK, Hongisto V, Edgren H, et al. The HER2 amplicon includes several genes required for the growth and survival of HER2 positive breast cancer cells. *Mol Oncol.* 2012; 7(3):392–401.

15. Marotta M, Onodera T, Johnson J, et al. Palindromic amplification of the ERBB2 oncogene in primary HER2-positive breast tumors. *Sci Rep.* 2017;7:41921.

16. Vanden Bempt I, Van Loo P, Drijkoningen M, et al. Polysomy 17 in breast cancer: clinicopathologic significance and impact on HER-2 testing. *J Clin Oncol.* 2008;26(30): 4869–4874.

17. Slamon DJ, Godolphin W, Jones LA, et al. Studies of the HER-2/neu proto-oncogene in human breast and ovarian cancer. *Science.* 1989;244(4905):707–712.

18. Beerli RR, Hynes NE. Epidermal growth factor-related peptides activate distinct subsets of erbb receptors and differ in their biological activities. *J Biol Chem.* 1996;271(11): 6071–6076.

19. Finn RD, Coggill P, Eberhardt RY, et al. The Pfam protein families database: towards a more sustainable future. *Nucleic Acids Res.* 2015;44(D1):D279–D285.

20. Cho HS. Structure of the extracellular region of HER3 reveals an interdomain tether. *Science.* 2002;297(5585): 1330–1333.

21. Bouyain S, Longo PA, Li S, Ferguson KM, Leahy DJ. The extracellular region of ErbB4 adopts a tethered conformation in the absence of ligand. *Proc Natl Acad Sci.* 2005; 102(42):15024–15029.

22. Ferguson KM, Berger MB, Mendrola JM, Cho H-S, Leahy DJ, Lemmon MA. EGF activates its receptor by removing interactions that autoinhibit ectodomain dimerization. *Mol Cell.* 2003;11(2):507–517.

23. Bublil EM, Yarden Y. The EGF receptor family: spearheading a merger of signaling and therapeutics. *Curr Opin Cell Biol.* 2007;19(2):124–134.

24. Holbro T, Hynes NE. ERBB receptors: directing key signaling networks throughout life. *Annu Rev Pharmacol Toxicol.* 2004;44(1):195–217.

25. Cho H-S, Mason K, Ramyar KX, et al. Structure of the extracellular region of HER2 alone and in complex with the Herceptin Fab. *Nature.* 2003;421(6924):756–760.

26. Garrett TPJ, McKern NM, Lou M, et al. The crystal structure of a truncated ErbB2 ectodomain reveals an active conformation, poised to interact with other erbb receptors. *Mol Cell.* 2003;11(2):495–505.

27. Beerli RR, Graus-Porta D, Woods-Cook K, Chen X, Yarden Y, Hynes NE. Neu differentiation factor activation of ErbB-3 and ErbB-4 is cell specific and displays a differential requirement for ErbB-2. *Mol Cell Biol.* 1995; 15(12):6496–6505.

28. Graus-Porta D. ErbB-2, the preferred heterodimerization partner of all ErbB receptors, is a mediator of lateral signaling. *EMBO J.* 1997;16(7):1647–1655.

29. Karunagaran D, Tzahar E, Beerli RR, et al. ErbB-2 is a common auxiliary subunit of NDF and EGF receptors: implications for breast cancer. *EMBO J.* 1996;15(2): 254–264.

30. Brix D, Clemmensen K, Kallunki T. When good turns bad: regulation of invasion and metastasis by ErbB2 receptor tyrosine kinase. *Cells.* 2014;3(1):53–78.

31. Negro A. Essential roles of Her2/erbB2 in cardiac development and function. *Recent Prog Horm Res.* 2004;59(1): 1–12.

32. Olayioye MA. New embo members' review: the erbb signaling network: receptor heterodimerization in development and cancer. *EMBO J.* 2000;19(13):3159–3167.

33. Lonardo F, Di Marco E, King CR, et al. The normal erbB-2 product is an atypical receptor-like tyrosine kinase with constitutive activity in the absence of ligand. *New Biol.* 1990;2(11):992–1003.

34. Iqbal N. Human epidermal growth factor receptor 2 (HER2) in cancers: overexpression and therapeutic implications. *Mol Biol Int.* 2014;2014:1–9.

35. Ross JS, Slodkowska EA, Symmans WF, Pusztai L, Ravdin PM, Hortobagyi GN. The HER-2 receptor and breast cancer: ten years of targeted anti-HER-2 therapy and personalized medicine. *Oncologist.* 2009;14(4): 320–368.

36. Trastuzumab. In: *Micromedex (Columbia Basin College Library ed.) [Electronic version].* Greenwood Village, CO: Truven Health Analytics; 2017.

37. Pertuzumab. In: *Micromedex (Columbia Basin College Library ed.) [Electronic version].* Greenwood Village, CO: Truven Health Analytics; 2017.

38. Fuentes G, Scaltriti M, Baselga J, Verma CS. Synergy between trastuzumab and pertuzumab for human epidermal growth factor 2 (Her2) from colocalization: an in silico-based mechanism. *Breast Cancer Res.* 2011;13(3).

39. Carson WE, Parihar R, Lindemann MJ, et al. Interleukin-2 enhances the natural killer cell response to Herceptin-coated Her2 /neu-positive breast cancer cells. *Eur J Immunol.* 2001;31(10):3016–3025.

40. Clynes RA, Towers TL, Presta LG, Ravetch JV. Inhibitory Fc receptors modulate in vivo cytotoxicity against tumor targets. *Nat Med.* 2000;6(4):443–446.

41. Shi Y, Fan X, Meng W, Deng H, Zhang N, An Z. Engagement of immune effector cells by trastuzumab induces HER2/ERBB2 downregulation in cancer cells through STAT1 activation. *Breast Cancer Res.* 2014;16(2).

42. Olivier Jr KJ, Hurvitz SA. *Antibody-Drug Conjugates: Fundamentals, Drug Development, and Clinical Outcomes to Target Cancer.* John Wiley & Sons; 2016.

43. Trastuzumab emtansine. In: *Micromedex (Columbia Basin College Library ed.) [Electronic version].* Greenwood Village, CO: Truven Health Analytics; 2017.

44. Druker BJ, Talpaz M, Resta DJ, et al. Efficacy and safety of a specific inhibitor of the bcr-abl tyrosine kinase in chronic myeloid leukemia. *N Engl J Med.* 2001;344(14): 1031–1037.

45. Joensuu H, Roberts PJ, Sarlomo-Rikala M, et al. Effect of the tyrosine kinase inhibitor STI571 in a patient with a metastatic gastrointestinal stromal tumor. *N Engl J Med.* 2001;344(14):1052–1056.

46. Kris MG, Natale RB, Herbst RS, et al. Efficacy of gefitinib, an inhibitor of the epidermal growth factor receptor tyrosine kinase, in symptomatic patients with non–small cell lung cancer. *JAMA.* 2003;290(16):2149.

47. Lynch TJ, Bell DW, Sordella R, et al. Activating mutations in the epidermal growth factor receptor underlying responsiveness of non–small-cell lung cancer to gefitinib. *N Engl J Med.* 2004;350(21):2129–2139.

48. Paez JG. EGFR mutations in lung cancer: correlation with clinical response to gefitinib therapy. *Science.* 2004; 304(5676):1497–1500.

49. Sordella R. Gefitinib-sensitizing EGFR mutations in lung cancer activate anti-apoptotic pathways. *Science.* 2004; 305(5687):1163–1167.

50. Lapatinib. In: *Micromedex (Columbia Basin College Library ed.) [Electronic version].* Greenwood Village, CO: Truven Health Analytics; 2017.

51. Neratinib. In: *Micromedex (Columbia Basin College Library ed.) [Electronic version].* Greenwood Village, CO: Truven Health Analytics; 2017.

52. Moulder SL, Borges VF, Baetz T, et al. Phase I study of ONT-380, a HER2 inhibitor, in patients with HER2(+)-advanced solid tumors, with an expansion cohort in HER2(+) metastatic breast cancer (MBC). *Clin Cancer Res.* 2017;23(14): 3529–3536.

53. Bose R, Kavuri SM, Searleman AC, et al. Activating HER2 mutations in HER2 gene amplification negative breast cancer. *Cancer Discov.* 2012;3(2):224–237.

54. Vogel CL. Efficacy and safety of trastuzumab as a single agent in first-line treatment of HER2-Overexpressing metastatic breast cancer. *J Clin Oncol.* 2002;20(3):719–726.

55. Chen FL, Xia W, Spector NL. Acquired resistance to small molecule ErbB2 tyrosine kinase inhibitors. *Clin Cancer Res.* 2008;14(21):6730–6734.

56. Menyhart O, Santarpia L, Gyorffy B. A comprehensive outline of trastuzumab resistance biomarkers in HER2 overexpressing breast cancer. *Curr Cancer Drug Targets.* 2015;15(8):665–683.

57. Xia W, Liu L-H, Ho P, Spector NL. Truncated ErbB2 receptor (p95ErbB2) is regulated by heregulin through heterodimer formation with ErbB3 yet remains sensitive to the dual EGFR/ErbB2 kinase inhibitor GW572016. *Oncogene.* 2004;23(3):646–653.

58. Gril B, Palmieri D, Bronder JL, et al. Effect of lapatinib on the outgrowth of metastatic breast cancer cells to the brain. *J Natl Cancer Inst.* 2008;100(15):1092–1103.

59. Blackwell KL, Burstein HJ, Storniolo AM, et al. Randomized study of lapatinib alone or in combination with trastuzumab in women with ErbB2-positive, trastuzumab-refractory metastatic breast cancer. *J Clin Oncol.* 2010;28(7):1124–1130.

60. Network NCC. NCCN Clinical Practice Guidelines in Oncology (NCCN Guidelines®) for Breast Cancer (Version 1.2017). http://www.nccn.org. Accessed October 1, 2017.

61. Slamon DJ. Proto-oncogenes and human cancers. *N Engl J Med.* 1987;317(15):955–957.

62. Pegram MD, Konecny G, Slamon DJ. The molecular and cellular biology of HER2/neu gene amplification/overexpression and the clinical development of herceptin (trastuzumab) therapy for breast cancer. *Cancer Treat Res.* 2000; 103:57–75.

63. Pietras RJ, Arboleda J, Reese DM, et al. HER-2 tyrosine kinase pathway targets estrogen receptor and promotes hormone-independent growth in human breast cancer cells. *Oncogene.* 1995;10(12):2435–2446.

64. Slamon DJ, Leyland-Jones B, Shak S, et al. Use of chemotherapy plus a monoclonal antibody against HER2 for metastatic breast cancer that overexpresses HER2. *N Engl J Med.* 2001;344(11):783–792.

65. Pegram MD, Pienkowski T, Northfelt DW, et al. Results of two open-label, multicenter phase II studies of docetaxel, platinum salts, and trastuzumab in HER2-positive advanced breast cancer. *J Natl Cancer Inst.* 2004;96(10): 759–769.

66. Pegram MD, Lipton A, Hayes DF, et al. Phase II study of receptor-enhanced chemosensitivity using recombinant humanized anti-p185HER2/neu monoclonal antibody plus cisplatin in patients with HER2/neu-overexpressing metastatic breast cancer refractory to chemotherapy treatment. *J Clin Oncol.* 1998;16(8):2659–2671.

67. Hudis CA. Trastuzumab – mechanism of action and use in clinical practice. *N Engl J Med.* 2007;357:39–51.

CHAPTER 2

HER2 Testing in the Era of Changing Guidelines

MICHAEL F. PRESS, MD, PHD • GRACE NAMJUNG KIM, MD •
MAHDI KHOSHCHEHREH, MD, MS • YANLING MA, MD, MS • DENNIS J. SLAMON, MD, PHD

BACKGROUND

Breast cancer, like other cancers, is a genetic disease, resulting from a combination of inherited and acquired genetic alterations, depending on the individuals and their background. A wide variety of alterations have been identified in human breast cancers[1,2]; however, relatively few of these have proven to be useful for therapeutic intervention in the disease. Of the genetic alterations, including genomic amplifications, and modifications in gene expression as well as sequence mutations that have been reported in literally hundreds of cancer-related genes in breast carcinomas, only five breast cancer markers currently play an important role in therapeutic decision-making. These include estrogen receptor-alpha (ER) expression, progesterone receptor (PR) expression, human epidermal growth factor receptor 2 (HER2) gene amplification/overexpression, and BRCA1/BRCA2-inherited mutations. The latter of these, BRCA1 and BRCA2 mutations, has recently played key roles in decisions related to prophylactic mastectomies for women in families with hereditary breast and ovarian cancer. In addition, olaparib, a PARP (poly ADP ribose polymerase) inhibitor, has recently been approved for treatment of women with metastatic BRCA1-mutated breast cancers. Three markers, ER, PR, and HER2, are required for decision-making with adjuvant or neoadjuvant therapeutics.

Antihormonal therapies as well as anti-HER2-targeted therapies have resulted in significant improvements in both disease-free survival (DFS) and overall survival (OS) among patients whose breast carcinomas express ER or have HER2 gene amplification/overexpression. Although ER and PR are well-established biomarkers for therapeutic decision-making and only those women whose cancers express these receptors experience therapeutic benefit from antiestrogen therapies, the clinical laboratory assays used to identify these receptors in breast cancer tissue are primarily laboratory-developed assays and these assays have shown marked variability in sensitivity and specificity for ER and PR as illustrated by problematic laboratory testing.[3] The use of laboratory-developed assays for ER and PR contrasts with the diagnostic testing conducted for the evaluation of HER2 gene amplification and overexpression. HER2 status is predominantly assessed with companion diagnostic assays that were approved for this purpose by the US Food and Drug Administration (FDA) (Table 2.1).

Not only is amplification and overexpression of the human epidermal growth factor receptor 2 gene (HER2, also known as ERBB2) associated with shortened disease-free and overall survival in patients whose breast cancers contain this alteration,[4-6] but this alteration is also targeted by such therapies as anti-HER2 humanized monoclonal antibodies (trastuzumab[7-9] and pertuzumab[10]), small molecule inhibitors of the HER2 kinase,[11-13] and antibody-drug conjugates, such as trastuzumab emtansine (TDM1),[14,15] which have proven to be efficacious in the treatment of patients with HER2-positive breast cancer. As a result, this alteration is both a prognostic and predictive biomarker. Consequently, assessment of HER2 gene amplification status is critically important for patient selection for treatment with these targeted therapeutics. To facilitate appropriate selection of patients for treatment with HER2-targeted therapies, the US FDA required the use of a companion diagnostic for approval of these drugs.

COMPANION DIAGNOSTICS AND US FOOD AND DRUG ADMINISTRATION DIAGNOSTIC CRITERIA

The HER2/ERBB2 gene encodes a membrane receptor protein that is expressed at low levels on the basal

TABLE 2.1
Companion Diagnostics Approved by the FDA for HER2 Testing

Year	Method	Assay Name	Indication	Approval Process	Company
1997	FISH	INFORM HER2[a]	Risk of early recurrence or death	Concordance Study and Cohort Study	Oncor, Inc.[a] Ventana Med Systems, Inc.
1998	IHC	HercepTest	Trastuzumab	Concordance Study with CTA	Dako, Inc.[b]
2012			Pertuzumab		
2013			Adotrastuzumab Emtansine		
2000	IHC	Pathway anti-HER2/neu (CB11)	Trastuzumab	Concordance study with HercepTest	Ventana Medical Systems[c]
2001	FISH	PathVysion	Trastuzumab	Retrospective assessment of breast cancer in trastuzumab H0648 trial compared with outcomes	Vysis, Inc.[d]
2004	IHC	InSite HER2/neu (CB11) Kit	Trastuzumab	Concordance study with HercepTest	Biogenex Laboratories, Inc.[e]
2005	FISH	Her2 FISH pharmDX Kit	Trastuzumab	Concordance Study with PathVysion and HercepTest	Dako, Inc.[b]
2012			Pertuzumab		
2013			Adotrastuzumab Emtansine		
2008	CISH	SPOT-Light HER2 CISH Kit	Trastuzumab	Concordance Study with PathVysion and HercepTest	Introgen, Inc.[f]
2011	Dual ISH	INFORM HER2	Trastuzumab	Concordance Study with PathVysion	Ventana Medical Systems
2011	Dual ISH	HER2 CISH pharmDx Kit	Trastuzumab	Concordance Study with PathVysion and PharmDx	Dako, Inc.
2012	IHC	Bond Oracle HER2 IHC	Trastuzumab	Concordance Study with PathVysion and HercepTest	Leica Biosystems
2017	NGS	FoundationOne CDx	Trastuzumab Pertuzumab Adotrastuzumab Emtansine	Concordance Study with F1 LDT	Foundation Medicine, Inc.

CISH, chromogenic in situ hybridization; *CTA*, clinical trials assay (4D5 and CB11); *FISH*, fluorescence in situ hybridization; *HER2*, human epidermal growth factor receptor type 2; *IHC*, immunohistochemical; *LDT*, laboratory-developed IHC test; *NGS*, next generation sequencing.

[a] INFORM HER-2/neu FISH assay, originally approved in 1997 by Oncor, Inc. through a Pre-Market Approval (PMA) as an "aid to stratify breast cancer patients according to risk for recurrence or disease-related death" and was, subsequently, acquired by Ventana Medical Systems, Inc., in 2000 and withdrawn from the market on October 22, 2007. The currently approved "INFORM HER2" has been revised as a bright-field microscopy dual ISH assay using a different HER2 DNA probe and chromosome 17 centromere probe. It is now approved for selection of patients to trastuzumab therapy.
[b] Acquired by Agilent, Inc.
[c] Ventana is now a subsidiary of F. Hoffmann-La Roche Ltd.
[d] Acquired by Abbott Laboratories, now Abbott-Molecular, Inc.
[e] InSite HER2/neu (C B11) kit was withdrawn from the market in 2006.
[f] Now Life Technologies, Inc.
Reference: https://www.fda.gov/MedicalDevices/ProductsandMedicalProcedures/InVitroDiagnostics/ucm301431.htm

and lateral membranes of essentially all normal grandular epithelial cells.[16] Because HER2 membrane protein overexpression is a direct consequence of *HER2* amplification, a variety of companion diagnostics are used to identify either *HER2* gene amplification or protein overexpression for selection of patients who might benefit from these targeted therapies. The FDA has used data submitted as part of the clinical trial evaluation process that was related to specific drugs to determine testing procedures for HER2 status.

INFORM HER2 FISH Assay

The first approval for HER2 testing was for a HER2 fluorescence in situ hybridization (FISH) assay with a clinical indication to identify breast cancers that placed patients at "high-risk for recurrence or disease-related death," not for selection of any therapeutic agent (Table 2.1). The study for this initial FDA approval of an HER2 FISH assay (Oncor, Inc.) was conducted in two phases. The first phase was a concordance study of 140 archival breast cancers evaluated independently for *HER2* gene amplification by Southern hybridization or dot blot hybridization compared with the HER2 FISH assay results in the same 140 cancers.[4] This comparison demonstrated a 98% sensitivity and a 100% specificity with the solid matrix blotting methodologies considered to be the established standard. In the second phase the *HER2* FISH assay was used to determine the *HER2* status of 324 axillary lymph node-negative invasive breast cancers from women with long-term (10-year) clinical outcome information. Gene amplification was observed in 57 of the 324 (18%) node-negative breast carcinomas. Among these patients, treated by surgery alone without radiation therapy, adjuvant chemotherapy, or hormone therapy except after development of recurrent disease, the relative risks (relative hazard) of early recurrence (recurrent disease within 24 months of diagnosis), recurrent disease (at any time), and disease-related death were significantly associated with amplification. The prognostic information contributed by *HER2* amplification was independent of the other traditional prognostic markers studied, including age at diagnosis, tumor size, histopathological grade, ER and PR status.[4] *HER2* amplification was associated with a more than threefold increased risk of early recurrence, recurrence at any time, and disease-related death. *HER2* was considered to be amplified in this study when either the average *HER2* gene copy number was greater than or equal to ($\geq$) 4.0 per tumor cell nucleus or when the ratio of the average *HER2* gene copy number divided by the average of an internal control genomic site at the centromere for

chromosome 17 (CEP17) per tumor cell was ≥ 2.0. Based on this, and other data, the FDA approved these criteria for *HER2* gene amplification by FISH for the Oncor INFORM HER2 assay (Table 2.2). These scoring criteria were similar to those used by us[19,20] and others[21,22] for FISH in research settings.

HercepTest and Other IHC Companion Diagnostic Assays

The first FDA HER2-targeted therapeutic drug approval was for trastuzumab and used the HercepTest (DAKO Corporation, Carpinteria, CA) as a companion diagnostic immunohistochemical (IHC) assay (Table 2.1) to identify "HER2-positive" breast cancer patients for treatment of metastatic disease. The clinical trial had been conducted by the use of a laboratory-developed IHC, the "Clinical Trials Assay" (CTA), which was composed of a primary anti-HER2 antibody (4D5), the murine precursor that was humanized to create the drug trastuzumab (Herceptin).[23,24] Both 4D5 and trastuzumab bind to an extracellular epitope of the HER2 protein in the juxtamembrane region. Although the initial assay used only 4D5, the assay was subsequently modified to use each of the two different anti-HER2 antibodies, 4D5 and CB11, in an avidin-biotin-peroxidase IHC format, incubated separately on two different slides, which were subjectively scored separately for the amount of IHC staining.[25] The CB11 antibody binds to an intracellular epitope near the C-terminus of the HER2 protein. The 4D5 and CB11 IHC assays differ in antigen retrieval methods, but both use a similar visualization method involving a biotinylated horse antimouse antibody and a standard avidin-biotin horseradish peroxidase complex.[25] Because Genentech, Inc., the pharmaceutical manufacturer of the drug and sponsor of the trial, was not prepared to commercialize the CTA as a companion diagnostic, they partnered with another company, Dako, Inc., to develop a HER2 IHC assay that could be similarly used to identify women whose breast cancers had "HER2-positive" disease. The DAKO HercepTest was approved by the FDA, based on a direct comparison of immunostaining obtained with the CTA and HercepTest in 548 breast cancer specimens, provided by the National Cancer Institute Cooperative Breast Cancer Tissue Resource, from patients who did not have clinical outcome information. Although these cases lacked outcome information, paraffin-embedded tissue blocks were available. The FDA required at least a 75% concordance rate between the two assays. An agreement or concordance rate of 79% was observed, and the FDA approval was granted on this basis.

TABLE 2.2
Comparison of Diagnostic Criteria and Categories Used by the FDA, 2007 ASCO-CAP Guidelines, 2013/2014 ASCO-CAP Guidelines, and the USC/TRIO Breast Cancer Analysis Laboratory

Assay Method/ Interpretation	FDA		2007 ASCO-CAP[a]		2013 ASCO-CAP[b]			USC BCAL/TRIO		
HER2 by IHC[c]								**Interpretation**		
Negative	0, 1+		0, 1+			0, 1+		Low expression	0, 1+	
Equivocal	2+*		2+**			2+*		Increased expression[d]	2+	
Positive	3+ (>10%)*		3+ (>30%)**			3+ (>10%)*		Overexpression[e]	3+[f]	
HER2 by ISH[f]	HER2/ CEP17 = Ratio	Average HER2 gene copies	HER2/ CEP17 = Ratio	Average HER2 gene copies	Group	HER2/ CEP17 = Ratio	Average HER2 gene copies	USC/TRIO interpretation by category	HER2/ CEP17 = Ratio	Average HER2 gene copies
Negative	Ratio <2.0	NA	Ratio <1.8	NA	5	Ratio <2.0	<4.0	Not amplified	Ratio <2.0	<4.0
Equivocal	NA	NA	Ratio 1.8 to 2.2	NA	4	Ratio <2.0	4.0 to <6.0	Not amplified	Ratio <2.0	4.0 to <6.0
Negative	Ratio <2.0	NA	Ratio <1.8	NA	3	Ratio <2.0	≥6.0	Mixed	Ratio <2.0	≥6.0
Positive	Ratio ≥2.0	NA	Ratio ≥2.2	NA	2	Ratio ≥2.0	<4.0	Not amplified	Ratio ≥2.0	<4.0
Positive	Ratio ≥2.0	NA	Ratio ≥2.2	NA	1	Ratio ≥2.0	≥4.0	Amplified	Ratio ≥2.0	≥4.0

HER2, human epidermal growth factor receptor type 2; ISH, in situ hybridization; NA, not applicable.

* At least 10% of tumor cells with IHC positive membranes.

** At least 30% of tumor cells with IHC positive membranes.

a Using IHC requires previous concordance of 95% or greater in each IHC category to be used for assessment.

b Using IHC no longer requires the previous concordance rate of 95% or greater in each IHC category to be used for assessment. Now Laboratories are responsible for ensuring the reliability and accuracy of their testing results, by compliance with accreditation and proficiency testing requirements for HER2 testing assays. Specific concordance requirements are not required (Data Supplement 11).[17,18]

c HER2 by IHC: HER2 protein expression by immunohistochemistry assay interpretations.

d Increased expression: Laboratory-developed 10H8-IHC assay is expected to be "HER2-positive" because from 65% (unpublished quality control for 2017) to 80%[13] of cases show HER2 gene amplification. Dako HercepTest might be "HER2-positive" because 50%[13] of cases show HER2 gene amplification.

e Overexpression: Laboratory-developed 10H8-IHC assay is expected to be "HER2-positive" because 99%[13] of cases show HER2 gene amplification. Dako HercepTest is expected to be "HER2-positive" because 97%[13] of cases show HER2 gene amplification.

f Percentage of positively stained tumor cells is considered to be greatly affected by fixation conditions because tumor cells in frozen tissues have been observed to have the same staining level throughout the tumor.[6] After fixation, this monotonous uniformity of IHC is altered to more variable IHC staining levels as described.[6]

Although commercial development of the CTA was considered impractical, it did serve as the prototype assay for both the HercepTest and an additional IHC assay, the Ventana Pathway (Ventana Medical Systems, Tucson, AZ) IHC assay. The initial Ventana Pathway assay used one of the anti-HER2 antibodies, CB11, from the original CTA and was compared with the FDA-approved HercepTest to show concordance. This PATHWAY assay using CB11 demonstrated equivalent results with the HercepTest to gain its FDA approval.

Subsequently, the mouse monoclonal CB11 anti-HER2 antibody was replaced with a rabbit monoclonal anti-HER2 antibody, 4B5, which could also be used on a Ventana-automated slide and immunohistochemistry staining platform. Approval for this second PATHWAY assay with the new anti-HER-2/neu (4B5) involved a comparison with the Ventana Medical Systems' (Ventana) PATHWAY HER2 (clone CB11) primary antibody on an independent sample, which demonstrated an 83% agreement rate and was interpreted as acceptably concordant. The actual correlation of PATHWAY anti-HER-2/neu (4B5) to clinical outcome was never established. The FDA has also approved the use of a computerized image analysis system, the Ventana Image Analysis System (VIAS), to score the IHC staining results from the 4B5 Pathway assay.

The scoring system used in these FDA-approved IHC assays was based on the CTA interpretative strategy, which itself was based on IHC scoring schemes used in a number of laboratory-developed research protocols described previously both by us[6,26,27] and others.[28–31] Patients were deemed eligible for the Genentech sponsored H0648 clinical trial of trastuzumab in women with metastatic disease if their biopsy specimen scored 2+ or 3+ by either 4D5 or CB11 in the CTA assay. The human breast cancer cell lines MDA-MB-231, MDA-MB-175, and SK-BR-3 served as performance control standards in each of these assays with corresponding IHC staining scores of 0, 1+, and 3+, respectively. Each of these IHC staining scores in tissue samples were subjectively assessed based on the intensity of membrane staining ranging from none (IHC 0) to detectable but weak (IHC 1+), moderate (IHC 2+), and strong (IHC 3+).[25]

PathVysion HER2 FISH Assay

Subsequently, additional FISH assays were approved by the FDA with trastuzumab treatment as an indication. In the first of these approved FISH assays to select patients for trastuzumab therapy, outcome data and tissue samples were characterized by FISH using a FISH assay from Vysis, Inc. with tissue from the initial pivotal H0648 clinical trial,[24] the study had been used for FDA approval of trastuzumab. This study was pursued in collaboration with Genentech investigators and some of the same investigators who had previously obtained approval for the Oncor INFORM HER2 assay. The study formed the basis for approval of a companion FISH assay, the HER2 PathVysion assay, for selection of patients with metastatic HER2-positive breast cancer for a trastuzumab clinical indication[32] (Table 2.1). The criteria for *HER2* gene amplification was similar in this study to those previously approved for the Oncor INFORM HER2 FISH assay, i.e., a ratio of the average *HER2* gene copy number divided by the average of an internal control genomic site at the centromere for chromosome 17 (CEP17) per tumor cell equal to or exceeding 2.0, the breast cancer was considered to have *HER2* gene amplification. This FISH assay used both a directly labeled HER2 DNA probe (red) and a directly labeled CEP17 probe (green) (Fig. 2.1).

Importantly, FDA-approved recommendations were followed near the cutoff ratio of 2.0 (or average *HER2* copy number of 4.0). When the *HER2*-to-CEP17 ratio is between 1.80 and 2.20, the FDA recommends a minimum of 20 additional cells be scored by the initial scorer and a second scorer counts a minimum of 40 additional cells. When ratios from these two individuals are in agreement, the FISH result is reported. If the ratios are not in agreement, the entire assay is repeated and the specimen is rescored. This additional attention is warranted because the increased number of tumor cells evaluated by two individuals will increase the precision of the estimated ratio and improve diagnostic accuracy at this critical cutoff point. Subsequently, each of the ASCO-CAP guidelines made changes to the FDA-approved criteria for FISH testing without significant data supporting the need for their recommended changes in either 2007 or 2013/2014.[17,18,34,35]

Additional revisions to FISA scoring were made in 2018[119] (see "Expectations" below).

The testing and interpretive criteria developed for these initial IHC and FISH assays went on to serve as the prototypes for subsequent HER2 IHC and in situ hybridization (ISH) assays (Table 2.1). As recommended by the initial FDA approval for the HercepTest, IHC was interpreted as "HER2-negative" for immunostaining scores of "0" or "1+" (no immunostaining or weak, discontinuous membrane staining, respectively) and "HER2-positive" when more than 10% of the invasive carcinoma cells showed strong, complete membrane staining, or "IHC 3+" staining. Although "IHC 2+" (moderate, complete membrane staining) was considered overexpression for accrual to the pivotal clinical trials of trastuzumab for metastatic breast cancer, the H0648, H0649, and H0650 trials,[24,32,36,37]

Schematic diagram of the ASCO-CAP algorithm for *HER2* testing by fluorescent in situ hybridization (FISH) and Examples of Breast Cancers in each *HER2* FISH Group

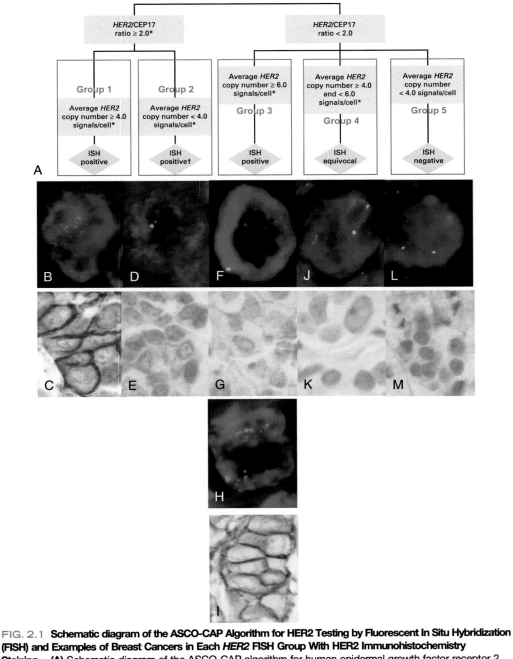

FIG. 2.1 **Schematic diagram of the ASCO-CAP Algorithm for HER2 Testing by Fluorescent In Situ Hybridization (FISH) and Examples of Breast Cancers in Each *HER2* FISH Group With HER2 Immunohistochemistry Staining.** **(A)** Schematic diagram of the ASCO-CAP algorithm for human epidermal growth factor receptor 2 (HER2) testing by FISH as published by the ASCO-CAP HER2 testing guidelines committee,[17,18] modified here by introduction of the group numbers, group 1 to group 5 to identify the various ASCO-CAP FISH groups categorized. Breast cancers with *HER2*-to-chromosome 17 centromere (CEP17) ratios ≥2.0 are divided in two groups, one with an average *HER2* gene copy number per tumor cell ≥4.0 (in situ hybridization [ISH] positive; our group 1) and one with an average HER2 gene copy number per tumor cell <4.0 (ISH positive; our group 2). Breast cancers with *HER2*-to-CEP17 ratios <2.0 are separated into three additional groups: one with average *HER2* gene copy

number per tumor cell ≥6.0 (ISH positive; our group 3), another with average *HER2* gene copy number per tumor cell ≥4.0 but <6.0 (ISH equivocal; our group 4), and one with breast cancers that contained an average *HER2* gene copy number per tumor cell <4.0 (ISH negative; our group 5). According to the ASCO-CAP guidelines,[17,18] breast cancers in groups 1, 2, and 3 are interpreted as "ISH-positive," group 4 as "ISH-equivocal," and group 5 as "ISH-negative." (B–M) ASCO-CAP guidelines algorithm ISH groups compared with observed *HER2* gene amplification status by FISH and HER2 protein expression status by IHC staining using the DAKO HercepTest IHC assay. ASCO-CAP guidelines algorithm identification of subdivisions by *HER2* FISH ratios and average *HER2* gene copy number into group 1 is categorized as ISH-positive, with results as illustrated in panels B (FISH) and C (IHC); group 2 is also categorized as "ISH-positive" but with our contradictory results as illustrated in panels D (FISH) and E (IHC); group 3 is categorized as "ISH-positive" but with mixed results as illustrated in panels F (FISH), G (IHC), H (FISH), and I (IHC); group 4 is categorized as "ISH-equivocal" but with contradictory results as illustrated in panels J (FISH) and K (IHC); and group 5 is categorized as ISH-negative, with confirmatory results as illustrated in panels L (FISH) and M (IHC). (B) ASCO-CAP group 1 breast cancer with *HER2* gene amplification by FISH, consistent with the ASCO-CAP guidelines designation of ISH-positive (and Breast Cancer International Research Group [BCIRG] designation of *HER2*-amplified). Average *HER2* gene copy number for this case was 16.85 copies per tumor cell, and the CEP17 copy number per cell was 2.28 with a *HER2*-to-CEP17 FISH ratio of 7.38. *HER2* signals are sufficiently numerous and are not captured in a single plain of focus in this photomicrograph so that some appear out of focus. Computer enhancement was not used for any image (BCIRG01661, original photomicrograph at 1,000×). (C) ASCO-CAP group 1 breast cancer case with HER2 protein overexpression, IHC3+ by HercepTest IHC assay (BCIRG01661, original magnification, 400×). (D) ASCO-CAP group 2 breast cancer. Average *HER2* gene copy number for this breast cancer was 3.75 copies per tumor cell, with a CEP17 copy number of 1.80 per cell and a *HER2*-to-CEP17 FISH ratio of 2.08. This breast cancer was evaluated in the BCIRG/Translational Research in Oncology (TRIO) central laboratory as *HER2*-not-amplified by FISH, which contradicted the ASCO-CAP guidelines designation of "ISH-positive" and the patient was accrued to the BCIRG-005 trial. Of the 52 patients whose breast cancers were in this group, 3 were accrued to BCIRG-005 and 46 were accrued to BCIRG-006 (BCIRG02899, original magnification, 1,000×). (E) ASCO-CAP group 2 breast cancer, corresponding to the breast cancer in panel D, with HER2 protein expression determined as IHC 0 with the HercepTest IHC assay, which contradicted the ASCO-CAP guidelines designation of "ISH-positive" (BCIRG02899, original magnification, 400×). (F) ASCO-CAP group 3 breast cancer. One of our group 3N cases was reported to have a lack of *HER2* gene amplification by FISH in the BCIRG/TRIO central laboratory, contrary to the current ASCO-CAP guidelines designation of "ISH-positive." Average *HER2* gene copy number for this breast cancer was 7.35 copies per tumor cell, average CEP17 copy number was 4.20 per cell, and, therefore, there was a *HER2*-to-CEP17 FISH ratio of 1.75 (BCIRG04086, original magnification, 1,000×). (G) ASCO-CAP group 3 breast cancer. Our group 3N, with low HER2 protein expression by IHC (IHC 0/1+), reported previously as *HER2*-not-amplified, contrary to the current ASCO-CAP guidelines designation of "ISH-positive" (BCIRG04086, original magnification, 400×). (H) ASCO-CAP group 3 breast cancer, one of the BCIRG group 3A cases, with an average *HER2* gene copy number of 27.50 per tumor cell, an average CEP17 copy number of 20.67 per tumor cell, and, therefore, a *HER2* FISH ratio of only 1.33. Please note that the *HER2* gene signals (orange) and CEP17 signals (green) are aggregated together in a limited geographic area of the nucleus, making assessment of individual signals challenging without the aid of single band-pass filters (see Fig. 3 for another example[33]). This breast cancer was reported as *HER2*-amplified in the BCIRG/TRIO central laboratory, and the patient was accrued to BCIRG-006. This case is consistent with the ASCO-CAP guidelines designation of "ISH-positive" (BCIRG00575, original magnification, 1,000×). (I) ASCO-CAP group 3 breast cancer, the same group 3A in panel H, with HER2 protein overexpression by IHC (IHC3+ by HercepTest), consistent with the ASCO-CAP guidelines designation of "ISH-positive" (BCIRG00575, original magnification, 400×). (J) ASCO-CAP group 4 breast cancer, referred to by the current ASCO-CAP guidelines as "ISH-equivocal." BCIRG/TRIO central laboratory reported the case as *HER2*-not-amplified by FISH, with an average *HER2* gene copy number of 4.22 per tumor cell, an average CEP17 copy number of 2.23 per tumor cell, and, therefore, an *HER2*-to-CEP17 FISH ratio of 1.89. The patient was randomly assigned in BCIRG-005 (BCIRG01911, original magnification, 1,000×). (K) ASCO-CAP group 4 breast cancer, as in panel J, with low HER2 protein expression by HercepTest (IHC 0; BCIRG01911, original magnification, 400×). (L) ASCO-CAP group 5 breast cancer, consistent with the guidelines designation of "ISH-negative," which was reported by the BCIRG/TRIO central laboratory as *HER2*-not-amplified by FISH. The case had an average *HER2* gene copy number of 1.35 per tumor cell, with 1.50 CEP17 copies per cell and an *HER2*-to-CEP17 ratio of 0.90 (BCIRG04095, original magnification 1,000×). (M) ASCO-CAP group 5 breast cancer, see panel L, with low HER2 protein expression by IHC with HercepTest (IHC 0), consistent the ASCO-CAP guidelines designation of "ISH-negative" (BCIRG04095, original magnification, 400×). (Reproduction with permission of Fig. 2 from Press MF, Sauter G, Buyse M, Fourmanoir H, Quinaux E, Eiermann W, Robert N, Pienkowski T, Crown J, Martin M, Valero V, Mackey JR, Bee V, Ma Y, Villalobos I, Campeau A, Mirlacher M, Lindsay MA, Slamon DJ. *HER2* Gene Amplification Testing by Fluorescence in situ Hybridization (FISH): Comparison of the American Society of Clinical Oncology {ASCO}-College of American Pathologists {CAP} Guidelines with FISH Scores used for enrollment in Breast Cancer International Research Group {BCIRG} Clinical Trials. *J Clin Oncol* 2016;34(29):3518–3528.) (*) Group 2 was revised to be "ISH-negative" by the Clinical Practice Focused update" in 2018[119] in agreement with our findings,[33,75] depending on the results of IHC.

IHC 2+ was later designated as "equivocal" for those carcinomas with more than 10% of the carcinoma cells showing weak to moderate, circumferential membrane staining. Subsequently, only IHC3+ was considered "HER2-positive" (strong, complete, circumferential membranous reactivity in greater than 10% of tumor cells) (https://www.accessdata.fda.gov/cdrh_docs/pdf/P980018S010b.pdf).

In Situ HER2 Assays Using Bright-Field Microscopy

Likewise, subsequent ISH assays were approved with interpretive criteria for *HER2* gene amplification using either an average greater than or equal to ($\geq$) 4.0 *HER2* gene copies per tumor cell nucleus for single probe assays, such as the chromogenic in situ hybridization (CISH) assay, or an average *HER2* gene copy number-to-chromosome 17 centromere (CEP17) ratio $\geq$2.0 for dual ISH assays (Table 2.2). Those breast cancers with HER2-to-CEP17 ratio within 10% of the 2.0 ratio, i.e., 1.80 to 2.20, required the assessment of an additional 40 tumor cells by each of two different observers. After assessment of 80 tumor cell nuclei in such cases, if both observers had ratios greater than or less than 2.0, the case was considered "HER2-positive" or "HER2-negative," respectively. There was no "equivocal" (i.e., "undecided") category. These scoring criteria were similar to those used for *HER2* gene amplification by FISH in research settings,[19-22] but they were changed in subsequent guidelines developed by ASCO-CAP (Table 2.2).

NGS and Foundation One CDx

Until 2017, all assays approved by the FDA for HER2 testing were either IHC assays or ISH assays (Table 2.1). In 2017, Foundation Medicine obtained approval for evaluation of *HER2* gene amplification using a next-generation (massively parallel DNA) sequencing (NGS) approach using formalin-fixed paraffin-embedded samples. This study involved 6300 samples (4200 analytical samples, inclusive of cell lines, and 2100 clinical samples). The F1CDx test is validated for solid tumors, including non–small cell lung carcinoma; breast, ovary, colorectal carcinomas; and melanoma. The assay tests across all four classes of genomic alterations (substitutions, insertions, deletions, and copy number alterations) in 324 genes and some gene rearrangements and also includes microsatellite instability (MSI) and tumor mutational burden analysis. With regard to breast cancers, the test detects amplification of *HER2/ERBB2* to identify patients with breast carcinomas that may be responsive to trastuzumab, ado-trastuzumab-emtansine, or pertuzumab. An *HER2/ERBB2* amplification result with copy number equal to 4 (baseline ploidy of tumor +2) should be reflexed to an alternative test for confirmation. The F1CDx study results were concordant with the FDA-approved Dako Her2 PharmDx FISH Kit from DAKO (positive-percent agreement 89.4%, negative-percent agreement 98.4%), other next-generation sequencing methods, and the FoundationOne test (reference: https://www.foundationmedicine.com/genomic-testing/foundation-one-cdx#cdx-claims).

2007 ASCO-CAP GUIDELINES FOR HER2 TESTING

Although concordance between HER2 IHC and FISH results is statistically significant,[25,38-44] the difficulties of standardizing IHC in paraffin-embedded tissue specimens have clearly been a problem. Initial reported frequencies of IHC positivity ranged from 2% to almost 50%.[45-48] It was thought that the use of a standardized test with standardized control cell lines would solve this problem; however, this approach did not circumvent scoring errors.[38,49,50] Frequencies of HER2 positivity ranging from 30% to 60% in large cohort studies were reported in studies using the FDA-approved HercepTest IHC assay (DAKO).[48] It became clear that variable fixation, especially ethanol exposure, and differing antigen retrieval methods led to incorrect IHC results.[38,49]

To address these issues related to HER2 assessment, the American Society of Clinical Oncology (ASCO) and the College of American Pathologists (CAP) published guidelines specifying criteria to be used for clinical assessment of HER2 status.[17,18,34,35,119] The initial 2007 ASCO-CAP guidelines committee was assembled to address reports of considerable variation among HER2 testing results. As reported in the 2007 guidelines,[34,35] "Prospective sub-studies from two of the adjuvant randomized trials of trastuzumab versus nil have demonstrated that approximately 20% of HER2 assays performed in the field (at the primary treatment site's pathology department) were incorrect when the same specimen was re-evaluated in a high volume, central laboratory.[51,52] Such a disorganized practice and high rate of inaccuracy, for such an important test that dictates a critically effective yet potentially life-threatening and expensive treatment, is not acceptable."

The ASCO-CAP guidelines stated, "Despite attempts within the international pathology community to improve the status of HER2 testing in routine practice,[53–57] testing inaccuracy remains a major issue with both IHC and FISH.[42,51,52"] However, HER2 testing irregularities had been reported almost exclusively with IHC testing,[25,39,43,44,52,58–69] as opposed to FISH testing. Among other problems, the critical area of subjectivity in IHC interpretation represents a major issue for IHC analyses, and numerous studies have documented this. For example, even when experienced pathologists are involved, kappa correlation statistics of only 0.67 and 0.74 were achieved for two IHC-based tests, whereas a kappa of 0.97 for FISH was observed in the same material.[70]

In contrast, the testing for *HER2* gene amplification by FISH was largely concordant from institution to institution[71] and had been demonstrated to be significantly more accurate than IHC.[72] Interlaboratory agreement for FISH assays were reported to show high concordance rates, ranging from 92% to 99%,[25,43,51] if unselected groups of patients were analyzed. An analysis of the CAP proficiency testing survey results showed that FISH assay comparisons between clinical laboratories demonstrated the highest level of interlaboratory agreement that CAP had observed for a test performed as part of its proficiency testing program.[50,54,73] When CAP published the initial results of its proficiency testing program for HER2 FISH assays, they found that 100% of the laboratories participating in the program correctly classified the unknown samples using FISH.[54] This initial publication reported results from the first two survey years with 35 and 63 laboratories participating. Moreover, subsequent published reports from the CAP proficiency testing program have consistently shown a high rate of agreement among the 139 laboratories participating in the FISH testing program.[73] Similar findings were reported for the proficiency testing programs in the United Kingdom.[55]

Since 2004, the number of laboratories performing FISH assays and participating in the CAP HER2 proficiency testing program has increased only modestly (174 laboratories in 2004; 317 laboratories in 2011[74]; and 330 laboratories in 2016), whereas the number of laboratories performing IHC assays and participating in the CAP HER2 IHC proficiency testing program has increased dramatically (125 laboratories in 2004; 1150 laboratories in 2011[74]; and 1399 laboratories in 2016). FISH external quality assurance schemes suggest that FISH is much more consistent in external quality audits. Finally, responses to HER2-targeted therapies, both trastuzumab and lapatinib therapies in the setting of metastatic disease, was more strongly associated with HER2 status determined by FISH than by IHC.[13,32]

IHC Changes From the FDA-Approved Requirements

Nevertheless, the 2007 ASCO-CAP guidelines for HER2 testing recommended changes in HER2 testing for both IHC and FISH. The 2007 guidelines codified an "optimal testing algorithm" (Fig. 2.2) for the assessment of HER2 status with IHC as the primary assay method, provided a clinical laboratory had performed a concordance assay comparing the HER2 IHC scoring with a second method, such as FISH, that demonstrated a 95% agreement rate for each immunostaining category, typically IHC 0, IHC 1+, and IHC 3+, which would be used in the laboratory for reporting and treatment decisions. The IHC 2+ category was referred to as "equivocal" with such breast cancers "reflexed" for HER2 testing by FISH.

The 2007 ASCO-CAP guidelines also arbitrarily, without providing any supportive data, required a minimum of 30% immunostaining among carcinoma cells at a particular level, rather than the FDA requirement of 10%, to assign HER2 immunostaining at the subjectively assessed level (1+/2+/3+) of positivity. Unfortunately, for those trying to adhere to the guidelines, neither of these percentages has been established to be important. In frozen tissue samples, HER2 protein has been established to be relatively uniformly expressed at low levels throughout all epithelial cells in both fetal and adult normal tissues.[16] Similarly, among breast cancers that lack *HER2* gene amplification, a similar low level of expression is also present in essentially all invasive carcinoma cells throughout the tumor.[6] Among breast cancers that have *HER2* gene amplification, an increased and uniform level of HER2 membrane protein immunostaining is observed throughout the entire population of cancer cells.[6] It is only when these frozen tissues are formalin-fixed and paraffin-embedded (FFPE) that variability in the level of immunostaining is observed among the tumor cell population within a given cancer as well as the normal epithelium.[6,16] This variability in immunostaining within a specimen is clearly a result of fixation artifacts and has little to do with actual variability in gene expression levels among tumor cells in the vast majority of tissue samples. Of note, this fixation-induced variability in FFPE tissue does not occur with FISH analyses.[13,32,33,75,76]

FISH Changes From FDA-Approved Requirements

The 2007 ASCO-CAP guidelines[34,35] also recommended changes in the FISH scoring criteria that differ from the FDA-approved FISH scoring. These guidelines

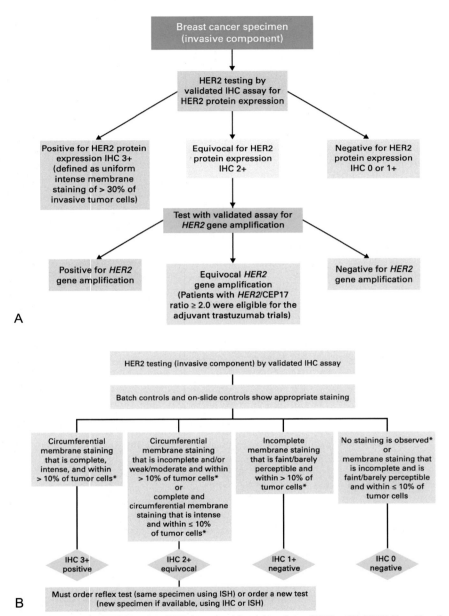

A

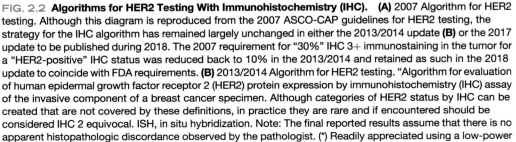

B

FIG. 2.2 **Algorithms for HER2 Testing With Immunohistochemistry (IHC).** **(A)** 2007 Algorithm for HER2 testing. Although this diagram is reproduced from the 2007 ASCO-CAP guidelines for HER2 testing, the strategy for the IHC algorithm has remained largely unchanged in either the 2013/2014 update **(B)** or the 2017 update to be published during 2018. The 2007 requirement for "30%" IHC 3+ immunostaining in the tumor for a "HER2-positive" IHC status was reduced back to 10% in the 2013/2014 and retained as such in the 2018 update to coincide with FDA requirements. **(B)** 2013/2014 Algorithm for HER2 testing. "Algorithm for evaluation of human epidermal growth factor receptor 2 (HER2) protein expression by immunohistochemistry (IHC) assay of the invasive component of a breast cancer specimen. Although categories of HER2 status by IHC can be created that are not covered by these definitions, in practice they are rare and if encountered should be considered IHC 2 equivocal. ISH, in situ hybridization. Note: The final reported results assume that there is no apparent histopathologic discordance observed by the pathologist. (*) Readily appreciated using a low-power

defined a range of 1.8–2.2 for *HER2*-to-CEP17 ratios and of 4.0–6.0 for average HER2 copy number per tumor cell nucleus as equivocal for *HER2* gene amplification. Approximately, 2% of breast cancers have HER2 FISH ratios in this 1.8 to 2.2 range.[71] However, because HER2 status is used by clinicians and patients to make a bimodal decision (to treat or not to treat), the recommendation to have three diagnostic ranges (amplified, equivocal, and not amplified) creates patient management challenges in the context of a dichotomous treatment decision. We do not believe that creation of this equivocal range was justified because no data exist demonstrating that the FDA-approved evaluation criteria, as already recommended by the manufacturer, were insufficient. Apparently, the 2013/2014 ASCO-CAP guidelines committee came to similar conclusions about the 1.8 to 2.2 ratio and changed their criteria for "equivocal" status, as described below.

Challenges With the 2007 ASCO-CAP Guidelines

One of the unstated IHC challenges of these 2007 guidelines was that few laboratories had such high agreement rates between IHC and FISH as required for use of IHC as the primary testing modality (Table 2.3). Among 19 published studies reported between 2000 and 2007, containing at least 100 breast cancers with blinded comparison of IHC and FISH, only two demonstrated the required 95% agreement for IHC 0, IHC 1+, and IHC 3+ with FISH in the same cohort (Table 2.3). In fact, this challenge did not improve after publication of the 2007 guidelines, given that in 18 papers published between 2008 and 2014, only two additional studies achieved this 95% concordance level. Moreover, this problem with IHC testing should have been expected because it had been reported in multiple studies, beginning in 1989, that IHC was associated with a variable number of false-negative results that

are dependent on the specific anti-HER2 antibody used[6,13,26,27,43,71,72] (see amplification rate among IHC 0/1+ breast cancers in Table 2.3). In addition, IHC also demonstrated a variable number of false-positive results that appear to be primarily related to the method or duration of fixation and/or the antigen retrieval method used in the assay[13,32,43,72] (note amplification rates less than 100% among IHC 3+ breast cancers in Table 2.3). Nevertheless, IHC became codified by the 2007 ASCO-CAP guidelines as the primary HER2 testing modality.

Why would IHC be favored over FISH when, as summarized above, HER2 testing by FISH had been consistently reported to be both more accurate and reproducible between laboratories? Probably, because IHC with bright-field microscopy is almost universally available and used in pathology laboratories across the United States and pathologists have had remarkable resistance to adapting the more accurate method that requires the use of fluorescence microscopy after hybridization of fluorescently labeled DNA probes. The subsequent approval of two bright-field microscopy methods for ISH (Table 2.1) could potentially assist with acceptance in pathology laboratories. However, while these ISH methods do improve assessment of HER2 status compared with IHC, they have some limitations, the most notable of which is the inability to accurately enumerate the *HER2* gene copy number in more highly amplified breast (or upper GI) cancer cases. However, treatment decisions are not currently driven by the gene amplification levels but instead by a result of "amplified" versus "not amplified." While our experience indicates that these bright-field microscopy ISH methods have some technical limitations, we consider them superior to IHC as a modality for accurate HER2 testing.

The stated goal of the 2007 ASCO-CAP guidelines committee was "To develop a guideline to improve

---

objective and observed within a homogeneous and contiguous invasive cell population." This algorithm for IHC largely ignores both the IHC false-negative and IHC false-positive results tabulated from the world's literature between 2000 and 2017 in Table 2.3. (Reproduction with permission of testing algorithm (Fig. 1) from Wolff AC, Hammond ME, Schwartz JN, Hagerty KL, Allred DC, Cote RJ, Dowsett M, Fitzgibbons PL, Hanna WM, Langer A, McShane LM, Paik S, Pegram MD, Perez EA, Press MF, Rhodes A, Sturgeon C, Taube SE, Tubbs R, Vance GH, van de Vijver M, Wheeler TM, Hayes DF. American Society of Clinical Oncology/College of American Pathologists guideline recommendations for human epidermal growth factor receptor 2 testing in breast cancer. *J Clin Oncol* 2007;25(1):118–145 and Reproduction with permission of testing algorithm (Fig. 1) from Wolff A, Hammond MEH, Hicks DG, Dowsett M, McShane L, Allison KH, Allred DC, Bartlett JMS, Bilous M, Fitzgibbons P, Hanna W, Jenkins RB, Mangu P, Paik S, Perez E, Press MF, Spears PA, Vance GH, Viale G, Hayes D. Recommendations for human epidermal growth factor receptor 2 testing in breast cancer: American Society of Clinical Oncology - College of American Pathologists {ASCO/CAP} clinical practice guideline update. *J Clin Oncol*. 2013;31:3997–4013.)

TABLE 2.3

Concordance Between IHC and FISH: Prevalence of HER2 Gene Amplification (%) in Each IHC Immunostaining Category (0, 1+, 2+, and 3+) by Study

HER2 GENE AMPLIFICATION RATE (%) ACCORDING TO IHC SCORE						
IHC 0	IHC 1+	IHC 2+	IHC 3+	Number	IHC Method	References
0%	0%	17%	89%	100	Dako HercepTest (FDA)	Hoang et al. [61]
	1.8%	35.9%	100%	750	Dako Ab (LDT)	Ridolfi et al. [67,b]
3.5%	66.2%	97%	99%	2857	Dako HercepTest (FDA)	Simon et al. [67]
0%	2.2%	38.2%	91.4%	189	Dako A0485 (LDT)	Wang et al. [69]
0%	5.7%	18.5%	100%	170	LDT	Kobayashi et al. [62]
3.8%	8.5%	42.2%	100%	198	Dako HercepTest (FDA)	McCormick et al. [65]
0%	0%	0%	89.8%	119	Dako HercepTest (FDA)	Roche et al. [52]
	0.7%	48.1%	94.1%	426	Dako HercepTest (FDA)	Dowsett et al. [58]
	4.2%	6.1%	48.8%	102	Dako HercepTest (FDA)	Hammock et al. [60]
1.1%	3.1%	26.5%	89.7%	2279	Dako HercepTest (FDA)	Lal et al. [63]
	0%	20%	90%	360	Dako HercepTest (FDA)	Mrozkowiak et al. [66]
	0%	11.6%	80.4%	788	Dako HercepTest (FDA)	Varshney et al. [68]
	2.8%	17%	91.6%	2913	Dako A0485 (LDT)	Yaziji et al. [44]
3%	7%	24%	89%	529	Clinical Trials Assay (LDT)	Dybdal et al. [25]
	6.9%	31.8%	90%	114	Dako HercepTest (FDA)	Ellis et al. [59]
	2.4%	72%	100%	215	Dako HercepTest (FDA)	Lottner et al. [64]
3.6%	5.3%	16.9%	78.2%	842	Dako HercepTes (FDA)t	Press et al. [43]
12.5%	6.7%	7%	52.4%	108	Dako HercepTest (FDA)	Ciampa et al. [39]
0%	0%	12.2%	91.6%	289	Dako HercepTest (FDA)	Hofmann et al. [77]
0%	8.3%	22.9%	56.3%	661	Dako HercepTest (FDA)	Rasmussen et al. [78]
	1.6%	29.1%	86.4%	697	A0485 (Dako)	Grimm et al. [79]
	12.2%	66.6%	93.9%	175	3B5 antibody (LDT)	Panjwani et al. [80]
	3.3%	57.9%	95.2%	100	Dako HercepTest (FDA)	Tsuda et al. [81,b]
0%	3.3%	15.2%	84.1%	200	4B5 antibody LDT	Lambein et al. [82]
0%	3.2%	21.5%	91%	681	Dako HercepTest (FDA)	Jorgenson [83]
	12.8%	43.8%	97.8%	291	A0485 (Dako) LDT	Bernasconi et al. [84]
0%	23%	38.8%	100%	216	CB11 antibody	Martin et al. 2012[85]
3.3%	7.1%	49.2%	88.4%	543	CB11 antibody	Lee et al. 2012[86]
0%	12.5%	76.5%	97.3%	125	Dako HercepTest (FDA)	Kiyose et al. [87]
	2.4%	39.9%	98.1%	1437	Dako HercepTest (FDA)	Vergara-Lluri et al. [88,b]
	9.6%	38.9%	87.2%	396	CB11 (Biogenix)	Kokate et al. [89]
2.6%	4.8%	28.1%	93.8%	950	A0485 (Dako) LDT	Park et al. [90]
0%	1%	19%	92%	154	Dako HercepTest (FDA)	Minot et al. [91]
10%	5%	13%	69%	2546	CB11 (Ventana)	Varga et al. [92]
0%	2.6%	29.4%	100%	150	4B5 (Ventana) (FDA)	Lambein et al. [93,b]
9.4%	6.4%	13.5%	55.1%	628	A0485 (Dako) LDT	Fasching et al. [75]

1.7%	3.3%	12.4%	81.1%	2590	Dako HercepTest (FDA)	Schalper et al. [94]
0.8%	0.7%	5.8%	84.3%	1528	Dako HercepTest (FDA)	Varga et al. [95]
	1.5%	16.4%	98.9%	811	4B5 (Ventana)	Green IF et al., Hum Pathol, 2015[96,b]
	31.3%	50.5%	95.2%	175	A0485 (Dako) (LDT)	Pu et al. [97]
	2%	53%	45.0%	943	A0485 (Dako) (LDT)	Pennacchia et al. [98]
	2.90%	13.3%	51.7%	93	4B5 (Ventana)	Layfield et al. [99]
	26.8%	33.3%	59.09%	180	Dako HercepTest (FDA)	Onguru et al. [100]
1%	0.6%	16.8%	49.1%	3605	Dako HercepTest (FDA)	Morey et al. [101]
	5.6%	40.3%	100%	314	4B5 rabbit monoclonal, Ventana (FDA)	Overcast et al. [102,b]
5.8%	6.2%	36.0%	96.4%	368	4B5 rabbit monoclonal, Ventana (FDA)	Solomon et al. [103]
0%	3.3%	23.5%	100%	129	4B5 rabbit monoclonal, Ventana (FDA)	Qi et al. [104,b]
	0.5%	47%	91.8%	240	Dako HercepTest (FDA)	Hyeon et al. [105]
	4.2%	31.1%	93%	432	Dako HercepTest (FDA)	Eswarachary et al. [106]
	3.2%	37.0%	97.8%	498	Dako HercepTest (FDA)	Furrer et al. [107,b]
2.5%	7.4%	31.3%	85.4%		Averages by studies with 4 IHC categories	
	3.9%	36.5%	91.5%		Averages by studies with 3 IHC categories	

LDT: laboratory-developed IHC test; FDA: FDA-approved IHC assay.

Overall the average prevalence of HER2-amplification by FISH in each immunohistochemical staining category among these studies are as follows: IHC0/1: 3.2%; IHC0: 2.5%; IHC1+: 7.4%; IHC2+: 33.9%; IHC3+: 88.4%. If weighted by the number of cases in each study the averages are slightly different: IHC0/1+: 3.2%; IHC0: 2.1%; IHC1+: 4.6%; IHC2+: 23.4%; IHC3+: 84.5%. If one considers only studies using FDA-approved assays the weighted averages for HER2-amplification are as follows: IHC0/1+: 3.1%; IHC0: 2.0%; IHC1+: 4.6%; IHC2+: 21.1%; IHC3+: 83.0%. If one considers only studies using laboratory-developed IHC assays the weighted average prevalence rates for HER2-amplification are as follows: IHC0/1+: 3.9%; IHC0: 3.7%; IHC1+: 4.8%; IHC2+: 24.7%; IHC3+: 89.5%.

[a] IHC and FISH comparisons of at least 100 cases.

[b] Studies which achieve 95% concordance for each IHC 0, IHC 1+, and IHC 3+ in a single study.

the accuracy of human epidermal growth factor receptor 2 (HER2) testing in invasive breast cancer and its utility as a predictive marker."[34,35] However, it is a matter of some debate whether or not the 2007 guidelines accomplished this goal.[71,94] Importantly, however, these guidelines did standardize preanalytical tissue processing of breast cancer specimens by designating formalin as the exclusive fixative of use. The 2007 guidelines also defined optimal required formalin fixation from 6 to 48 h, although this requirement was subsequently changed to 6–72 h in the 2013/2014 ASCO-CAP guidelines. The 2007 guidelines also led to a much wider adoption of the HER2 proficiency testing program provided by CAP and required by these guidelines.[74]

2013/2014 ASCO-CAP GUIDELINES FOR HER2 TESTING

The ASCO-CAP guidelines were modified in concurrent papers with publication dates in 2013[17] and 2014[18] "to improve the accuracy of HER2 testing and its utility as a predictive marker in invasive breast cancer." Although there were minor changes made to the 2007 guidelines for testing with IHC, the changes made to the guidelines for testing with ISH were more substantial.

IHC Testing

Immunohistochemistry remained as the primary testing modality for HER2 assessments in the 2013/2014 ASCO-CAP guidelines and the four immunostaining categories were maintained; however, the requirement for >30% of the tumor cells to show a particular level of staining was decreased to the previous >10% originally required by the FDA and kit manufacturers in 1998.

The IHC algorithm for HER2 testing was maintained with IHC considered the acceptable primary testing modality. IHC 2+ breast cancers were reflexed to ISH for assessment of HER2 gene amplification (Fig. 2.1). Interestingly, the guidelines still recommend clinical laboratories using IHC to engage in a concordance study with ISH before implementation of IHC as their primary testing modality. However, the percentage of agreement with ISH, formerly 95%, was no longer explicitly stated, rather the new guidelines were more generalized and stated that "Laboratories are responsible for ensuring the reliability and accuracy of their testing results, by compliance with accreditation and proficiency testing requirements for HER2 testing assays. Specific concordance requirements are not required (Data Supplement 11)."[17,18]

The 2013/2014 guidelines also required strong and complete membrane staining in >10% of tumor cells for a IHC 3+ score. However, this has been modified following a "Letter to the Editor," which points out that micropapillary breast cancers with HER2 gene amplification have strong membrane staining of only the lateral and basal membranes but not of the apical membranes.[108]

Although this is true for micropapillary breast carcinomas, it is also true for all other adenocarcinomas, including breast,[109] and all normal epithelial cells lining glandular structures, such as breast, gastrointestinal tract, respiratory tract, female reproductive tract, and the choroid plexus of the brain.[16] The likely reason this is not more widely appreciated, including by the ASCO-CAP guidelines, is related to the relative infrequency or relative lack of glandular lumens in grade 2 and grade 3 breast cancers, which are the cancers that most frequently have HER2 gene amplification and overexpression. Therefore, breast cancers with HER2 gene amplification only "appear" to have circumferential strong immunostaining. In fact, if the pseudoglandular lumens are sought and identified, they lack HER2 membrane staining.[109]

Although the 2013/2014 ASCO-CAP guidelines recommend reflex FISH analysis in equivocal IHC 2+ breast cancers to identify the approximately 15%–48% of "IHC 2+" breast cancers that have HER2 gene amplification (Table 2.3), the guidelines continue to make no recommendation about identification of the critical 2%–8% of IHC 0/1+ breast cancers[75] that also have HER2 gene amplification or the 5%–22% of IHC 3+

breast cancers[13,32] that lack HER2 gene amplification (Table 2.3).

ISH Testing

The 2013/2014 guidelines were designed to address both FISH and bright-field in situ hybridization (CISH, SISH, DISH) assays. In these guidelines, the assessment of HER2 ISH status was substantially changed. Instead of having three categories based on ISH ratios, "positive" (ISH ratio ≥2.2), "equivocal" (ISH ratio 1.8 to 2.2), and "negative" (ISH ratio <1.8), as recommended in 2007, the 2013/2014 guidelines created five different ISH categories, three of which were "ISH-positive," one "ISH-equivocal," and one "ISH-negative." These five categories are based on a combination of average HER2 gene copy number and HER2-to-CEP17 ratio (Fig. 2.1). Breast cancers with HER2-to-CEP17 ratios ≥2.0 are composed of two groups: one with an average HER2 gene copy number ≥4.0 per tumor cell (our "group 1") and one with an average HER2 gene copy number <4.0 per tumor cell (our "group 2"). Breast cancers with HER2-to-CEP17 ratios <2.0 are composed of three additional groups: one with average HER2 gene copy number ≥6.0 per tumor cell (our "group 3"), which is also classified as "ISH-positive;" another with average HER2 gene copy number ≥4.0 but <6.0 signals/tumor cell (our "group 4"), which is classified as the new "ISH-equivocal" cases; and one additional category with breast cancers containing an average HER2 gene copy number <4.0 signals/tumor cell (our "group 5"), which is classified as "ISH-negative." According to these ASCO-CAP guidelines,[17,18] breast cancers in groups 1, 2, and 3 are interpreted as "ISH-positive," group 4 as "ISH-equivocal," and group 5 as "ISH-negative" (Fig. 2.1).

Problems With ISH Testing according to the 2013/2014 Guidelines

At the time these guidelines were published, no clinical or demographic data were available using this revised classification schema and basic information such as the prevalence of each FISH group in the general breast cancer population was unknown. Moreover, data regarding whether these new ASCO-CAP groups correlated with HER2 protein expression or, more importantly, clinical outcomes were also not available. To better address these questions, we conducted two retrospective studies of breast cancer specimens previously characterized for HER2 status in our laboratories: one set was from a cohort of an academic consultation practice,[76] and the other set was from breast cancers screened for entry to Breast Cancer International Research Group (BCIRG)/Translational Research in

TABLE 2.4
Prevalence of Breast Cancer for Each ASCO-CAP HER2 FISH Group

Group	Description of FISH Category	BCIRG/TRIO TRIALS[33]		CONSULTATION PRACTICE[76]	
		Number of Cases	Overall (%)	Number of Cases	Overall (%)
1	Ratio ≥2.0; HER2 average ≥ 4.0	4269	40.8	1328	17.7
2	Ratio ≥2.0; HER2 average < 4.0	71	0.7	31	0.4
3	Ratio <2.0; HER2 average ≥ 6.0	55	0.5	48	0.6
4	Ratio <2.0; HER2 average ≥ 4.0, <6.0	432	4.1	345	4.6
5	Ratio <2.0; HER2 average < 4.0	5641	53.9	5774	76.7
Total		10,468	100	7526	100

ASCO, American Society of Clinical Oncology; BCIRG, Breast Cancer International Research Group; CAP, College of American Pathologists; FISH, fluorescence in situ hybridization; HER2, human epidermal growth factor receptor 2; TRIO, Translational Research in Oncology. Reproduced as a combined single table using data from Table 1 in each of two studies Press MF, Sauter G, Buyse M, et al. HER2 gene amplification testing by fluorescent in situ hybridization (FISH): comparison of the ASCO-College of American pathologists guidelines with FISH scores used for enrollment in breast cancer international research group clinical trials. *J Clin Oncol* 2016;**34**:3518–3528; Press MF, Villalobos I, Santiago A, et al: Assessing the new American Society of Clinical Oncology/College of American Pathologists Guidelines for HER2 testing by fluorescence in situ hybridization: experience of an academic consultation practice. *Arch Pathol Lab Med* 2016;**140**:1250–1258.

Oncology (TRIO) clinical trials.[33] From these studies, we were able to determine the prevalence of each group in the general breast cancer patient population (Table 2.4).

Although the 2013/2014 ASCO-CAP guidelines[17,18] had retained the designation of "equivocal" for ISH, the definition of what constituted a "HER2-equivocal" breast cancer was modified. Based on the data from our studies and those of others, it became clear that the number of "equivocal" cases had increased from approximately 2%[71] to between 4% and 12%.[33,76,95,102,110–113] This expanded use of the HER2-equivocal category by the ASCO-CAP "reaffirms its 2013 intent to err on the side of sensitivity rather than specificity in view of the known benefits and low risks associated with anti-HER2 therapy such as trastuzumab."[114] However, no data or analyses were provided to justify this "intent to err."

Based on our studies of the USC academic consultation practice and the BCIRG/TRIO breast cancer trials, we respectfully disagree with the ASCO-CAP about the designations assigned to three of the five ISH categories (Table 2.2). Although we agree with the designation of only group 1 as "ISH-positive" and only group 5 as "ISH-negative," we estimate that these two groups contain between 90% and 95% of all breast carcinomas (Table 2.4). Therefore, our disagreement impacts multiple ISH categories but only approximately 5%–10% of breast cancer patients.

USC/BCIRG-TRIO CENTRAL LABORATORY

In FISH analyses, each copy of the HER2 gene and its centromere 17 (CEP17) reference are visible and can be counted in the tumor cell nuclei using a tissue section (Fig. 2.1). To define amplification, the presence of at least twice as many HER2 signals as CEP17 signals per tumor cell has been recommended by us[4,19,20,27] and others[21,22] based on previous studies with DNA analysis using Southern blot hybridization.[4] This cutoff value, later used in clinical trials, was subsequently accepted by the FDA as the value to differentiate HER2-amplified from HER2-not-amplified breast cancers. Use of this cutoff has correlated well with overexpression of the gene product as assessed by either mRNA or protein analyses,[6,41,72] with more aggressive disease behavior[4,6,27] and with responsiveness to HER-2–targeted therapy.[7–9,24,32,37] Although we recommend the use of an internal control, such as CEP17, we have shown that similar conclusions are generally reached with either the HER2-to-CEP17 ratio, as originally formulated using the Oncor INFORM FISH assay, or the average HER2 copy number alone, as subsequently used in the Oncor/Ventana INFORM FISH assay.[4] However, there are some breast cancers that may be misclassified using this latter approach. Those breast cancers (approximately 6%–9% of cases) with increased CEP17 copy number (four copies or more per tumor cell) but without HER2 gene amplification may be incorrectly considered as HER2 amplified (false positive) if no CEP17 control is included in the FISH assay.[115] Despite the fact that the different FISH assessment strategies generally yield similar results, for these less frequent breast cancers the use of an internal control probe from the same chromosome but outside the HER2 amplicon is important. The FISH ratio is also useful to assist with decision-making near the cutoff of 2.0. For example, near this cutoff ratio (2.0), the average HER2 copy number (numerator) should be increased above an average of 4.0 copies per tumor cell nucleus. In addition, the use of a ratio with a control gene on the same chromosome is consistent with the approach used to originally assess gene amplification by Southern blot hybridization.[5,6,72,113] We consider the use of both HER2 and CEP17 copy numbers to determine a FISH ratio as the optimal and most biologically appropriate approach to identify HER2-amplified tumors.

From this perspective, the current use of both the average HER2 gene copy number as well as HER2-to-CEP17 FISH ratio to categorize various HER2 groups appears reasonable. However, in the absence of data, associating these ASCO-CAP HER2 FISH groups with HER2 protein overexpression or clinical outcome was problematic. Therefore, we performed two studies to assess these associations.[33,76]

Association of Each ASCO-CAP FISH Group With HER2 Protein Expression Level

Because the primary biologic consequence of HER2 gene amplification is HER2 protein overexpression, we evaluated the association of each ASCO-CAP FISH group with HER2 protein expression levels determined by IHC to assess agreement between ASCO-CAP FISH guidance and the protein expression category by IHC. As expected, we found that ASCO-CAP FISH group 1 breast cancers were significantly associated with increased protein expression (IHC 2+ and IHC 3+). Also, as expected, ASCO-CAP FISH group 5 breast cancers were significantly associated with low HER2 protein expression (IHC 0 and IHC 1+). Contrary to the ASCO-CAP designations, we found that ASCO-CAP group 2 was significantly associated with low HER2 protein expression, rather than overexpression as would be expected for an ISH-positive breast cancer (Fig. 2.1D and E). Likewise, ASCO-CAP group 4 "ISH-equivocal" breast cancers were significantly associated with low HER2 protein expression (IHC 0/1+) (Fig. 2.1J and K). The ASCO-CAP group 3 breast cancers appeared to be composed of two different subgroups, a more numerous subgroup of cases that we have previously reported as "HER2-not-amplified" (our group 3N) that show an association with low expression (IHC 0/1+) (Fig. 2.1F and G). Another less numerous subgroup (our group 3A) had

been previously reported as "HER2-amplified" and had an association with HER2 protein overexpression (IHC 2+/3+) (Figs. 2.1H,I and 2.3). Therefore, we considered the ASCO-CAP FISH group 3 breast cancers to be a mixed group, composed of at least two subgroups.

Association of Each ASCO-CAP FISH Group With Clinical Outcomes

Human breast cancer cell lines engineered to overexpress HER2 have an increased proliferative rate, migrate further and more rapidly, and have increased angiogenesis and greater invasive capacity in model systems. Likewise, breast cancers with HER2 gene amplification/overexpression clinically behave more aggressively than breast cancers lacking this alteration as reflected in shorter patient DFS and OS. In addition, only those breast cancers with HER2 amplification/overexpression respond to HER2-targeted therapies in preclinical model systems and in patient clinical trials.[7–9,13,24,32,116] Using these clinical behavioral criteria, we investigated whether the ASCO-CAP guidelines HER2 FISH groups behave clinically in a fashion consistent with or, alternatively, inconsistent with the group designation of either "ISH HER2-positive" or "ISH HER2-negative." This analysis was performed using data from two large randomized clinical trials, the BCIRG-005 (trial of adjuvant chemotherapy in "HER2-not-amplified" disease treated without HER2-targeted therapy) and BCIRG-006 (trial of "HER2-amplified" disease treated with HER2-targeted therapy in the adjuvant setting).[33]

As expected for "ISH-positive" disease, ASCO-CAP group 1 breast cancer patients from the BCIRG-006 trial had a significantly improved DFS and OS, among those randomized to trastuzumab compared with those who received standard AC-T chemotherapy alone. Although the number of patients with ASCO-CAP group 2 breast cancers enrolled in BCIRG-006 were limited, as expected from the approximately 1% frequency of these cases, patients whose cancers were in group 2 showed no significant improvement in either DFS or OS when randomized to trastuzumab compared with those randomized to standard AC-T chemotherapy alone. This is what would be expected for "ISH-negative" disease, not "ISH-positive," as designated by the 2013/2014 ASCO-CAP guidelines. The 2018 Clinical Practice Guideline Focused Update has re-classified Group 2 as "ISH-negative" provided IHC assay is *not* IHC 3+ for these causes.[119]

HER2 ASCO-CAP FISH group 4 ("ISH HER2-equivocal") breast cancer patients were enrolled in the BCIRG-005 trial with other "HER2-not-amplified" cases, not in the BCIRG-006 trial. Had these patients had more aggressive disease than the ASCO-CAP group

5 patients, enrolled in BCIRG-005, one would have predicted that separate identification of these patients as a subgroup of the trial would have found this subgroup to have shorter DFS and shorter OS; however, this was not observed. As expected for a subgroup of patients who also have "ISH HER2-negative" breast cancers, ASCO-CAP group 4 breast cancer patients had a DFS and OS that was not significantly different from ASCO-CAP group 5 breast cancer patients who were also enrolled in the same trial.[33]

Confirmation of this "*HER2*-not-amplified" status in ASCO-CAP FISH group 4 or "ISH-equivocal" breast cancers is also supported by recent findings from investigators at MD Anderson Cancer Center.[113] In this study, alternative control probes were used as suggested by the 2013/2014 ASCO-CAP guidelines to separate the "ISH HER2-equivocal" breast cancers into "ISH HER2-positive" and "ISH HER2-negative" subgroups for making HER2-targeted therapy treatment decisions. These investigators used alternative control probes other than chromosome 17 centromere to identify a subgroup of patients having breast cancers with *HER2*-to-alternative control ratios ≥ 2.0 and another subgroup of patients with *HER2*-to-alternative control ratio < 2.0. The DFS and OS of patients in these two "ISH HER2-equivocal" subgroups were not significantly different from one another[113] (Fig. 2.4). These findings highlight a shortcoming of this approach. This pitfall is the lack of recognition that these alternative control genomic regions, especially those on the p-arm of chromosome 17, may frequently undergo heterozygous deletion leading to an increased *HER2*-to-control probe ratio ≥ 2.0 based exclusively on the heterozygous deletion of the control genomic locus rather than true gene amplification (unpublished data). This independent study from MD Anderson Cancer Center shows that those breast cancer cases that were changed from "ISH HER2-equivocal" to "ISH HER2-positive," based on the use of p-arm alternative controls to convert a HER2 FISH ratio from < 2.0 to ≥ 2.0 have DFS and OS rates similar to those of patients whose cancers continued to have a HER2 FISH ratio < 2.0 after evaluation with these same alternative controls (Fig. 2.4).[113]

The small numbers of patients with ASCO-CAP group 3 tumors, and the requirement to further subdivide them into ASCO-CAP group 3N tumors and ASCO-CAP group 3A tumors, created subgroups too small for meaningful outcome analyses.[33]

In aggregate, the analyses of both HER2 protein expression and clinical outcomes data led to a consistent interpretive pattern as follows: ASCO-CAP FISH group 1: *HER2*-amplified; ASCO-CAP FISH group 2: *HER2*-not-amplified; ASCO-CAP FISH group 3: mixed group with both *HER2*-not-amplified ("group 3N") and *HER2*-amplified ("group 3A") tumors; ASCO-CAP group 4: *HER2*-not-amplified; and ASCO-CAP group 5: *HER2*-not-amplified (Table 2.2).

EXPECTATIONS

As indicated by the title of this chapter, the guidelines for HER2 testing have been in a state of change for more than a decade. We think this flux is likely to continue for the foreseeable future. Based on the studies summarized in the previous sections and studies published by others,[117,118] the ASCO-CAP guidelines committee decided to "update" the HER2 testing recommendations during late 2016 and 2017 to address five clinical questions.[119] These questions are as follows: (1) What is the most appropriate definition for IHC 2+ (IHC Equivocal)? (2) Must HER2 testing be repeated on a surgical specimen if initially negative test on core biopsy? (3) Should invasive cancers with a *HER2*/CEP17 ratio ≥ 2.0 but an average *HER2* copy number < 4.0 signals/cell be considered ISH HER2-positive? (4) Should invasive cancers with an average *HER2* copy number ≥ 6.0 signals/cell but a *HER2*/CEP17 ratio < 2.0 be considered ISH HER2-positive? and (5) What is the appropriate diagnostic work-up for invasive cancers with an average *HER2* copy number ≥ 4.0 but < 6.0 signals/cell and a *HER2*/CEP17 ratio < 2.0 and initially deemed to have an equivocal *HER2* ISH test result?

The committee answered these questions as follows: (1) Define IHC 2+ "as invasive breast cancer with weak to moderate complete membrane straining observed in $> 10\%$ of tumor cells". However, the committee did not recognize that HER2 protein is not expressed on the luminal membranes of either normal or malignant glandular epithelium, only lateral and basal membranes, as reported elsewhere[16,71,109]; (2) Recommended that additional HER2 testing is optional as would have been expected, considering the histopathological grade of many "triple-negative" (ER-negative, PR-negative, and HER2-not-amplified) breast cancers; (3) Ironically, required additional testing by a less accurate[6,26,43,72] IHC approach to resolve the status of these already evidence-based *HER2*-not-amplified "group 2" and "group 4" breast cancers "to arrive at the most accurate HER2 status determination (positive or negative) based on combined interpretation of the ISH and IHC assays"; (4) Again, recommend additional testing with IHC rather than the previous "ISH-positive" designation which is unsupported by any data; and (5) Once

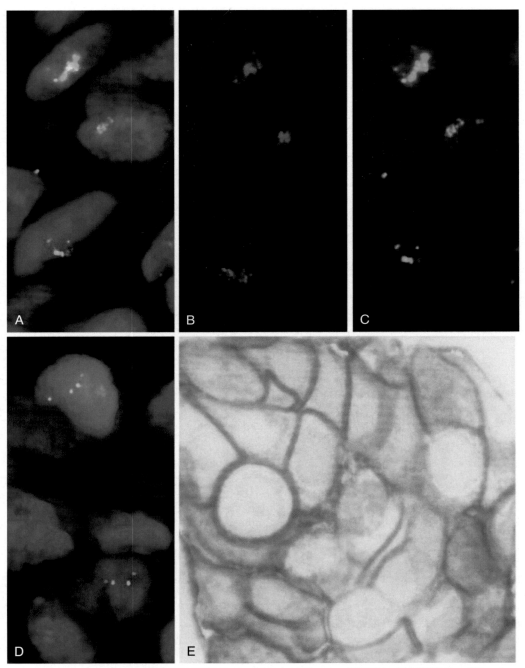

FIG. 2.3 **Assessment of ASCO-CAP FISH Group 3A Breast Cancers (*HER2*-to-CEP17 Ratio <2.0 and an Average *HER2* Gene Copy Number ≥6.0 Per Tumor Cell Nucleus).**   A minority of American Society of Clinical Oncology/College of American Pathologists (ASCO-CAP) group 3 breast cancers, referred to here as "group 3A," show both *HER2* gene amplification and HER2 protein overexpression. **(A)** An ASCO-CAP group 3 breast cancer, one of our group 3A cases. This breast cancer has an average *HER2* gene copy number of 23.2 per tumor cell and an average chromosome 17 centromere (CEP17) copy number of 15.75 per tumor cell. It therefore has a *HER2* FISH ratio of only 1.47. This triple bandpass image shows the composite (blue/orange/green) image with *HER2* gene copies (orange) and CEP17 copies (green) arranged together in a limited geographic area of tumor cell nuclei

again, recommend additional testing with IHC rather than an unsupported-by-data "ISH-positive" or "ISH-negative" designation, based on the result of testing with alternative control gene probes, as described by others.[113,120−122] While these responses represent an advancement over the confusion created in HER2 FISH testing by the 2013/2014 ASCO-CAP HER2 testing guidelines, they still do not take full advantage of well-established data, both recent and old, to adjust the designations so they coincide with the known associations described using correlative science and clinical outcomes. As a result, we expect continued fluidity and confusion in the application of the guidelines.

CONCLUSION

A strength of the original FDA-related guidelines is that they are based on data submitted with the companion diagnostic to obtain approval. One can take issue with the amount or quality of the data provided for some tests, but these applications and approvals are based on analyses of the submitted data. A few of these applications, for example, the first two FISH assays, have used clinical outcome information in the application process, which requires substantial investment and more time and effort, often within a clinical trial, to support the review process. Other applications have used primarily concordance studies in the application process. These require less data, are much less costly, but have often been deemed sufficient. As a result, those companion diagnostics based on concordance data alone have some vulnerabilities because their diagnostic interpretative criteria are not related to clinical outcomes (Table 2.1).

In our opinion, the ASCO-CAP guidelines are at their best when they adhere to benchmarks established by data submitted to the FDA and published in the literature. Changes to HER2 testing guidelines that differ from the FDA criteria and/or those based on opinions of committee members, without published data, such as the use of a FISH ratio of 2.2 in 2007 or the separation of HER2 FISH assay results into five categories based on both average HER2 copy number and HER2 FISH ratios without any published data, are problematic. Those instances where ASCO-CAP guidelines contradict published data are potentially even more challenging to resolve because erroneous approaches to testing become entrenched in practice. For example, the continued use of IHC as an acceptable sole screening procedure is recommended in each of the ASCO-CAP guidelines, yet the world's literature demonstrates the presence of both "false-negative" (IHC 0 and IHC 1+/FISH-amplified) and "false-positive" (IHC 3+/FISH-not-amplified) breast cancers with this approach

---

(blue). Please note that the HER2 gene signals (orange) and CEP17 signals (green) are aggregated together in the same limited geographic area of nuclei, making assessment of individual signals challenging without the aid of single bandpass filters, as illustrated in B and C. HER2 gene (orange) and CEP17 (green) are identified using the Abbott-Molecular PathVysion HER2 DNA probe kit (Vysis LSI HER-2/neu SpectrumOrange/CEP17 SpectrumGreen) FISH assay. Consultation case number C20906. **(B)**. This single bandpass image (orange filter) shows the distribution of HER2 gene copies in the same tumor cell nuclei illustrated in A and C. HER2 gene copies (orange) are identified using the Abbott-Molecular PathVysion HER2 DNA probe kit (Vysis LSI HER-2/neu SpectrumOrange/CEP17 SpectrumGreen) FISH assay. Consultation case number C20906. **(C)** This single bandpass image (green filter) shows the distribution of alpha satellite DNA of CEP17 (green) in the same tumor cell nuclei illustrated in A and B. Abbott-Molecular PathVysion HER2 DNA probe kit (Vysis LSI HER-2/neu SpectrumOrange/CEP17 SpectrumGreen) FISH assay. Consultation case number C20906. **(D)** FISH of alternative control probes located on chromosome 17 remote from the HER2 locus. The use of retinoic acid receptor alpha (RARA) gene probe (green) in this breast cancer demonstrated an average of 2.55 RARA copies per tumor cell by FISH, providing a HER2/RARA ratio of 9.1. Similarly, using the Smith-Magenis Syndrome (SMS) region FISH probe (orange) as an alternative control gene probe, there were 1.85 copies per tumor cell, providing a HER2/SMS ratio of 12.54. This breast cancer was reported as "HER2-amplified" in our consultation practice, consistent with the ASCO-CAP guidelines' designation of "ISH-positive." RARA gene (green) and SMS (orange) are identified using the Abbott-Molecular Vysis Smith-Magenis Region LSI SMS SpectrumOrange/RARA SpectrumGreen probes. Consultation case number C20906. **(E)** ASCO-CAP group 3 breast cancer, corresponding to our "group 3A" cases, with HER2 protein overexpression by immunohistochemistry (IHC; IHC 3+ by HercepTest) consistent with the ASCO-CAP guidelines' designation of "ISH-positive." Similar results were obtained with our 10H8-IHC assay (IHC 3+, data not shown). Consultation case number C20906 (original magnifications 1000× [A through D] and 400× [E]). (Reproduction with permission of Fig. 3 from Press MF, Villalobos I, Santiago A, Guzman R, Estrada MC, Gasparyan A, Campeau A, Ma Y, Tsao-Wei D, Groshen SL. Assessing the New American Society of Clinical Oncology/College of American Pathologists Guidelines for HER2 testing by fluorescence in situ hybridization: experience of an academic consultation practice. Arch Pathol Lab Med 2016;140(11):1250−1258.)

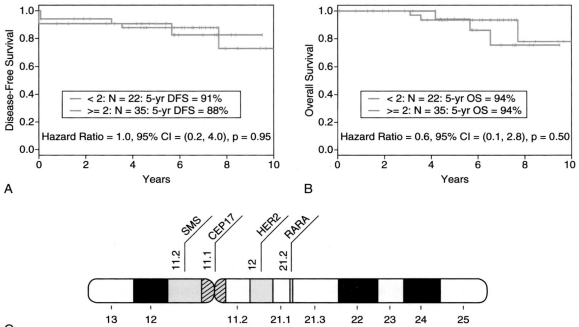

FIG. 2.4 **Clinical Outcomes of ASCO-CAP FISH Group 4 ("HER2-equivocal") Breast Cancer Patients Whose Cancers Were Evaluated with Alternative Control Probes and Reported as Either "ISH-positive" or "ISH-negative" Depending on the Ratios Greater Than or Equal to 2.0 or Less Than 2.0.** **(A)** Kaplan–Meier DFS curves according to the HER2/alternative chromosome 17 gene ratio in 57 patients with equivocal HER2 results (22 with ratios<2 and 35 with ratios ≥2). *CI,* confidence interval; *DFS,* disease-free survival; *HER2,* human epidermal growth factor receptor 2. **(B)** Kaplan–Meier OS curves according to the HER2/alternative chromosome 17 gene ratio in 57 patients with equivocal HER2 results (22 with ratios <2 and 35 with ratios ≥2). *CI,* confidence interval; *HER2,* human epidermal growth factor receptor 2; *OS,* overall survival. **(C)** Location of alternative control gene sites (SMS and RARA) relative to chromosome 17 centromere (CEP17) and *HER2* gene on chromosome 17 p- and q-arms. (Reproduced with permission, Figs. 4, 5 and 6 from Sneige N, Hess KR, Multani AS, Gong Y, Ibrahim NK. Prognostic significance of equivocal human epidermal growth factor receptor 2 results and clinical utility of alternative chromosome 17 genes in patients with invasive breast cancer: a cohort study. *Cancer* 2017;123(7):1115–1123. doi:10.1002/cncr.30460.)

(Table 2.3). As a result, this entrenched approach to testing is not likely to change in the near future.

In the BCIRG/TRIO and the USC Breast Cancer Analysis Laboratory, we have used established disease-related characteristics to assess the appropriateness of the 2013/2014 ASCO-CAP FISH interpretative guidelines for HER2.[33,76] As we previously reported, in the absence of HER2 protein overexpression, one has to question whether the ASCO-CAP FISH group 2, group 3N, or group 4 breast cancers could be anything other than *HER2*-not-amplified. These interpretations are also supported by the clinical outcome findings for ASCO-CAP group 2 and group 4 breast cancer patients. In the case of group 4 ("ISH HER2-equivocal") breast cancers, patient outcomes in the absence of HER2-targeted

therapies are not significantly different from group 5 (ISH HER2-negative) breast cancer patients.[33] In the case of ASCO-CAP group 2 ("ISH HER2-positive" with ratio ≥2.0 but an average HER2 copy number <4.0) breast cancers, patients randomized to trastuzumab in the BCIRG-006 trial of adjuvant trastuzumab with 10 years of clinical follow-up did not show an improvement in either DFS or OS compared with similar patients randomized to treatment with chemotherapy alone.

HER2 gene amplification is directly associated with HER2 protein overexpression. In the nearly three decades since the initial demonstration of this association,[6] there has been no other mechanism for pathologic HER2 protein overexpression identified. Breast cancers originally thought to be *HER2*-not-amplified by solid matrix blotting, but to have HER2 overexpression,[6] have since been demonstrated to be *HER2*-amplified by FISH.[71,109,123] Numerous studies demonstrate that patients whose breast cancers have *HER2* amplification/overexpression and are not treated with HER2-targeted therapies experience significantly worse DFS and OS when compared with similar patients whose cancers lack this alteration. We have used these known biological associations of *HER2* gene amplification status in the BCIRG/TRIO trials and USC consultation practice to assess the classification and interpretation of the five 2013/2014 ASCO-CAP FISH groups.[33,76] This has led us to strongly question the interpretations of the ASCO-CAP guidelines committee for three of the five groups.[17,18] Although breast cancers in these three groups (our ASCO-CAP groups 2, 3, and 4) represent only approximately 5%–12% of all invasive breast cancers, they nevertheless represent significant numbers of patients who, in our opinion, are potentially being subjected to inappropriate treatment based on these erroneous interpretations of *HER2* FISH status. Although some oncologists and pathologists will require results from randomized clinical trials that include HER2-targeted therapy to confirm the correctness of our assertions, we can offer limited clinical trials data for only one of the ASCO-CAP groups, group 2 (average HER2 gene copy number <4.0 and HER2-to-CEP17 ratio ≥2.0). In our studies, ASCO-CAP group 2 breast cancers have significant associations with low HER2 protein expression, not overexpression.[33,76] In addition, among the limited number of such patients accrued to the BCIRG-006 trial of trastuzumab in the adjuvant setting, those randomized to trastuzumab with chemotherapy did not show a significant benefit from this HER2-targeted treatment.

Our assessments of HER2 status are supported by laboratory data from human breast cancer cell lines, clinically annotated human breast cancer tissue samples (both frozen and fixed, paraffin-embedded), and outcomes for various interpretative groups in clinical trials and large cohort studies. As may be apparent from this summary of HER2 testing issues, our approach differs from the ASCO-CAP HER2 testing guidelines in several ways, including the use of both FISH and IHC with FISH established as the primary, more accurate method. In addition, our interpretative designations, particularly for HER2 FISH groups 2, 3, and 4, differ substantially from those specified by the 2013/2014 ASCO-CAP guidelines.

To date, no data have been provided to contradict our reported findings or our classifications.[33,76] Some oncologists and pathologists may want additional outcome data from randomized clinical trials of HER2-targeted therapies for patients in each of these ASCO-CAP FISH groups, much like the NSABP-B47 trial which recently reported absolutely no benefit from trastuzumab among 3270 randomized women whose breast cancers lacked *HER2* amplification and had low expression of HER2 with IHC 1+ or IHC 2+ IHC staining.[116] Such clinical trials require patients to make commitments with their lives to these studies and are extremely costly undertakings. We think clinicians are well advised to treat their patients according to the preponderance of current data until such specialized clinical trials demonstrate our findings to be in error.

The HER2 alteration, as initially described in 1987, is *amplification* of the *HER2* gene.[5] Use of indirect assessments of the effects of *HER2*-amplification such as the measurement of HER2 messenger-RNA or protein levels resulting from the alteration remain a full step away from a direct and accurate assessment of the central event itself, i.e., gene amplification. In fact, they do little more than provide additional technical challenges that make effective indirect assessment of the effects of DNA amplification even more problematic. Assessment of tumor DNA for the presence or absence of *HER2* gene amplification should be based on evidence supported by actual molecular biologic findings, clinical outcomes known to be associated with *HER2* amplification in the pre-trastuzumab era and/or preferably, clinical response data to effective and approved HER2 targeting agents rather than estimates of what might or might not constitute actual gene amplification. We believe that the methods and analyses described in this chapter for effective *HER2* gene amplification assessment provide such evidence.

SUPPORT

Supported in part by grants from the Breast Cancer Research Foundation, Tower Cancer Research Foundation (Jessica M. Berman Senior Investigator Award), a gift from Dr. Richard Blach, and Entertainment Industry Foundation as well as an endowed chair, the Harold E. Lee Chair for Cancer Research. Support for BCIRG/TRIO trials was provided to the Breast Cancer International Research Group (BCIRG), now Translational Research in Oncology. The BCIRG-005 trial was sponsored by Sanofi.

ACKNOWLEDGMENTS

We thank the patients who enrolled in the BCIRG-005 trial and gave their consent as well as the Translational Research in Oncology (previously known as Breast Cancer International Research Group), investigators who recruited these patients at each of the clinical sites, and staff at those sites who supported the trial. We would also like to thank Angela Santiago (University of Southern California central laboratory), Armen Gasparyan (USC central laboratory), Jian-Yuan Zhou, MD (USC central laboratory), Rooba Wardeh, MD (USC central laboratory), Yong-Tian (Brandon) Li, MD (USC central laboratory), Hedvika Novotny (Central laboratory, Basel, Switzerland), Sandra Schneider (Central laboratory, Basel, Switzerland), and Rosemarie Chaffard (Central laboratory, Basel, Switzerland) for technical assistance; Sandra Swain, MD, chair of the data and safety monitoring committee; and all steering committee and translational research committee members.

DISCLOSURE STATEMENT

Disclosure of any relationship with a commercial company that has a direct financial interest in subject matter or materials discussed in the article or with a company making a competing product.

REFERENCES

1. Cancer Genome Atlas N. Comprehensive molecular portraits of human breast tumours. *Nature.* 2012;490: 61−70.
2. Curtis C, Shah SP, Chin SF, et al. The genomic and transcriptomic architecture of 2,000 breast tumours reveals novel subgroups. *Nature.* 2012;486:346−352.
3. Hede K. Breast cancer testing scandal shines spotlight on black box of clinical laboratory testing. *J Natl Cancer Inst.* 2008;100, 836−837, 844.
4. Press MF, Bernstein L, Thomas PA, et al. HER-2/neu gene amplification characterized by fluorescence in situ hybridization: poor prognosis in node-negative breast carcinomas. *J Clin Oncol.* 1997;15:2894−2904.
5. Slamon DJ, Clark GM, Wong SG, et al. Human breast cancer: correlation of relapse and survival with amplification of the HER-2/neu oncogene. *Science.* 1987;235: 177−182.
6. Slamon DJ, Godolphin W, Jones LA, et al. Studies of the HER-2/neu proto-oncogene in human breast and ovarian cancer. *Science.* 1989;244:707−712.
7. Piccart-Gebhart MJ, Procter M, Leyland-Jones B, et al. Trastuzumab after adjuvant chemotherapy in HER2-positive breast cancer. *N Engl J Med.* 2005;353: 1659−1672.
8. Romond EH, Perez EA, Bryant J, et al. Trastuzumab plus adjuvant chemotherapy for operable HER2-positive breast cancer. *N Engl J Med.* 2005;353:1673−1684.
9. Slamon D, Eiermann W, Robert N, et al. Adjuvant trastuzumab in HER2-positive breast cancer. *N Engl J Med.* 2011;365:1273−1283.
10. Swain SM, Baselga J, Kim SB, et al. Pertuzumab, trastuzumab, and docetaxel in HER2-positive metastatic breast cancer. *N Engl J Med.* 2015;372:724−734.
11. Geyer CE, Forster J, Lindquist D, et al. Lapatinib plus capecitabine for HER2-positive advanced breast cancer. *N Engl J Med.* 2006;355:2733−2743.
12. Piccart-Gebhart M, Holmes E, Baselga J, et al. Adjuvant lapatinib and trastuzumab for early human epidermal growth factor receptor 2-positive breast cancer: results from the randomized phase III adjuvant lapatinib and/or trastuzumab treatment optimization trial. *J Clin Oncol.* 2016;34:1034−1042.
13. Press MF, Finn RS, Cameron D, et al. HER-2 gene amplification, HER-2 and epidermal growth factor receptor mRNA and protein expression, and lapatinib efficacy in women with metastatic breast cancer. *Clin Cancer Res.* 2008;14:7861−7870.
14. Perez EA, Barrios C, Eiermann W, et al. Trastuzumab emtansine with or without pertuzumab versus trastuzumab plus taxane for human epidermal growth factor receptor 2-positive, advanced breast cancer: primary results from the phase III MARIANNE study. *J Clin Oncol.* 2017;35:141−148.
15. Verma S, Miles D, Gianni L, et al. Trastuzumab emtansine for HER2-positive advanced breast cancer. *N Engl J Med.* 2012;367:1783−1791.
16. Press MF, Cordon-Cardo C, Slamon DJ. Expression of the HER-2/neu proto-oncogene in normal human adult and fetal tissues. *Oncogene.* 1990;5:953−962.
17. Wolff AC, Hammond ME, Hicks DG, et al. Recommendations for human epidermal growth factor receptor 2 testing in breast cancer: American Society of Clinical Oncology/College of American Pathologists clinical practice guideline update. *J Clin Oncol.* 2013;31: 3997−4013.
18. Wolff AC, Hammond ME, Hicks DG, et al. Recommendations for human epidermal growth factor receptor 2 testing in breast cancer: American Society of Clinical Oncology/College of American Pathologists clinical practice guideline update. *Arch Pathol Lab Med.* 2014;138: 241−256.
19. Press MF, Pike MC, Hung G, et al. Amplification and overexpression of HER-2/neu in carcinomas of the salivary gland: correlation with poor prognosis. *Cancer Res.* 1994;54:5675−5682.
20. Saffari B, Jones LA, el-Naggar A, et al. Amplification and overexpression of HER-2/neu (c-erbB2) in endometrial cancers: correlation with overall survival. *Cancer Res.* 1995;55:5693−5698.
21. Kallioniemi OP, Kallioniemi A, Kurisu W, et al. ERBB2 amplification in breast cancer analyzed by fluorescence in situ hybridization. *Proc Natl Acad Sci USA.* 1992;89: 5321−5325.
22. Sauter G, Moch H, Moore D, et al. Heterogeneity of erbB-2 gene amplification in bladder cancer. *Cancer Res.* 1993; 53:2199−2203.

23. Carter P, Presta L, Gorman CM, et al. Humanization of an anti-p185HER2 antibody for human cancer therapy. *Proc Natl Acad Sci USA.* 1992;89:4285–4289.
24. Slamon DJ, Leyland-Jones B, Shak S, et al. Use of chemotherapy plus a monoclonal antibody against HER2 for metastatic breast cancer that overexpresses HER2. *N Engl J Med.* 2001;344:783–792.
25. Dybdal N, Leiberman G, Anderson S, et al. Determination of HER2 gene amplification by fluorescence in situ hybridization and concordance with the clinical trials immunohistochemical assay in women with metastatic breast cancer evaluated for treatment with trastuzumab. *Breast Cancer Res Treat.* 2005;93:3–11.
26. Press MF, Hung G, Godolphin W, et al. Sensitivity of HER-2/neu antibodies in archival tissue samples: potential source of error in immunohistochemical studies of oncogene expression. *Cancer Res.* 1994;54:2771–2777.
27. Press MF, Pike MC, Chazin VR, et al. Her-2/neu expression in node-negative breast cancer: direct tissue quantitation by computerized image analysis and association of overexpression with increased risk of recurrent disease. *Cancer Res.* 1993;53:4960–4970.
28. Gullick WJ, Love SB, Wright C, et al. c-erbB-2 protein overexpression in breast cancer is a risk factor in patients with involved and uninvolved lymph nodes. *Br J Cancer.* 1991;63:434–438.
29. Lovekin C, Ellis IO, Locker A, et al. c-erbB-2 oncoprotein expression in primary and advanced breast cancer. *Br J Cancer.* 1991;63:439–443.
30. O'Reilly SM, Barnes DM, Camplejohn RS, et al. The relationship between c-erbB-2 expression, S-phase fraction and prognosis in breast cancer. *Br J Cancer.* 1991;63:444–446.
31. Winstanley J, Cooke T, Murray GD, et al. The long term prognostic significance of c-erbB-2 in primary breast cancer. *Br J Cancer.* 1991;63:447–450.
32. Mass RD, Press MF, Anderson S, et al. Evaluation of clinical outcomes according to HER2 detection by fluorescence in situ hybridization in women with metastatic breast cancer treated with trastuzumab. *Clin Breast Cancer.* 2005;6:240–246.
33. Press MF, Sauter G, Buyse M, et al. HER2 gene amplification testing by fluorescent in situ hybridization (FISH): comparison of the ASCO-College of American pathologists guidelines with FISH scores used for enrollment in breast cancer international research group clinical trials. *J Clin Oncol.* 2016;34:3518–3528.
34. Wolff AC, Hammond ME, Schwartz JN, et al. American Society of Clinical Oncology/College of American Pathologists guideline recommendations for human epidermal growth factor receptor 2 testing in breast cancer. *J Clin Oncol.* 2007;25:118–145.
35. Wolff AC, Hammond ME, Schwartz JN, et al. American Society of Clinical Oncology/College of American Pathologists guideline recommendations for human epidermal growth factor receptor 2 testing in breast cancer. *Arch Pathol Lab Med.* 2007;131:18–43.
36. Cobleigh MA, Vogel CL, Tripathy D, et al. Multinational study of the efficacy and safety of humanized anti-HER2 monoclonal antibody in women who have HER2-overexpressing metastatic breast cancer that has progressed after chemotherapy for metastatic disease. *J Clin Oncol.* 1999;17:2639–2648.
37. Vogel CL, Cobleigh MA, Tripathy D, et al. Efficacy and safety of trastuzumab as a single agent in first-line treatment of HER2-overexpressing metastatic breast cancer. *J Clin Oncol.* 2002;20:719–726.
38. Jacobs TW, Gown AM, Yaziji H, et al. Comparison of fluorescence in situ hybridization and immunohistochemistry for the evaluation of HER-2/neu in breast cancer. *J Clin Oncol.* 1999;17:1974–1982.
39. Ciampa A, Xu B, Ayata G, et al. HER-2 status in breast cancer: correlation of gene amplification by FISH with immunohistochemistry expression using advanced cellular imaging system. *Appl Immunohistochem Mol Morphol.* 2006;14:132–137.
40. Owens MA, Horten BC, Da Silva MM. HER2 amplification ratios by fluorescence in situ hybridization and correlation with immunohistochemistry in a cohort of 6556 breast cancer tissues. *Clin Breast Cancer.* 2004;5:63–69.
41. Pauletti G, Dandekar S, Rong H, et al. Assessment of methods for tissue-based detection of the HER-2/neu alteration in human breast cancer: a direct comparison of fluorescence in situ hybridization and immunohistochemistry. *J Clin Oncol.* 2000;18:3651–3664.
42. Perez EA, Suman VJ, Davidson NE, et al. HER2 testing by local, central, and reference laboratories in specimens from the North Central Cancer Treatment Group N9831 intergroup adjuvant trial. *J Clin Oncol.* 2006;24:3032–3038.
43. Press MF, Sauter G, Bernstein L, et al. Diagnostic evaluation of HER-2 as a molecular target: an assessment of accuracy and reproducibility of laboratory testing in large, prospective, randomized clinical trials. *Clin Cancer Res.* 2005;11:6598–6607.
44. Yaziji H, Goldstein LC, Barry TS, et al. HER-2 testing in breast cancer using parallel tissue-based methods. *JAMA.* 2004;291:1972–1977.
45. Barnes DM, Lammie GA, Millis RR, et al. An immunohistochemical evaluation of c-erbB-2 expression in human breast carcinoma. *Br J Cancer.* 1988;58:448–452.
46. Baselga J, Tripathy D, Mendelsohn J, et al. Phase II study of weekly intravenous trastuzumab (Herceptin) in patients with HER2/neu-overexpressing metastatic breast cancer. *Semin Oncol.* 1999;26:78–83.
47. De Potter CR, Beghin C, Makar AP, et al. The neu-oncogene protein as a predictive factor for haematogenous metastases in breast cancer patients. *Int J Cancer.* 1990;45:55–58.
48. Roche PC, Ingle JN. Increased HER2 with U.S. Food and Drug Administration-approved antibody. *J Clin Oncol.* 1999;17:434.

49. Jacobs TW, Gown AM, Yaziji H, et al. Specificity of HercepTest in determining HER-2/neu status of breast cancers using the United States Food and Drug Administration-approved scoring system. *J Clin Oncol.* 1999;17:1983–1987.

50. Tubbs RR, Pettay JD, Roche PC, et al. Discrepancies in clinical laboratory testing of eligibility for trastuzumab therapy: apparent immunohistochemical false-positives do not get the message. *J Clin Oncol.* 2001;19:2714–2721.

51. Paik S, Bryant J, Tan-Chiu E, et al. Real-world performance of HER2 testing—national surgical adjuvant breast and bowel project experience. *J Natl Cancer Inst.* 2002;94:852–854.

52. Roche PC, Suman VJ, Jenkins RB, et al. Concordance between local and central laboratory HER2 testing in the breast intergroup trial N9831. *J Natl Cancer Inst.* 2002;94:855–857.

53. Bilous M, Dowsett M, Hanna W, et al. Current perspectives on HER2 testing: a review of national testing guidelines. *Mod Pathol.* 2003;16:173–182.

54. Cell Markers and Cytogenetics Committees, College of American Pathologists. Clinical laboratory assays for HER-2/neu amplification and overexpression: quality assurance, standardization, and proficiency testing. *Arch Pathol Lab Med.* 2002;126:803–808.

55. Ellis IO, Bartlett J, Dowsett M, et al. Best practice No 176: updated recommendations for HER2 testing in the UK. *J Clin Pathol.* 2004;57:233–237.

56. Hanna W, O'Malley F. Updated recommendations from the HER2/neu consensus meeting. *Curr Oncol.* 2002;9(suppl. 1):S18–S19.

57. Zarbo RJ, Hammond ME. Conference summary, Strategic Science symposium. Her-2/neu testing of breast cancer patients in clinical practice. *Arch Pathol Lab Med.* 2003;127:549–553.

58. Dowsett M, Bartlett J, Ellis IO, et al. Correlation between immunohistochemistry (HercepTest) and fluorescence in situ hybridization (FISH) for HER-2 in 426 breast carcinomas from 37 centres. *J Pathol.* 2003;199:418–423.

59. Ellis CM, Dyson MJ, Stephenson TJ, et al. HER2 amplification status in breast cancer: a comparison between immunohistochemical staining and fluorescence in situ hybridisation using manual and automated quantitative image analysis scoring techniques. *J Clin Pathol.* 2005;58:710–714.

60. Hammock L, Lewis M, Phillips C, et al. Strong HER-2/neu protein overexpression by immunohistochemistry often does not predict oncogene amplification by fluorescence in situ hybridization. *Hum Pathol.* 2003;34:1043–1047.

61. Hoang MP, Sahin AA, Ordonez NG, et al. HER-2/neu gene amplification compared with HER-2/neu protein overexpression and interobserver reproducibility in invasive breast carcinoma. *Am J Clin Pathol.* 2000;113:852–859.

62. Kobayashi M, Ooi A, Oda Y, et al. Protein overexpression and gene amplification of c-erbB-2 in breast carcinomas: a comparative study of immunohistochemistry and

fluorescence in situ hybridization of formalin-fixed, paraffin-embedded tissues. *Hum Pathol.* 2002;33:21–28.

63. Lal P, Salazar PA, Hudis CA, et al. HER-2 testing in breast cancer using immunohistochemical analysis and fluorescence in situ hybridization: a single-institution experience of 2,279 cases and comparison of dual-color and single-color scoring. *Am J Clin Pathol.* 2004;121:631–636.

64. Lottner C, Schwarz S, Diermeier S, et al. Simultaneous detection of HER2/neu gene amplification and protein overexpression in paraffin-embedded breast cancer. *J Pathol.* 2005;205:577–584.

65. McCormick SR, Lillemoe TJ, Beneke J, et al. HER2 assessment by immunohistochemical analysis and fluorescence in situ hybridization: comparison of HercepTest and PathVysion commercial assays. *Am J Clin Pathol.* 2002;117:935–943.

66. Mrozkowiak A, Olszewski WP, Piascik A, et al. HER2 status in breast cancer determined by IHC and FISH: comparison of the results. *Pol J Pathol.* 2004;55:165–171.

67. Ridolfi RL, Jamehdor MR, Arber JM. HER-2/neu testing in breast carcinoma: a combined immunohistochemical and fluorescence in situ hybridization approach. *Mod Pathol.* 2000;13:866–873.

68. Varshney D, Zhou YY, Geller SA, et al. Determination of HER-2 status and chromosome 17 polysomy in breast carcinomas comparing HercepTest and PathVysion FISH assay. *Am J Clin Pathol.* 2004;121:70–77.

69. Wang S, Saboorian MH, Frenkel EP, et al. Assessment of HER-2/neu status in breast cancer. Automated Cellular Imaging System (ACIS)-assisted quantitation of immunohistochemical assay achieves high accuracy in comparison with fluorescence in situ hybridization assay as the standard. *Am J Clin Pathol.* 2001;116:495–503.

70. Bartlett JM, Going JJ, Mallon EA, et al. Evaluating HER2 amplification and overexpression in breast cancer. *J Pathol.* 2001;195:422–428.

71. Sauter G, Lee J, Bartlett JM, et al. Guidelines for human epidermal growth factor receptor 2 testing: biologic and methodologic considerations. *J Clin Oncol.* 2009;27:1323–1333.

72. Press MF, Slamon DJ, Flom KJ, et al. Evaluation of HER-2/neu gene amplification and overexpression: comparison of frequently used assay methods in a molecularly characterized cohort of breast cancer specimens. *J Clin Oncol.* 2002;20:3095–3105.

73. Persons DL, Tubbs RR, Cooley LD, et al. HER-2 fluorescence in situ hybridization: results from the survey program of the College of American Pathologists. *Arch Pathol Lab Med.* 2006;130:325–331.

74. Wolff AC, Hammond ME, Hayes DF. Re: predictability of adjuvant trastuzumab benefit in N9831 patients using the ASCO/CAP HER2-positivity criteria. *J Natl Cancer Inst.* 2012;104:957–958.

75. Fasching PA, Weihbrecht S, Haeberle L, et al. HER2 and TOP2A amplification in a hospital-based cohort of breast cancer patients: associations with patient and tumor characteristics. *Breast Cancer Res Treat.* 2014;145:193–203.

76. Press MF, Villalobos I, Santiago A, et al. Assessing the new American Society of Clinical Oncology/College of American Pathologists Guidelines for HER2 testing by fluorescence in situ hybridization: experience of an academic consultation practice. *Arch Pathol Lab Med.* 2016;140:1250−1258.

77. Hofmann M, Stoss O, Gaiser T, et al. Central HER2 IHC and FISH analysis in a trastuzumab (Herceptin) phase II monotherapy study: assessment of test sensitivity and impact of chromosome 17 polysomy. *J Clin Pathol.* 2008;61:89−94.

78. Rasmussen BB, Andersson M, Christensen IJ, et al. Evaluation of and quality assurance in HER2 analysis in breast carcinomas from patients registered in Danish Breast Cancer Group (DBCG) in the period of 2002−2006. A nationwide study including correlation between HER-2 status and other prognostic variables. *Acta Oncol.* 2008; 47:784−788.

79. Grimm EE, Schmidt RA, Swanson PE, et al. Achieving 95% cross-methodological concordance in HER2 testing: causes and implications of discordant cases. *Am J Clin Pathol.* 2010;134:284−292.

80. Panjwani P, Epari S, Karpate A, et al. Assessment of HER-2/neu status in breast cancer using fluorescence in situ hybridization & immunohistochemistry: experience of a tertiary cancer referral centre in India. *Indian J Med Res.* 2010;132:287−294.

81. Tsuda H, Kurosumi M, Umemura S, et al. HER2 testing on core needle biopsy specimens from primary breast cancers: interobserver reproducibility and concordance with surgically resected specimens. *BMC Cancer.* 2010;10:534.

82. Lambein K, Praet M, Forsyth R, et al. Relationship between pathological features, HER2 protein expression and HER2 and CEP17 copy number in breast cancer: biological and methodological considerations. *J Clin Pathol.* 2011;64:200−207.

83. Jorgensen JT, Moller S, Rasmussen BB, et al. High concordance between two companion diagnostics tests: a concordance study between the HercepTest and the HER2 FISH pharmDx kit. *Am J Clin Pathol.* 2011;136: 145−151.

84. Bernasconi B, Chiaravalli AM, Finzi G, et al. Genetic heterogeneity in HER2 testing may influence therapy eligibility. *Breast Cancer Res Treat.* 2012;133:161−168.

85. Martin V, Camponovo A, Ghisletta M, et al. Internal quality assurance program for ERBB2 (HER2) testing improves the selection of breast cancer patients for treatment with trastuzumab. *Pathol Res Int.* 2012;2012: 261857.

86. Lee Y, Ryu Y, Jeong H, et al. Effectiveness of silver-enhanced in situ hybridization for evaluating HER2 gene status in invasive breast carcinoma: a comparative study. *Arch Med Res.* 2012;43:139−144.

87. Kiyose S, Igarashi H, Nagura K, et al. Chromogenic in situ hybridization (CISH) to detect HER2 gene amplification in breast and gastric cancer: comparison with immunohistochemistry (IHC) and fluorescence in situ hybridization (FISH). *Pathol Int.* 2012;62:728−734.

88. Vergara-Lluri ME, Moatamed NA, Hong E, et al. High concordance between HercepTest immunohistochemistry and ERBB2 fluorescence in situ hybridization before and after implementation of American Society of Clinical Oncology/College of American Pathology 2007 guidelines. *Mod Pathol.* 2012;25:1326−1332.

89. Kokate P, Sawaimoon S, Bhatia S, et al. Evaluation of genetic status of HER-2/neu and aneusomy 17 by fluorescence in situ hybridization and comparison with immunohistochemistry assay from Indian breast cancer patients. *Genet Test Mol Biomark.* 2012;16:239−245.

90. Park S, Park HS, Koo JS, et al. Breast cancers presenting luminal B subtype features show higher discordant human epidermal growth factor receptor 2 results between immunohistochemistry and fluorescence in situ hybridization. *Cancer.* 2012;118:914−923.

91. Minot DM, Voss J, Rademacher S, et al. Image analysis of HER2 immunohistochemical staining. Reproducibility and concordance with fluorescence in situ hybridization of a laboratory-validated scoring technique. *Am J Clin Pathol.* 2012;137:270−276.

92. Varga Z, Noske A, Ramach C, et al. Assessment of HER2 status in breast cancer: overall positivity rate and accuracy by fluorescence in situ hybridization and immunohistochemistry in a single institution over 12 years: a quality control study. *BMC Cancer.* 2013;13:615.

93. Lambein K, Van Bockstal M, Vandemaele L, et al. Distinguishing score 0 from score 1+ in HER2 immunohistochemistry-negative breast cancer: clinical and pathobiological relevance. *Am J Clin Pathol.* 2013; 140:561−566.

94. Schalper KA, Kumar S, Hui P, et al. A retrospective population-based comparison of HER2 immunohistochemistry and fluorescence in situ hybridization in breast carcinomas: impact of 2007 American Society of Clinical Oncology/College of American Pathologists criteria. *Arch Pathol Lab Med.* 2014;138:213−219.

95. Varga Z, Noske A. Impact of modified 2013 ASCO/CAP guidelines on HER2 testing in breast cancer. One year experience. *PLoS One.* 2015;10:e0140652.

96. Green IF, Zynger DL. Institutional quality assurance for breast cancer HER2 immunohistochemical testing: identification of outlier results and impact of simultaneous fluorescence in situ hybridization cotesting. *Hum Pathol.* 2015;46:1842−1849.

97. Pu X, Shi J, Li Z, et al. Comparison of the 2007 and 2013 ASCO/CAP evaluation systems for HER2 amplification in breast cancer. *Pathol Res Pract.* 2015;211:421−425.

98. Pennacchia I, Vecchio FM, Carbone A, et al. HER2 immunohistochemical assessment with A0485 polyclonal antibody: is it time to refine the scoring criteria for the "2+" category? *Appl Immunohistochem Mol Morphol.* 2015;23: 31−35.

99. Layfield LJ, Frazier S, Esebua M, et al. Interobserver reproducibility for HER2/neu immunohistochemistry: a comparison of reproducibility for the HercepTest and the 4B5 antibody clone. *Pathol Res Pract.* 2016;212: 190−195.

100. Onguru O, Zhang PJ. The relation between percentage of immunostained cells and amplification status in breast cancers with equivocal result for Her2 immunohistochemistry. *Pathol Res Pract.* 2016;212:381–384.

101. Morey AL, Brown B, Farshid G, et al. Determining HER2 (ERBB2) amplification status in women with breast cancer: final results from the Australian in situ hybridisation program. *Pathology.* 2016;48:535–542.

102. Overcast WB, Zhang J, Zynger DL, et al. Impact of the 2013 ASCO/CAP HER2 revised guidelines on HER2 results in breast core biopsies with invasive breast carcinoma: a retrospective study. *Virchows Arch.* 2016;469:203–212.

103. Solomon JP, Dell'Aquila M, Fadare O, et al. Her2/neu status determination in breast cancer: a single institutional experience using a dual-testing approach with immunohistochemistry and fluorescence in situ hybridization. *Am J Clin Pathol.* 2017;147:432–437.

104. Qi L, Zhou L, Lu M, et al. Development of a highly specific HER2 monoclonal antibody for immunohistochemistry using protein microarray chips. *Biochem Biophys Res Commun.* 2017;484:248–254.

105. Hyeon J, Cho SY, Hong ME, et al. NanoString nCounter(R) approach in breast cancer: a comparative analysis with quantitative real-time polymerase chain reaction, in situ hybridization, and immunohistochemistry. *J Breast Cancer.* 2017;20:286–296.

106. Eswarachary V, Mohammed IG, Jayanna PK, et al. HER2/neu testing in 432 consecutive breast cancer cases using FISH and IHC - a comparative study. *J Clin Diagn Res.* 2017;11:EC01–EC05.

107. Furrer D, Jacob S, Caron C, et al. Concordance of HER2 immunohistochemistry and fluorescence in situ hybridization using tissue microarray in breast cancer. *Anticancer Res.* 2017;37:3323–3329.

108. Rakha EA, Pigera M, Shaaban A, et al. National guidelines and level of evidence: comments on some of the new recommendations in the American Society of Clinical Oncology and the College of American Pathologists human epidermal growth factor receptor 2 guidelines for breast cancer. *J Clin Oncol.* 2015;33:1301–1302.

109. Press MF, Ma Y, Sauter G, et al. Controversies in HER2 oncogene testing: what constitutes a true positive result in breast cancer patients? *Am J Hematol/Oncol.* 2017;13: 18–28.

110. Long TH, Lawce H, Durum C, et al. The new equivocal: changes to HER2 FISH results when applying the 2013 ASCO/CAP guidelines. *Am J Clin Pathol.* 2015;144: 253–262.

111. Muller KE, Marotti JD, Memoli VA, et al. Impact of the 2013 ASCO/CAP HER2 guideline updates at an academic medical center that Performs primary HER2 FISH testing: increase in equivocal results and utility of reflex immunohistochemistry. *Am J Clin Pathol.* 2015;144: 247–252.

112. Sapino A, Maletta F, Verdun di Cantogno L, et al. Gene status in HER2 equivocal breast carcinomas: impact of distinct recommendations and contribution of a polymerase chain reaction-based method. *Oncologist.* 2014;19:1118–1126.

113. Sneige N, Hess KR, Multani AS, et al. Prognostic significance of equivocal human epidermal growth factor receptor 2 results and clinical utility of alternative chromosome 17 genes in patients with invasive breast cancer: a cohort study. *Cancer.* 2017;123:1115–1123.

114. Wolff AC, Hammond ME, Hicks DG, et al. Reply to E.A. Rakha et al. *J Clin Oncol.* 2015;33:1302–1304.

115. Downey L, Livingston RB, Koehler M, et al. Chromosome 17 polysomy without human epidermal growth factor receptor 2 amplification does not predict response to lapatinib plus paclitaxel compared with paclitaxel in metastatic breast cancer. *Clin Cancer Res.* 2010;16: 1281–1288.

116. Fehrenbacher L, Cecchini RS, Geyer CE, et al. NSABP B-47 (NRG oncology): phase III randomized trial comparing adjuvant chemotherapy with adriamycin (A) and cyclophosphamide (C) → weekly paclitaxel (WP), or docetaxel (T) and C with or without a year of trastuzumab (H) in women with node-positive or high-risk node-negative invasive breast cancer (IBC) expressing HER2 staining intensity of IHC 1+ or 2+ with negative FISH (HER2-Low IBC). In: *Cancer Research San Antonio Breast Cancer Symposium.* 2017.

117. Ballard M, Jalikis F, Krings G, et al. 'Non-classical' HER2 FISH results in breast cancer: a multi-institutional study. *Mod Pathol.* 2017;30:227–235.

118. Stoss OC, Scheel A, Nagelmeier I, et al. Impact of updated HER2 testing guidelines in breast cancer—re-evaluation of HERA trial fluorescence in situ hybridization data. *Mod Pathol.* 2015;28:1528–1534.

119. Wolff AC, Hammond MEH, Allison KH, et al. HER2 testing in breast cancer: American Society of Clinical Oncology/College of American Pathologists Clinical Practice Guideline Focused Update. *J Clin Oncol.* 2018; 36. https://doi.org/10.1200/JCO.2018.77.8738.

120. Donaldson AR, Shetty S, Wang Z, et al. Impact of an alternative chromosome 17 probe and the 2013 American Society of Clinical Oncology and College of American Pathologists guidelines on fluorescence in situ hybridization for the determination of HER2 gene amplification in breast cancer. *Cancer.* 2017;123:2230–2239.

121. Shah MV, Wiktor AE, Meyer RG, et al. Change in pattern of HER2 fluorescent in situ hybridization (FISH) results in breast cancers submitted for FISH testing: experience of a reference laboratory using US Food and Drug Administration Criteria and American Society of Clinical Oncology and College of American Pathologists Guidelines. *J Clin Oncol.* 2016;34: 3502–3510.

122. Tse CH, Hwang HC, Goldstein LC, et al. Determining true HER2 gene status in breast cancers with polysomy by using alternative chromosome 17 reference genes: implications for anti-HER2 targeted therapy. *J Clin Oncol.* 2011; 29:4168–4174.

123. Pauletti G, Godolphin W, Press MF, et al. Detection and quantitation of HER-2/neu gene amplification in human breast cancer archival material using fluorescence in situ hybridization. *Oncogene.* 1996;13:63–72.

CHAPTER 3

Optimal First-Line Treatment of Advanced HER2-Positive Breast Cancer

RUTA RAO, MD • MELODY COBLEIGH, MD

INTRODUCTION

Approximately, 20% of breast cancers have overexpression of the HER2 protein and/or amplification of the *HER2* gene, which has been associated with aggressive tumor behavior and poor disease-free survival (DFS) and overall survival (OS) rates. A seminal study by Slamon and colleagues published in 1987[1] reported on 189 primary human breast cancers, 30% of which had *HER2* gene amplification. *HER2* gene amplification was a significant predictor of decreased time to relapse and decreased OS. A number of subsequent studies confirmed the correlation of HER2 status with disease outcomes.

Treatment options and outcomes for this disease have been revolutionized with the introduction of HER2-targeted therapies, including monoclonal antibodies against HER2, tyrosine kinase inhibitors, and antibody-drug conjugates (ADCs). These therapies have improved the prognosis of women with HER2-positive (HER2+) metastatic disease in terms of progression-free survival (PFS) and OS. The subsequent use of these targeted therapies in the early-stage setting has led to significant improvements in DFS and OS for these patients. In this chapter, we will outline the options for first-line treatment of metastatic HER2+ breast cancer.

TRASTUZUMAB

Trastuzumab is a recombinant monoclonal antibody directed against subdomain IV of the extracellular portion of the HER2 receptor. Trastuzumab affects the HER2 receptor in a number of ways; but its major mechanism of action is thought to be antibody-dependent cellular cytotoxicity (ADCC). It can also trigger HER2 receptor internalization and degradation. Finally, trastuzumab interferes with dimerization of the HER2 receptor, which is required for activation. By doing so, it leads to inhibition of the downstream MAPK

(mitogen-activated protein kinase) and PI3K (phosphatidylinositol 3-kinase)/AKT (a serine/threonine kinase also known as protein kinase B) pathways, culminating in suppression of cell growth, proliferation, differentiation, motility, and survival.

THE ADDITION OF TRASTUZUMAB TO CHEMOTHERAPY

Before targeted therapies, chemotherapy was the mainstay of treatment for HER2+ metastatic breast cancer (MBC). A pivotal trial published by Slamon et al. in the *New England Journal of Medicine* in 2001 showed that treatment with trastuzumab, in addition to chemotherapy, significantly improved PFS and OS when compared with chemotherapy alone.[2] This trial enrolled women who had breast cancers that overexpressed HER2, defined as 2+ or 3+ on immunohistochemistry (IHC), and had received no prior chemotherapy for metastatic disease. They were randomized to receive chemotherapy alone or chemotherapy plus trastuzumab (Fig. 3.1). Chemotherapy consisted of either an anthracycline (doxorubicin 60 mg/m^2 or epirubicin 75 mg/m^2) and cyclophosphamide (600 mg/m^2) or paclitaxel (175 mg/m^2) if they had previously received anthracycline in the adjuvant setting. They were treated every 3 weeks for six cycles with additional cycles given at the investigator's discretion. Trastuzumab was given at a loading dose of 4 mg/kg followed by a dose of 2 mg/kg weekly until disease progression. The primary endpoints of the study were time to disease progression and the incidence of adverse events. Secondary endpoints were response rate (RR), duration of response, time to treatment failure, and OS. The study enrolled 469 patients and was published with a median follow-up of 30 months. The median time to tumor progression (TTP) was improved for

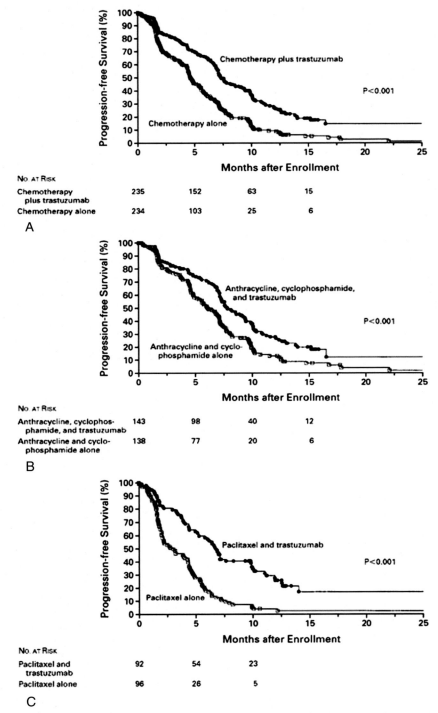

FIG. 3.1 Kaplan-Meier Estimates of Progression-Free Survival According to Whether Patients Were Randomly Assigned to Receive Chemotherapy Plus Trastuzumab or Chemotherapy Alone **(Panel A)** and Whether Chemotherapy Consisted of Either a Combination of an Anthracycline and Cyclophosphamide **(Panel B)** or Paclitaxel **(Panel C)**. (Slamon DJ, Leyland-Jones B, Shak S, et al. Use of chemotherapy plus a monoclonal antibody against HER2 for metastatic breast cancer that overexpresses HER2. *N Engl J Med*. 2001;344(11): 783–792.)

the patients receiving chemotherapy and trastuzumab versus those who received chemotherapy alone (7.4 months vs. 4.6 months; $P < .001$). This difference was seen in both the subgroup that received anthracycline and cyclophosphamide (7.8 months vs. 6.1 months; $P < .001$) and the subgroup that received paclitaxel and trastuzumab (6.9 months vs. 3.0 months; $P < .001$). The addition of trastuzumab to chemotherapy also improved the RR (50% vs. 32%; $P < .001$), duration of response (median 9.1 months vs. 6.1 months; $P < .001$), and time to treatment failure (6.9 months vs. 4.5 months; $P < .001$). Most strikingly, OS was improved to 25.1 months in the patients who received chemotherapy and trastuzumab compared with 20.3 months for the patients who received chemotherapy alone ($P = .046$). This difference was seen despite the crossover bias that may have diminished this benefit. Two-thirds of the patients who received chemotherapy alone went on to receive open-label trastuzumab (alone or with chemotherapy) upon disease progression; but as this was an intent-to-treat analysis, these patients were included in the chemotherapy-alone analysis. This trial enrolled patients with HER2 2+ and HER2 3+ diseases, but patients who were HER2 3+ received a greater degree of benefit from the addition of trastuzumab. This is consistent with the findings of other studies which showed that a significant benefit from trastuzumab was seen only in patients with tumors which were *HER2* gene amplified by fluorescence in situ hybridization (FISH) (Fig. 3.2).[3]

The benefit of adding trastuzumab to chemotherapy was confirmed in another trial, M77001.[4] This was an open-label randomized multicenter phase II trial comparing the efficacy and safety of first-line trastuzumab with docetaxel compared with docetaxel alone in patients with HER2+ MBC who had not received prior chemotherapy for metastatic disease. Initially, patients with HER2 IHC 2+ and 3+ were enrolled, but as data from trials showed that only IHC 3+ and gene-amplified patients received the greatest benefit from trastuzumab, a protocol amendment restricted enrollment to patients who were IHC 3+ and/or gene amplified by FISH. The trial enrolled 188 patients. In the intent-to-treat analysis, the overall RR in the combination arm was 61% compared with 34% in the docetaxel-only arm ($P = .0002$). All subgroups received a benefit from the addition of trastuzumab. Median OS was 31.2 months for trastuzumab plus docetaxel versus 22.7 months for docetaxel alone ($P = .0325$). The duration of response, TTP, and time to treatment failure were all superior for patients who received trastuzumab and docetaxel. In this trial, 57% of patients in the docetaxel-only arm crossed over to receive trastuzumab, either at disease progression, upon discontinuation of docetaxel for toxicity, or for other reasons.

The concordant results of these two trials clearly show the benefit of the addition of trastuzumab to chemotherapy, with improvements in all endpoints, including OS. They led to the use of trastuzumab plus a taxane as the first-line therapy for metastatic HER2+ breast cancer.

Trastuzumab has considerably altered the natural history of HER2+ MBC. This was demonstrated in a single institution study[5] that compared survival differences among women based on HER2 status and treatment. Patients were identified who were diagnosed with MBC between 1991 and 2007 with known HER2 status and had not received adjuvant trastuzumab. Of the 2019 patients, 118 (5.6%) had HER2+ disease and did not receive trastuzumab treatment in the metastatic setting and 191 (9.1%) had HER2+ disease and received trastuzumab for first-line treatment of their metastatic disease. With a median follow-up of 16.9 months, women with HER2+ disease who received trastuzumab had an improved prognosis compared with women with HER2-negative disease, and women with HER2+ disease who did not receive trastuzumab had the worst prognosis. The 1-year survival rates were 86.6%, 75.1%, and 70.2%, respectively.

THE ADDITION OF OTHER DRUGS TO THE TRASTUZUMAB AND TAXANE BACKBONE

A randomized phase III trial evaluated the clinical benefit and safety of adding carboplatin to trastuzumab and paclitaxel.[6] One hundred and ninety-six women with HER2+ (HER2 2+ and amplified by FISH or HER2 3+) MBC who had not received prior therapy for metastatic disease were randomized to either receive trastuzumab and paclitaxel (TP) or this same combination with carboplatin (TPC). The primary endpoint was objective RR with secondary endpoints of PFS and OS. Trastuzumab was dosed at 4 mg/kg loading dose on day 1, followed by 2 mg/kg weekly, paclitaxel was dosed at 175 mg/m^2, and carboplatin was given with an AUC of 6 every 3 weeks. The objective RR was slightly higher for the three drug combination (52% vs. 36%, $P = .04$) and median PFS was significantly longer in the patients receiving TPC (10.7 months vs. 7.1 months, HR 0.66, $P = .03$). There was a trend toward improved OS in the TPC patients (35.7 months vs. 32.2 months), but this was not statistically significant. As expected, the addition of carboplatin increased the rates of grade 4 neutropenia and grade 3 thrombocytopenia.

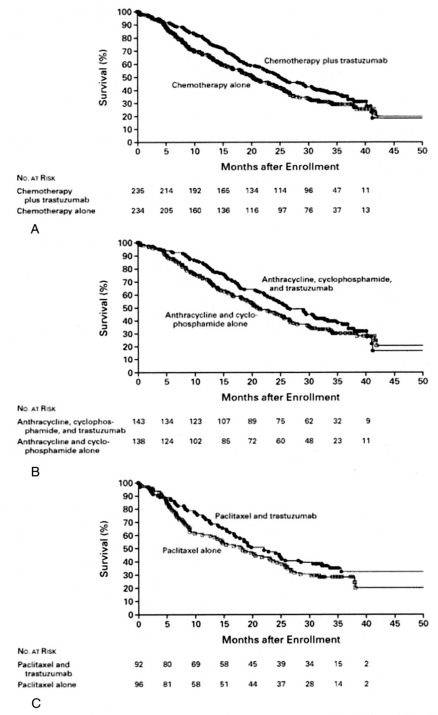

FIG. 3.2 Kaplan-Meier Estimates of Overall Survival According to Whether Patients Were Randomly Assigned to Receive Chemotherapy Plus Trastuzumab or Chemotherapy Alone **(Panel A)** and Whether Chemotherapy Consisted of Either a Combination of an Anthracycline and Cyclophosphamide **(Panel B)** or Paclitaxel **(Panel C)**. (Slamon DJ, Leyland-Jones B, Shak S, et al. Use of chemotherapy plus a monoclonal antibody against HER2 for metastatic breast cancer that overexpresses HER2. *N Engl J Med*. 2001;344(11): 783–792.)

Given these promising results, the BCIRG 007 trial was conducted.[7] This phase III trial randomized 263 patients with HER2+ (gene amplified by FISH) metastatic disease who had not been previously treated in the metastatic setting to receive docetaxel, carboplatin, and trastuzumab (TCH) or docetaxel and trastuzumab (TH). Trastuzumab was given weekly at a dose of 2 mg/kg. Docetaxel was given at 100 mg/m^2 on day 1 every 3 weeks for patients receiving TH or at 75 mg/m^2 with carboplatin AUC 6 every 3 weeks for patients receiving TCH. The primary endpoint of the study was TTP, defined as the interval from the day of randomization to disease progression, second primary malignancy, or death. Secondary endpoints were RR, duration of response, and OS. The median time to progression was not statistically different between the two groups at 11.07 months for TH versus 10.35 months for TCH ($P = .57$). The median OS was 37.1 months for TH and 37.4 months for TCH ($P = .99$), again with no statistically significant difference. The RR was 72% in each group, and the median duration of response was not significantly increased for the TCH patients. Based on these results, the standard of care for first-line metastatic HER2+ breast cancer became taxane and trastuzumab.

A randomized phase II trial examined the addition of capecitabine to the taxane and trastuzumab backbone.[8] Patients (n = 222) with HER2+, locally advanced or MBC, were randomized to receive either HT (trastuzumab plus docetaxel) or HTX (trastuzumab and docetaxel plus capecitabine). Trastuzumab was dosed at 8 mg/kg loading dose followed by 6 mg/kg every 3 weeks. Docetaxel was given every 3 weeks at 75 mg/m^2 in the three drug combination and 100 mg/m^2 in the two drug combination. Capecitabine was dosed at 950 mg/m^2 twice daily on days 1–14 of a 21-day cycle. The primary endpoint, overall RR, was not different between the two regimens (70.5% for HTX vs. 72.7% for HT; $P = .717$). HTX had a longer PFS with a median PFS of 17.9 months versus 12.8 months ($P = .045$). The toxicity profiles were different between the two regimens, as expected given the difference in docetaxel dose and the addition of capecitabine. The authors concluded that the HTX combination is an effective and feasible first-line regimen for metastatic HER2+ breast cancer. Caution should be used when interpreting this as such, as this was a randomized phase II trial, not a phase III trial, and OS was not improved.

Based on biological rationale for targeting both HER2 and VEGF pathways together, a phase III trial, AVEREL, evaluated the addition of bevacizumab to docetaxel and trastuzumab for the first-line treatment of HER2+, locally recurrent or MBC.[9] In this trial, 424 patients were randomized to TH (docetaxel 100 mg/m^2 + trastuzumab 8 mg/kg loading dose followed by 6 mg/kg) or BTH (TH plus bevacizumab 15 mg/kg) every 3 weeks. With a median follow-up of 26 months, the primary endpoint of investigator-assessed PFS was 13.7 months for TH and 16.5 months for BTH ($P = .0775$); the difference did not reach statistical significance. There were no differences in the overall RR or OS. The adverse events seen on the study were consistent with the known safety profile of bevacizumab. As the primary endpoint was not met, this study did not change the standard of care of taxane and trastuzumab.

Hyperactivation of the PIK/AKT/mTOR (mammalian target of rapamycin) pathway due to PTEN (phosphatase and tensin homolog) loss can lead to trastuzumab resistance. mTOR inhibitors may sensitize PTEN-deficient tumors to trastuzumab. This theory was tested in the BOLERO-1 trial.[10] In this phase III double-blind trial, 719 patients with HER2+ MBC who had not received previous trastuzumab or chemotherapy for advanced breast cancer within 12 months were randomized to everolimus (10 mg) or placebo with trastuzumab and paclitaxel weekly in a 2:1 ratio. With a median follow-up of 41.3 months, median PFS was not improved in the overall patient population (14.95 months for everolimus vs. 14.49 months for placebo, $P = .1166$). In the hormone receptor–negative subpopulation (n = 311), the median PFS was increased with everolimus to 20.27 months versus 13.08 months, but this was not statistically significant ($P = .0049$) as the protocol-specified significance threshold ($P = .0044$) was not crossed. Patients treated with everolimus had higher rates of stomatitis (67% vs. 32%), diarrhea (57% vs. 47%), and alopecia (47% vs. 53%). There was more grade 3 or 4 neutropenia (25% vs. 15%), stomatitis (13% vs. 1%), anemia (10% vs. 3%), and diarrhea (9% vs. 4%). There were 17 (4%) adverse event-related deaths in the everolimus group and none in the placebo group. Given the activity in the hormone receptor–negative HER2+ group, further studies could be considered.

TRASTUZUMAB WITH OTHER CHEMOTHERAPY AGENTS

For patients who cannot tolerate a taxane, other chemotherapy agents may be considered. A phase II trial showed that trastuzumab with vinorelbine was an effective and well-tolerated first-line treatment.[11] In this study, 55 patients with documented HER2 overexpression (3+ by IHC or gene amplification by FISH) were treated weekly with trastuzumab with a 4 mg/kg loading dose and 2 mg/kg weekly dosing along with vinorelbine 25 mg/m^2 weekly. An objective RR (complete or partial response) was seen in 37 patients (68%), and another 9 patients had stable disease for 6 months or longer. Nearly 40% of patients did not have disease progression at 1 year.

A prospective, multicenter, randomized trial[12] compared trastuzumab with vinorelbine versus taxane (paclitaxel or docetaxel, per investigator's choice) as first-line chemotherapy for patients with measurable MBC that was either HER2 3+ by IHC or gene amplified by FISH. The trial was closed early because of poor accrual. The primary endpoint was RR. In 81 evaluable patients, both regimens were active. The RR was 51% for the patients receiving trastuzumab and vinorelbine compared with 40% for the patients receiving trastuzumab and taxane, but this difference was not statistically significantly different ($P = .37$).

A phase III trial, the HERNATA study,[13] randomized 143 patients with HER2+ MBC who had not received treatment for advanced disease to docetaxel (100 mg/m^2, day 1) or vinorelbine (30–35 mg/m^2 on days 1 and 8). Both groups received trastuzumab every 3 weeks. There was no difference in the primary endpoint of TTP (12.4 months vs. 15.3 months, $P = .67$) or in the secondary endpoints of median OS (35.7 months vs. 38.7 months, $P = .98$), median time to treatment failure, or investigator-assessed overall RR. More patients in the docetaxel group discontinued treatment because of toxicity. The toxicities were consistent with the known profiles of the drugs. The authors concluded that although the vinorelbine and trastuzumab combination was not superior to docetaxel plus trastuzumab, it was better tolerated and should be considered as an alternative first-line treatment.

The combination of capecitabine and trastuzumab has been shown to be active and well tolerated for patients with HER2+ advanced and MBC. In an open-label, single-arm phase II study from Germany,[14] 27 patients with metastatic HER2+ breast cancer who had been treated with anthracycline and/or taxane were treated with this combination, and an RR of 45% was noted. A study from Japan[15] enrolled and treated 59 women with metastatic HER2+ breast cancer with this combination as well. Sixty-four percent had received prior chemotherapy for metastatic disease. An overall RR of 50% was noted with a higher RR of 65.0% in patients who were being treated with this combination as first-line therapy for metastatic disease. Patients receiving this therapy in the first line had longer

time to progression and OS than patients receiving it in later lines of therapy. Treatment-related adverse events were as expected.

TRASTUZUMAB AS A SINGLE AGENT

Trastuzumab as a single agent is a treatment option for first-line HER2+ metastatic disease for women who do not wish to receive cytotoxic chemotherapy.[16] A single-blind, multicenter study randomized 114 patients with HER2+ (IHC 2+ or 3+) MBC who had not yet received chemotherapy to two dose levels of trastuzumab as first-line treatment (loading dose of 4 mg/kg followed by 2 mg/kg weekly or loading dose of 8 mg/kg followed by 4 mg/kg weekly). This study had an objective RR of 26% and a clinical benefit rate of 38%. Responses were only seen in patients who overexpressed HER2 at the 3+ level. A retrospective analysis of HER2 gene amplification showed that the RR was 34% in patients with HER2-amplified tumors compared with 7% for those whose tumors were nonamplified. Similarly, the median TTP was greater for those with HER2 amplification (4.3 months vs. 1.7 months). This patient population was similar to that of the pivotal trial in which response rates of 56% for doxorubicin and cyclophosphamide with trastuzumab and 41% for paclitaxel plus trastuzumab were seen. The median duration of survival for all patients was 24.2 months. When compared with the OS results of the pivotal trial (25.1 months for chemotherapy and trastuzumab), the authors concluded that the patients did not have a survival disadvantage if they received trastuzumab alone as first-line therapy for metastatic disease.

A randomized phase III trial done in Japan[17] had conflicting results. This trial examined the efficacy and safety of sequential therapy with trastuzumab followed by trastuzumab plus docetaxel on progression versus the combination of trastuzumab plus docetaxel as first-line therapy. The hypothesis was that if the two were equivalent in OS, then starting with trastuzumab alone would improve quality of life. The joint primary endpoints were PFS and OS. The trial enrolled 112 of the 160 planned patients and was stopped early due to a difference in PFS between the two groups. The median PFS was 3.7 months for monotherapy and 14.6 months for the combination ($P < .01$). Overall survival was also worse for single-agent trastuzumab, although the significance level specified for the interim analysis (1%) was not reached. The median OS was not available because the number of deaths was small in both groups.

PERTUZUMAB

Pertuzumab is a monoclonal antibody that binds subdomain II of the HER2 receptors, whereas trastuzumab binds domain IV. Because trastuzumab and pertuzumab bind at different subdomains of HER2, they can provide a more comprehensive blockade of HER2 signaling when given together. Pertuzumab binding to HER2 also prevents HER2 dimerization with other members of the HER2 family, especially HER3. Dimerization is essential to the activation of the HER family of receptors. There can be dimerization between two molecules of the same receptor (homodimerization) or two different HER receptors (heterodimerization). The HER2-HER3 heterodimer is thought to be the most potent signaling pair. Dimerization leads to transphosphorylation of the tyrosine kinase domains of the receptor with signaling via downstream intracellular pathways leading to cell activation and proliferation. Disruption of dimerization can block this cell signaling, leading to inhibition of cell growth. Like trastuzumab, pertuzumab also stimulates antibody-dependent cell-mediated cytotoxicity (ADCC).

Results of the CLEOPATRA (Clinical Evaluation of Pertuzumab and Trastuzumab) trial[18,19] led to a change in first-line therapy for women with HER2+ MBC. In this phase 3, double-blind, placebo-controlled trial, 808 women with metastatic HER2+ breast cancer who had not received prior chemotherapy or anti-HER2 therapy for metastatic disease were randomized in a 1:1 ratio to receive placebo, trastuzumab and docetaxel, or pertuzumab plus trastuzumab plus docetaxel. The primary endpoint of the study was independently assessed PFS, which was defined as the time from randomization to the first documented radiographic evidence of progression disease or death from any cause after the last independent assessment of tumors. Patients were treated with standard loading doses (8 mg/kg) followed by maintenance doses of trastuzumab (6 mg/kg) and docetaxel 75 mg/m^2 every 3 weeks. Pertuzumab was given at a fixed loading dose of 840 mg followed by 420 mg every 3 weeks. If docetaxel chemotherapy was discontinued because of toxicity, the antibody therapy was continued until progression of disease or unacceptable toxicity. The addition of pertuzumab significantly improved PFS by a total of 6.1 months, from 12.4 months in the control group to 18.5 months in the pertuzumab group (HR 0.75, $P < .001$). A benefit was seen in all predefined subgroups, including those who had received prior neoadjuvant or adjuvant chemotherapy, and regardless of hormone receptor status. At the time of the initial

publication, the median follow-up was 19.3 months and survival data were not yet mature (Fig. 3.3).

A subsequent publication of the CLEOPATRA trial[19] showed that the addition of pertuzumab to the treatment regimen significantly improved not only PFS but also the secondary endpoint of OS. With a median of 50 months of follow-up, the median OS was improved from 40.8 months in the control group to 56.5 months in the pertuzumab group (HR 0.68, $P < .001$). Exploratory analyses showed a consistent benefit in all predefined subgroups. The median PFS remained unchanged from the prior analysis, from 12.4 months in the control group to 18.7 months in the pertuzumab group. As this was an intent-to-treat analysis, patients in the control group who crossed over to receive pertuzumab were still analyzed in the control group, adding to the strength of these findings (Fig. 3.4).

Based on the results of the CLEOPATRA trial, a phase II study of pertuzumab, trastuzumab, and weekly paclitaxel was conducted to evaluate the safety and efficacy of this regimen.[20] Patients with HER2+ (IHC 3+ or FISH *HER2/CEP17* ratio greater than or equal to 2) were treated with this regimen as first- or second-line therapy for metastatic disease. The primary objective was the proportion of patients who were free of progression at 6 months. The trial enrolled 69 patients, 51 of whom were receiving first-line treatment. With a median follow-up of 33 months, the 6-month PFS was 86%, the median PFS was 21.4 months, and the median OS was 44 months. This trial confirmed the activity of weekly paclitaxel with trastuzumab and pertuzumab and suggested that this is an alternative to docetaxel-based chemotherapy.

In 2012, based on the CLEOPATRA trial, the US Food and Drug Administration (FDA) approved pertuzumab in combination with trastuzumab and docetaxel chemotherapy for the treatment of patients with HER2+ MBC who have not received prior anti-HER2 therapy or chemotherapy for metastatic disease. The National Comprehensive Cancer Network (NCCN) added pertuzumab as a preferred first-line agent for HER2+ MBC with trastuzumab and taxane in 2013. According to the most recent version of these guidelines, NCCN version 2.2017,[21] this remains the first-line therapy for HER2+ MBC: pertuzumab + trastuzumab + docetaxel (category 1) or paclitaxel (category 2A). The current recommendation is to discontinue pertuzumab on disease progression, but trials are needed to clarify the most effective duration of pertuzumab therapy.

Independently Assessed Progression-free Survival

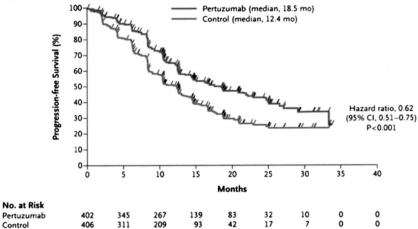

No. at Risk

Pertuzumab	402	345	267	139	83	32	10	0	0
Control	406	311	209	93	42	17	7	0	0

A

Progression-free Survival in Prespecified Subgroups

Subgroup	No. of Patients	Hazard Ratio (95% CI)	
All patients	808		0.63 (0.52–0.76)
Previous neoadjuvant or adjuvant chemotherapy			
No	432		0.63 (0.49–0.82)
Yes	376		0.61 (0.46–0.81)
Geographic region			
Europe	306		0.72 (0.53–0.97)
North America	135		0.51 (0.31–0.84)
South America	114		0.46 (0.27–0.78)
Asia	253		0.68 (0.48–0.95)
Age group			
<65 yr	681		0.65 (0.53–0.80)
≥65 yr	127		0.52 (0.31–0.86)
<75 yr	789		0.64 (0.53–0.78)
≥75 yr	19		0.55 (0.12–2.54)
Race or ethnic group			
White	480		0.62 (0.49–0.80)
Black	30		0.64 (0.23–1.79)
Asian	261		0.68 (0.49–0.95)
Other	37		0.39 (0.13–1.18)
Disease type			
Visceral disease	630		0.55 (0.45–0.68)
Nonvisceral disease	178		0.96 (0.61–1.52)
Hormone-receptor status			
ER-positive, PgR-positive, or both	388		0.72 (0.55–0.95)
ER-negative and PgR-negative	408		0.55 (0.42–0.72)
ER and PgR status unknown	12		—
HER2 status			
IHC 3+	721		0.60 (0.49–0.74)
FISH-positive	767		0.64 (0.53–0.78)

Pertuzumab Better   Placebo Better

B

FIG. 3.3 (A) Independently Assessed Progression-Free Survival and (B) Progression-Free Survival in Prespecified Subgroups, as Assessed at an Independent Review Facility. (Baselga J, Cortés J, Kim SB, et al. Pertuzumab plus trastuzumab plus docetaxel for metastatic breast cancer. *N Engl J Med*. 2012;366(2): 109–119.)

Overall Survival

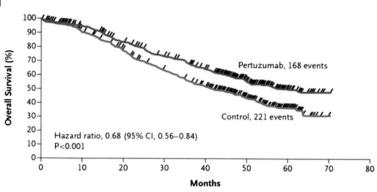

Subgroup Analysis of Overall Survival

Subgroup	No. of Patients	Hazard Ratio (95% CI)	Hazard Ratio (95% CI)	P Value for Interaction
All patients	808		0.67 (0.55–0.82)	
Previous adjuvant or neoadjuvant treatment				0.63
No	432		0.64 (0.48–0.85)	
Yes	376		0.70 (0.53–0.93)	
Region				0.36
Europe	306		0.65 (0.47–0.91)	
North America	135		0.63 (0.37–1.07)	
South America	114		0.50 (0.30–0.85)	
Asia	253		0.82 (0.57–1.16)	
Age				0.27
<65 yr	681		0.70 (0.56–0.87)	
≥65 yr	127		0.53 (0.31–0.90)	
Age				0.84
<75 yr	789		0.68 (0.55–0.83)	
≥75 yr	19		0.85 (0.26–2.73)	
Race or ethnic group				0.40
White	480		0.63 (0.49–0.82)	
Black	30		0.41 (0.11–1.45)	
Asian	261		0.82 (0.58–1.17)	
Other	37		0.37 (0.13–1.06)	
Disease type				0.03
Visceral	630		0.59 (0.48–0.74)	
Nonvisceral	178		1.11 (0.66–1.85)	
ER or PgR status				0.47
Positive	388		0.71 (0.53–0.96)	
Negative	408		0.61 (0.47–0.81)	
HER2 status				
IHC 3+	721		0.66 (0.53–0.81)	0.52
FISH-positive	767		0.69 (0.56–0.85)	0.14

0.2   0.4   0.6   1.0   2.0   3.0 4.0

B

← Pertuzumab Better   Placebo Better →

FIG. 3.4 (A) Overall Survival and (B) Subgroup Analysis of Overall Survival. (Swain SM, Baselga J, Kim SB, Ro J, Semiglazov V, Campone M, et al. Pertuzumab, trastuzumab, and docetaxel in HER2-positive metastatic breast cancer. *N Engl J Med*. 2015;372(8):724–734.)

For patients who cannot tolerate taxane chemotherapy, the combination of trastuzumab, pertuzumab, and vinorelbine is an option based on the VELVET trial.[22] In this open-label phase II study, Cohort 1 consisted of 106 patients with HER2+ locally advanced or MBC with no prior treatment for advanced disease who were treated with this combination. The investigator-assessed overall RR was 74.2%, and the median PFS was 14.3 months. Treatment was well tolerated with no unexpected toxicities.

Eribulin has also been tested in combination with trastuzumab and pertuzumab in a multicenter open-label phase II study of the three drug combination as first- and second-line therapy for HER2+ metastatic or advanced breast cancer.[23] All patients enrolled had previously received trastuzumab and a taxane, either as adjuvant therapy or in the first-line for metastatic disease. The primary endpoint was PFS. Out of the 50 patients who were enrolled, 8 were treated in the first-line metastatic setting. The median PFS has not yet been reached. The response rate was 56.5%. The authors' conclusion is that this combination was well-tolerated and could be an alternative to docetaxel-based combination therapy for HER2+ MBC.

Phase III trials of pertuzumab with chemotherapy without trastuzumab have not been reported.

TRASTUZUMAB EMTANSINE

Trastuzumab emtansine (T-DM1) is an ADC in which molecules of DM1, a cytotoxic microtubule polymerization inhibitor, are bound via a stable thioether linker to trastuzumab.[24] This unique mechanism allows the delivery of the cytotoxic drug directly into tumor cells. T-DM1 binds to the extracellular domain of the HER2 protein and carries out the previously described HER2 receptor–mediated effects of trastuzumab. In addition, the ADC is internalized by the cell, where the molecules of DM1 are released.

The EMILIA study[25] was a phase III trial showing an improvement in PFS for T-DM1 compared with the lapatinib and capecitabine combination in patients with HER2+ MBC who had been previously treated with trastuzumab and taxane therapy. Based on these results, a randomized phase II trial was done comparing T-DM1 every 3 weeks to docetaxel and trastuzumab (HT) every 3 weeks.[26] Patients (n = 137) with HER2+ (IHC 3+ or gene amplified by FISH) breast cancer who had not previously received treatment for their metastatic disease were randomized to one of these two treatment arms. The primary endpoints of the study were investigator-assessed PFS and safety. The PFS was 14.2 months for T-DM1 compared with 9.2 months for HT (hazard ratio 0.59, $P = .035$). The overall response rates and clinical benefit rates were similar between the two groups, but the duration of response for patients who achieved an objective response was longer with T-DM1. T-DM1 had a favorable safety profile, with fewer grade 3 and 4 adverse events than lapatinib plus capecitabine. Preliminary OS rates were similar between the two groups.

The phase III MARIANNE trial was designed to evaluate the efficacy and safety of T-DM1 and T-DM1 plus pertuzumab compared with trastuzumab plus taxane in patients with HER2+ advanced breast cancer who had no prior therapy for advanced disease.[27] The control arm of study was chosen because in 2009, when the study was designed, taxane and trastuzumab was the standard first-line regimen. Patients (n = 1095) were randomized in a 1:1:1 fashion to one of the three arms: trastuzumab plus taxane, T-DM1, or T-DM1 plus pertuzumab. The primary endpoint was independently assessed PFS. Median PFS was 13.7 months with trastuzumab plus taxane, 14.1 months with T-DM1, and 15.2 months with T-DM1 plus pertuzumab. Both T-DM1 groups had a noninferior PFS compared with taxane and trastuzumab, but neither PFS was superior. The toxicities seen in each arm were consistent with the known side effect profiles of the drugs. The addition of pertuzumab to T-DM1 did not improve PFS. Overall survival was 50.9 months for trastuzumab plus taxane, 53.7 months for T-DM1, and 51.8 months for T-DM1 plus pertuzumab. The authors of this study concluded that based on its improved tolerability, noninferior PFS, and similar OS, T-DM1 may provide an effective and tolerable treatment alternative to trastuzumab plus taxane for these patients (Fig. 3.5).

LAPATINIB

Lapatinib is a potent, oral, reversible, dual inhibitor of EGFR (epidermal growth factor receptor) and HER2 tyrosine kinases. It has been shown to be active in HER2+ breast cancer in combination with letrozole as first-line treatment (see section on endocrine therapy).

Lapatinib has no role with chemotherapy as a first-line treatment option for metastatic HER2+ breast cancer. Earlier trials[28,29] suggested that lapatinib alone or with chemotherapy had activity in this first-line setting, leading to the conduction of phase III trials. The COMPLETE trial was a randomized open-label phase III study of taxane-based chemotherapy with lapatinib or

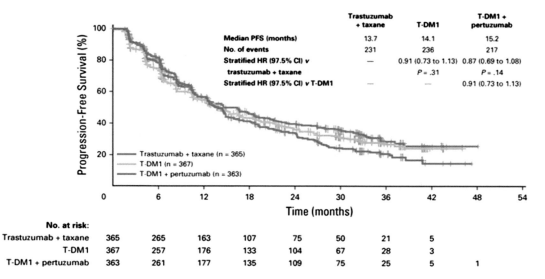

Baseline Risk Factors	Total No.	Trastuzumab + Taxane (n = 365) Median, Mo	T-DM1 (n = 367) Median, Mo	HR (97.5% CI)	← T-DM1 Better	Trastuzumab + Taxane Better →
All patients	732	13.7	14.1	0.94 (0.76 to 1.16)		
World region*						
Asia	153	17.2	11.9	1.16 (0.72 to 1.85)		
E. Europe	115	12.4	12.4	1.00 (0.59 to 1.69)		
W. Europe, Canada, Australia/Pacific	271	14.0	15.9	0.89 (0.63 to 1.25)		
United States	89	12.9	12.6	0.82 (0.45 to 1.49)		
Others	104	10.5	14.6	0.75 (0.44 to 1.29)		
Neoadjuvant/adjuvant therapy*						
Yes, trastuzumab or lapatanib	226	10.3	15.2	0.75 (0.52 to 1.09)		
Yes, not trastuzumab or lapatanib	182	16.5	18.0	0.86 (0.56 to 1.32)		
No	324	14.8	12.4	1.12 (0.82 to 1.54)		
Visceral involvement*						
Yes	492	12.5	12.4	0.92 (0.72 to 1.18)		
No	240	18.1	19.5	0.96 (0.64 to 1.42)		
Age group, years						
< 65	609	13.2	13.3	0.96 (0.77 to 1.21)		
≥ 65	123	14.6	19.5	0.82 (0.49 to 1.39)		
Hormonal status						
ER+ and/or PR+	402	13.7	13.4	0.94 (0.71 to 1.25)		
ER- and PR-	314	14.0	13.3	1.00 (0.73 to 1.37)		
Prior taxane						
Yes	233	10.8	15.2	0.69 (0.48 to 0.99)		
No	499	14.9	12.6	1.10 (0.85 to 1.41)		

0.2   0.5   1   2   5

B

FIG. 3.5 Progression-Free Survival, as Assessed by Independent Review. **(A)** Kaplan-Meier estimates of progression-free survival in the intention-to-treat population. Stratified hazard ratios and 97.5% CIs obtained from stratified Cox proportional hazards regression model and P values retrieved from stratified log-rank tests are shown. Stratification was according to world regions, prior neoadjuvant/adjuvant therapy, and presence of visceral disease. **(B)** Progression-free survival assessed in prespecified patient subgroups for

trastuzumab as first-line therapy for women with HER2+ MBC.[30] The study was discontinued early after an interim analysis in April 2012 showed that trastuzumab recipients had significantly longer PFS than lapatinib recipients. MA.31 compared a combination of HER2-targeted therapy (lapatinib or trastuzumab) with a taxane in the first-line treatment of 651 HER2+ breast cancer patients.[31] Patients were treated for 24 weeks with combination therapy followed by the same HER2-targeted therapy until disease progression. The primary endpoint was PFS. With a median follow-up of 21.5 months, the median intent-to-treat PFS was inferior for lapatinib at 9.0 months compared to 11.3 months for trastuzumab (HR 1.37, $P = .001$). In addition, more toxicity was seen with lapatinib.

NERATINIB

Neratinib is an oral, small molecule, irreversible tyrosine kinase inhibitor of EGFR1, HER2, HER3, and HER4, leading to sustained inhibition of intracellular signaling. NEfERT-T[32] was originally designed as a randomized phase III trial to determine whether neratinib plus paclitaxel was superior to trastuzumab plus paclitaxel in first-line, HER2+ MBC. The study was revised, and the accrual goal reduced from 1200 to 480 patients, so it was no longer powered as a randomized phase III trial. The trial enrolled 479 patients. The median PFS was 12.9 months in both groups ($P = .89$). The objective RR was similar (74.8% vs. 77.6%, $P = .52$), as was the clinical benefit rate (88.4% vs. 85.2%, $P = .24$). There was more diarrhea and nausea in the neratinib-treated patients. Three patients in the neratinib-treated group died because of treatment-related adverse events, and one patient died in the trastuzumab group. The authors suggested that because there were no statistically significant differences in PFS, overall RR, clinical benefit rate, and duration of response, the two regimens had similar efficacy with different toxicity profiles. Interestingly, there was a reduction in the frequency of symptomatic or progressive central nervous system (CNS) recurrences, a prospectively defined endpoint.

TRASTUZUMAB BIOSIMILARS

A biosimilar is a biologic product that has been shown to be highly similar to an FDA-approved biologic product, known as the reference product. It has no clinically meaningful efficacy or safety differences from the reference product. There are minor differences in the clinically inactive components. Biosimilars are being tested in cancer trials. Recently, a bevacizumab biosimilar was approved for the treatment of adult patients with certain colorectal, lung, brain, kidney, and cervical cancers.

HERITAGE[33] is a multicenter, international, double-blind, randomized phase III trial that compared the efficacy, safety and immunogenicity of a trastuzumab biosimilar (MYL-1401O; Mylan) given in combination with a taxane to trastuzumab plus a taxane for patients with HER2+ (IHC 3+ or IHC 2+ with FISH HER2/CEP17 ratio > 2) MBC with measurable disease who had received no previous treatment for their advanced disease. Patients were randomized 1:1 to receive trastuzumab or the trastuzumab biosimilar with a taxane of the investigator's choice (docetaxel 75 mg/m^2 every 3 weeks or paclitaxel 80 mg/m^2 weekly could omit 1 week every 4 weeks). Treatment was given for a minimum of 8 three-week cycles. If the patients had a response or stable disease, chemotherapy could be discontinued after 8 cycles with continuation of trastuzumab or the biosimilar until disease progression. The primary endpoint of the study was overall response rate, defined as complete or partial response at week 24. Secondary endpoints analyzed at 48 weeks included time to progression, PFS, and OS. Other endpoints included adverse events, laboratory assessments, left ventricular ejection fraction, and immunogenicity. The trial enrolled 500 patients, but after a protocol amendment to exclude patients who had already received first-line therapy, 42 patients were excluded from the primary ITT analysis. The overall RR was 69.6% for the biosimilar versus 64% for trastuzumab. The overall RR ratio (1.09; 90% CI 0.974–1.211) and overall RR difference (5.53; 95% CI −3.08 to 14.04) were within the equivalence boundaries. At 48 weeks, there was no statistically significant difference between the two for

trastuzumab emtansine (T-DM1) compared with trastuzumab plus taxane. Medians, unstratified hazard ratios, and 97.5% CIs for progression-free survival comparing T-DM1 and trastuzumab plus taxane in prespecified subgroups representing stratification factors and clinically important variables. Vertical dashed line indicates the hazard ratio for all patients. (*) Stratification factor. ER, estrogen receptor; HR, hazard ratio; PR, progesterone receptor. (Perez EA, Barrios C, Eiermann W, Toi M, Im YH, Conte P, Martin M, Pienkowski T, Pivot X, Burris H III, Petersen JA, Stanzel S, Strasak S, Patre M, Ellis P, *J Clin Oncol.* 2017;35:141–148. DOI: 10.1200/JCO.2016.67.4887, Copyright © 2016 American Society of Clinical Oncology.)

time to progression, PFS, or OS. Safety profiles were very similar between the two groups. The conclusion of the authors was that further studies are needed to evaluate safety and long-term clinical outcome of the biosimilar.

Other biosimilar studies are ongoing. One study is evaluating PF-05280014 (Trastuzumab-Pfizer) versus Herceptin (Trastuzumab-EU) plus paclitaxel in HER2+ first-line MBC (REFLECTIONS B327-02). Another study is comparing the safety and efficacy of BCD-022 with paclitaxel compared with Herceptin with paclitaxel.

ENDOCRINE THERAPY WITH HER2 THERAPY

Approximately, half of HER2+ breast cancers are also hormone receptor positive (HR+).[34-37] Trastuzumab is proven to be effective in patients with HER2+ disease, regardless of HR status.[4,34-36,38] There is cross talk between the pathways involving epidermal growth factor receptor (EGFR), HER2, and the estrogen receptor (ER), which has been implicated in the resistance of HR+ and HER2+ breast cancers to endocrine therapy. The discovery of this cross talk between the pathways led to trials of HER2 therapy with endocrine therapy.

The TAnDEM (Trastuzumab and Anastrozole Directed Against ER-Positive HER2-Positive Mammary Carcinoma) trial[39] was an open-label phase III trial that randomized 207 women with HER2+ (IHC 3+ or gene amplified by FISH), HR+ MBC to anastrozole or to trastuzumab weekly with anastrozole. The primary endpoint, PFS, was improved to a median of 4.8 months for the combination versus 2.4 months for anastrozole alone (P = .0016). A secondary endpoint of TTP was significantly improved as well. The median OS was 28.5 months in the trastuzumab and anastrozole arm and 23.9 months in the anastrozole alone arm, but this difference was not statistically significant(P = .325). The shorter-than-expected PFS for both arms could be explained by the aggressive nature of HER2+ tumors or by the fact that approximately two-thirds of the patients received prior tamoxifen, either as adjuvant treatment or in the metastatic setting. The patients who received anastrozole alone were allowed the option of switching to a trastuzumab-containing regimen on disease progression. This may have reduced any potential survival benefit of receiving trastuzumab up front.

The eLEcTRA study[40] compared the combination of letrozole plus trastuzumab to letrozole alone in 57 postmenopausal patients. A third cohort of 35 HER2-negative patients was enrolled and received letrozole

alone. The study accrued slowly and closed early before the planned 370 patients were enrolled. The results showed that the addition of trastuzumab to letrozole improved the time to progression from 3.3 months for letrozole alone to 14.1 months (P = .23) for the combination. In the HER2-negative group, the time to progression was 15.2 months. The clinical benefit rate (65% vs. 39%) was also improved for the patients receiving the combination.

In another randomized, double-blind, placebo-controlled, phase III trial,[41] women with advanced breast cancer (stage IIIB/IIIC or IV) that was ER and/or progesterone receptor (PR) positive (HR+) who had received no prior therapy for advanced or metastatic disease were randomized to letrozole 2.5 mg orally daily in combination with either lapatinib (1500 mg orally) or placebo. Therapy was given until disease progression or withdrawal from the study. The primary endpoint was investigator-assessed PFS, defined as time from randomization to disease progression or death from any cause. Of the 1286 patients with HR+ disease, 17% in each arm were confirmed to be HER2+ by central lab (n = 111 and n = 108 in lapatinib and placebo arms, respectively). For these 219 HER2+ patients and with a median follow-up of 1.8 years, median PFS increased from 3.0 months for the letrozole-placebo patients to 8.2 months for the letrozole-lapatinib patients (HR 0.71, P = .019). In this population of patients, the overall RR was improved from 15% to 28% for the patients treated with lapatinib (P = .021), and the clinical benefit rate was improved from 29% to 48% (P = .003). The OS was not significantly different at 33 months versus 32 months. There was a higher incidence of diarrhea and rash in the lapatinib-treated patients with 10% of the patients developing grade 3 or 4 diarrhea and 15% of those discontinuing therapy for that reason. The remainder was treated with dose reduction, dose interruption, or supportive intervention without treatment dose adjustment (Fig. 3.6).

Given the benefit of dual HER2-targeted therapy with chemotherapy, the open-label phase II PERTAIN trial was conducted to assess the benefit of dual-targeted therapy of trastuzumab and pertuzumab with an aromatase inhibitor (AI), either anastrozole or letrozole.[42] The trial enrolled 258 postmenopausal women with HER2+, HR+ locally advanced or MBC and randomized them to receive either pertuzumab with trastuzumab and an AI or trastuzumab alone with an AI, with or without induction chemotherapy. The primary endpoint of the trial, PFS, was improved by 3.09 months, from 15.80 months for the patients

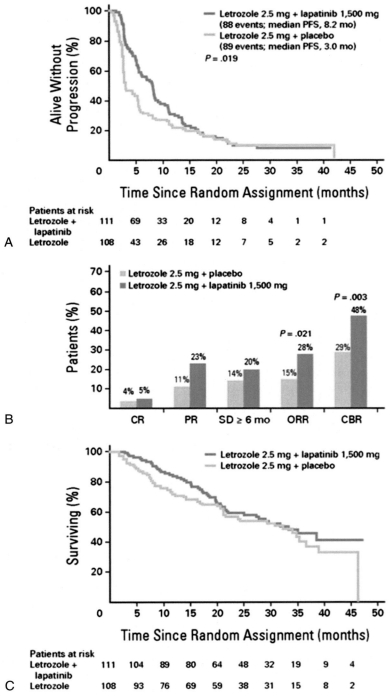

FIG. 3.6 Clinical Efficacy in Human Epidermal Growth Factor Receptor 2–Positive Population. **(A)** Kaplan-Meier estimates of progression-free survival (PFS), **(B)** response rates and clinical benefit rates (CBR), and **(C)** Kaplan-Meier estimates of overall survival. *CR*, complete response; *ORR*, overall response rate; *PR*, partial response; *SD*, stable disease. (Reproduced from Johnston S, Pippen J Jr, Pivot X, Lichinitser M, Sadeghi S, Dieras V, Gomez HL, Romieu G, Manikhas A, Kennedy MJ, Press MF, Maltzman J, Florance A, O'Rourke L, Oliva C, Stein S, Pegram M, *J Clin Oncol*. 2009;27:5538–5546. DOI: 10.1200/JCO.2009.23.3734, Copyright © 2009.)

treated with trastuzumab and an AI to 18.89 months for the patients treated with pertuzumab, trastuzumab, and an AI. There was a reduction in the risk of progression or death, an improvement in objective RR, and an improved median duration of response with the addition of pertuzumab. There were no new safety signals identified.

Comparisons cannot be made between these studies and those trials comparing first-line taxane with or without trastuzumab, as the patient populations were different. Specifically, all the patients were HR+ in these trials. Together, the trials show that patients fare better with HER2-targeted therapy in addition to standard chemotherapy or endocrine therapy. The combination of HER2-targeted therapy with endocrine therapy is superior to endocrine therapy alone for HR-positive, HER2+ MBC in improving PFS. These studies support the use of these combinations as a treatment option in appropriate patients. These treatments could potentially increase the amount of time before chemotherapy with HER2-directed antibodies required and provide treatment options for patients who are not candidates for or who decline chemotherapy.

AMERICAN SOCIETY OF CLINICAL ONCOLOGY GUIDELINES

In 2014, the American Society of Clinical Oncology published a Clinical Practice Guideline to address systemic therapy for patients with advanced HER2+ breast cancer.[43] These guidelines are formulated by a multidisciplinary group of experts using a review of phase III randomized controlled trials and their clinical experience. The guidelines that are relevant to first-line treatment are reviewed here.

HER2-targeted therapy combinations should be recommended for first-line treatment, except for highly selected patients with ER- and/or PR-positive breast cancers who may receive endocrine therapy alone (type: evidence based; evidence quality: high; strength of recommendations: strong). This recommendation is based on trials, including the pivotal trial by Slamon and colleagues,[2] which showed that HER2-targeted therapy in combination with chemotherapy in the first-line setting led to improvements in response rates, PFS, TTP, and OS compared with chemotherapy alone. In the endocrine therapy trials,[39,40] the addition of HER2-targeted therapy improved RR and PFS but not OS.

The combination of trastuzumab, pertuzumab, and taxane should be recommended for first-line treatment, unless the patient has a contraindication to taxane treatment (type: evidence based; evidence quality: high; strength of recommendations: strong). This recommendation is based on the CLEOPATRA trial,[18,19] which showed an improvement in PFS and OS. The panel felt that paclitaxel could be used in place of docetaxel. The data for other chemotherapy agents were more limited, and the panel felt that these should generally be avoided until more data are available.

The panel addressed the question of the duration of treatment. For patients receiving HER2-targeted therapy and chemotherapy, the chemotherapy should continue for approximately 4–6 months (or longer) and/or to the time of maximal response. When chemotherapy is stopped, HER2-targeted therapy should be continued, and no further changes are required until disease progression or unacceptable toxicity (type: evidence based; evidence quality: intermediate; strength of recommendation: moderate).

If a patient recurs more than 12 months after trastuzumab-based adjuvant therapy, first-line therapy recommendations should be followed (type: evidence based; evidence quality: intermediate; strength of recommendation: strong). The CLEOPATRA trial[18,19] allowed patients who received prior trastuzumab if there had been a ≥12 month interval between neoadjuvant or adjuvant trastuzumab and the diagnosis of MBC. If a patient recurs less than or equal to 12 months from trastuzumab-based adjuvant therapy, then second-line therapy recommendations should be followed (type: evidence based; evidence quality: intermediate; strength of recommendation: moderate).

If a patient's cancer is HR+ and HER2+, clinicians may recommend either HER2-targeted therapy plus chemotherapy (type: evidence based; evidence quality: high; strength of recommendation: strong), endocrine therapy with trastuzumab or lapatinib (type: evidence based; evidence quality: high; strength of recommendation: moderate), or endocrine therapy alone in selected cases (type: evidence based; evidence quality: intermediate; strength of recommendation: weak). In special cases, such as low disease burden, comorbidities, or contraindications to HER2-targeted therapy, and/or the presence of a long disease-free interval, clinicians may offer first-line endocrine therapy alone (type: informal consensus; evidence quality: intermediate; strength of recommendation: weak). The endocrine therapy trials have not shown an overall survival benefit,[39–41] whereas CLEOPATRA[18,19] did show an OS benefit for both ER-positive and ER-negative diseases. No studies, however, have compared HER2-targeted therapy with endocrine therapy versus HER2-targeted therapy with chemotherapy. Endocrine therapy can be considered for appropriate patients, such as those who have a long disease-free interval, have indolent disease, have significant comorbidities, are not good candidates for chemotherapy, or prefer to avoid chemotherapy. It can be given alone or with HER2-targeted therapy, as the trials showed no difference in overall survival. At this time, there are no methods for determining which patients would benefit from the addition of HER2-directed therapy to endocrine therapy alone.

If a patient has started with a HER2-targeted therapy and chemotherapy combination, clinicians may add endocrine therapy to the HER2-targeted therapy when chemotherapy ends and/or when the cancer progresses (type: informal consensus; evidence quality: insufficient; strength of recommendation: weak).

NATIONAL COMPREHENSIVE CANCER NETWORK GUIDELINES

The NCCN regularly publishes updated guidelines for the treatment of cancers by site.[21] The recommendations are published and rated according to the NCCN Guidelines Categories of Evidence and Consensus. Category 1 recommendations are based on high-level evidence and have uniform NCCN consensus that the intervention is appropriate. Category 2A recommendations are based on lower-level evidence, with uniform consensus that the intervention is appropriate. Category 2B recommendations are based on lower-level evidence and NCCN consensus, whereas Category 3 recommendations are based on any level of evidence with major disagreement that the intervention is appropriate. All recommendations are category 2A unless otherwise stated. The panel recommends treatment with HER2-targeted therapy for all tumors that are HER2+, defined as 3+ on IHC, or gene amplified by in situ hybridization. The HER2 testing recommendations are described in the guidelines.

According to the NCCN Guidelines Version 2.2017 for Invasive Breast Cancer (www.nccn.org), the preferred first-line agents for HER2+ disease include the following:

- Pertuzumab, trastuzumab, and docetaxel (Category 1)
- Pertuzumab, trastuzumab, and paclitaxel (Category 2A)

Other agents listed include the following:

- Ado-trastuzumab emtansine (T-DM1)
- Trastuzumab + paclitaxel ± carboplatin
- Trastuzumab + docetaxel
- Trastuzumab + vinorelbine
- Trastuzumab + capecitabine

Based on the MARIANNE trial,[27] which showed that T-DM1 and T-DM1 and pertuzumab were noninferior in efficacy and better tolerated than the trastuzumab and taxane regimen, T-DM1 was included as a first-line option for HER2+ MBC but should only be considered in patients not suitable for the preferred treatment of pertuzumab, trastuzumab, and a taxane according to NCCN guidelines.

TOXICITIES

The drugs mentioned above have well-known toxicity profiles that will be reviewed here.

Trastuzumab has the following boxed warnings: cardiomyopathy, serious and fatal infusion reactions and pulmonary toxicity, and embryo-fetal toxicity.

The use of trastuzumab can lead to subclinical and clinical heart failure. The incidence and severity are highest in patients receiving trastuzumab concurrently with anthracycline-based chemotherapy. In the trial of single-agent trastuzumab as first-line treatment,[16] 3 of the 114 women were determined to have had cardiac events. Two of these three patients had histories of significant cardiac disease, and one had received adjuvant anthracycline chemotherapy. The third patient had a cardiac event that was attributed to her underlying breast cancer. In the pivotal trial, 63 of 234 patients had symptomatic or asymptomatic cardiac dysfunction.[2] The incidence of New York Heart Association Class III or IV was highest in patients who had received trastuzumab with an anthracycline and cyclophosphamide (16%) compared with those who received an anthracycline and cyclophosphamide alone (3%), trastuzumab and paclitaxel (2%), or paclitaxel alone (1%). It is recommended that left ventricular function is evaluated in all patients before and during treatment with trastuzumab. For patients with metastatic disease, the risk of cardiotoxicity must be weighed against the life-prolonging benefits of trastuzumab.

In the pivotal trial,[2] 25% of patients had chills on infusion of trastuzumab, but this was reduced with slowing the infusion rate. Infections occurred in 47% of patients who received chemotherapy and trastuzumab, compared with 29% of patients who received chemotherapy alone. In the single-agent trastuzumab trial, the most common treatment-related adverse events were chills (25%), asthenia (23%), pain (18%), and nausea (14%).[16] Most adverse events were mild to moderate in intensity. Trastuzumab in combination with other chemotherapy drugs did not significantly add to the known toxicity profiles of those chemotherapy agents.

The addition of pertuzumab to trastuzumab and chemotherapy increased the incidence of diarrhea, rash, mucosal inflammation, febrile neutropenia, and dry skin.[18] The majority of these events were grade 1 and 2 and occurred during the period of concomitant docetaxel administration. An increased incidence of grade 3 febrile neutropenia and diarrhea were seen in the pertuzumab group. Left ventricular systolic dysfunction was not seen more frequently in the pertuzumab group. After the discontinuation of docetaxel, the side effects that differed by more than 5% between the two groups were diarrhea, rash, upper respiratory infections, and muscle spasm (Table 3.1).[19]

In the MARIANNE trial,[27] the most common grade ≥3 toxicities were increased aspartate aminotransferase (6.6%), thrombocytopenia (6.4%), and anemia (4.7%) with T-DM1, and thrombocytopenia (7.9%), anemia (6.0%), and increased alanine aminotransferase (5.2%) with T-DM1 plus pertuzumab. Except for an increase in grade ≥3 diarrhea (2.5% vs. 0.3% for T-DM1), the addition of pertuzumab to T-DM1 did not substantially increase toxicity.

Lapatinib was associated with the adverse events of diarrhea and rash when lapatinib was given alone or in addition to letrozole.[28,41] The addition of lapatinib to paclitaxel chemotherapy increased the rates of rash,

TABLE 3.1
Adverse Events After the Discontinuation of Docetaxel in the Safety Population.

Adverse Event	Control Group (N = 261)	Pertuzumab Group (N = 306)
MOST COMMON EVENTS OF ANY GRADE—NUMBER OF PATIENTS (%)[b]		
Alopecia	6 (2.3)	5 (1.6)
Diarrhea[c]	37 (14.2)	86 (28.1)
Neutropenia	13 (5.0)	10 (3.3)
Nausea	30 (11.5)	39 (12.7)
Fatigue	25 (9.6)	41 (13.4)
Rash[c]	21 (8.0)	56 (18.3)
Asthenia	23 (8.8)	41 (13.4)
Decreased appetite	14 (5.4)	22 (7.2)
Peripheral edema	32 (12.3)	28 (9.2)
Vomiting	17 (6.5)	30 (9.8)
Myalgia	19 (7.3)	25 (8.2)
Mucosal inflammation	4 (1.5)	11 (3.6)
Headache	32 (12.3)	52 (17.0)
Constipation	18 (6.9)	17 (5.6)
Upper respiratory tract infection[c]	32 (12.3)	56 (18.3)
Pruritus[c]	15 (5.7)	42 (13.7)
Febrile neutropenia	0	0
Dry skin	10 (3.8)	10 (3.3)
Muscle spasm[c]	6 (2.3)	24 (7.8)

[a] Data are for patients who received at least one dose of a study drug after completing docetaxel treatment. Data for overall adverse events are provided in Table S1 in the Supplementary Appendix.

[b] The most common events are those that occurred with a frequency of 25% or more overall (including during the docetaxel treatment period) or that differed by 5% points or more in frequency between the two groups overall.

[c] The frequency of this event was at least 5% points greater in the pertuzumab group, as compared with the control group.

Reproduced from Swain SM, Baselga J, Kim SB, Ro J, Semiglazov V, Campone M, et al. Pertuzumab, trastuzumab, and docetaxel in HER2-positive metastatic breast cancer. *N Engl J Med.* 2015;372(8):724–734.

diarrhea, mucositis, and vomiting.[29] In MA-31,[31] which compared lapatinib versus trastuzumab in combination with taxane therapy, there was an increased frequency of diarrhea and rash in the lapatinib arm. Decreased left ventricular ejection fraction of 20% was infrequent (2.3%) but only seen in the trastuzumab arm.

Neratinib has a known side effect profile of diarrhea. In the NEfERT-T trial,[32] diarrhea was seen at a rate of 92.5% in patients receiving neratinib and paclitaxel versus 33.3% for the patients receiving trastuzumab and paclitaxel only. Of note, primary prophylaxis for diarrhea was not mandatory in this trial. Nausea was also increased at 44.2% versus 30.3%. Alopecia, peripheral neuropathy, and fatigue were similar between the two groups. Three patients in the neratinib and paclitaxel group died because of treatment-related adverse events (one from septic shock, one from intestinal obstruction, and one from ascites) and one patient died in the trastuzumab and paclitaxel group from pneumonitis.

ONGOING PHASE III TRIALS IN THE FIRST-LINE SETTING

A number of phase III trials are ongoing comparing different drugs or combinations for the first-line treatment of HER2+ MBC.

- A phase III randomized, double-blind study of Pf-05280014 plus paclitaxel versus trastuzumab plus Paclitaxel for the first-line treatment of Patients with HER2+ MBC (REFLECTIONS B327-02).
- International multicenter randomized double-blind phase III clinical trial comparing safety and efficacy of BCD-022 (CJSC BIOCAD, Russia) used with paclitaxel to Herceptin (F. Hoffmann-La Roche Ltd, Switzerland) used with paclitaxel in the first-line treatment of HER2+ MBC patients.
- An open-label, randomized, multicenter phase III study in patients with HER2+ MBC responding to first-line treatment with intravenous trastuzumab for at least 3 years and investigating patient preference for subcutaneous trastuzumab.
- An open-label, multicentre, phase IIIb study with intravenous administration of pertuzumab, subcutaneous trastuzumab, and a taxane in patients with HER2+ MBC (SAPPHIRE).
- A phase IIIb study of pertuzumab in combination with trastuzumab (Herceptin) and a taxane (investigator's choice of docetaxel, paclitaxel or nab-paclitaxel) in first-line treatment in participants with human epidermal growth factor 2 (HER2)-positive advanced breast cancer (PERUSE).

- A randomized phase III trial of paclitaxel/trastuzumab/pertuzumab compared to paclitaxel/trastuzumab/pertuzumab/pembrolizumab in first-line HER2+ MBC.
- A randomized open-label phase III study of taxane-based chemotherapy with lapatinib or trastuzumab as first-line therapy for women with HER2/Neu positive MBC.
- Dasatinib in combination with trastuzumab and paclitaxel in the first-line treatment of HER2+ MBC patients by the Spanish Breast Cancer Research Group.
- A phase iii study comparing chemotherapy versus endocrine therapy in combination with dual HER2-targeted therapy with trastuzumab and pertuzumab for patients with HER2-positive/HR-positive MBC.

There are many novel molecules in clinical trials, mostly in later line settings:

- Tucatinib (ONT-380) is a highly selective small molecule inhibitor of HER2 kinase. Unlike other dual HER2/EGFR drugs, it does not inhibit EGFR at clinically relevant concentrations, leading to reduced potential for EGFR-related toxicities (severe skin rash and diarrhea). This is currently being evaluated in a phase II randomized double-blind study of tucatinib versus placebo in combination with capecitabine and trastuzumab in patients with unresectable locally advanced or metastatic HER2+ breast carcinoma who have received previous treatment with a taxane, trastuzumab, pertuzumab, and T-DM1 (HER2CLIMB).
- ZW25 is an anti-HER2 bispecific monoclonal antibody that targets two different epitopes of the extracellular portion of the HER2 receptor. It binds to the same extracellular domains of HER2 as trastuzumab and pertuzumab with increased binding and internalization compared with trastuzumab alone.
- PI3K-inhibitors:
  - Alpelisib is an oral phosphatidylinositol 3-kinase (PI3K) inhibitor that selectively inhibits the PI3Kα isoform. Constitutive activation of this signaling pathway is a mechanism of trastuzumab resistance in HER2+ MBC. A phase I study[44] showed that the combination of alpelisib and T-DM1 was safe in HER2+ MBC patients and had significant antitumor activity, even in patients previously treated with T-DM1.
  - Also ongoing is an open-label study evaluating the safety and tolerability of LJM716, BYL719, and trastuzumab in patients with metastatic HER2+ breast cancer.

- Margetuximab is an Fc-modified monoclonal antibody to HER2 that recognizes the same epitope on HER2 as trastuzumab does and with a similar affinity. It has increased affinity to the activating CD16A Fc-receptor found on NK cells and macrophages and decreased affinity to the inhibitory CD32B receptor compared with trastuzumab. SOPHIA is an ongoing phase III, randomized study of margetuximab plus chemotherapy versus trastuzumab plus chemotherapy (physician's choice: capecitabine, eribulin, gemcitabine, or vinorelbine) in patients with previously treated, HER2+ MBC.
- Patritumab (a human anti-HER3 monoclonal antibody) is being tested in a randomized placebo-controlled double-blind phase Ib/2 study in combination with trastuzumab plus paclitaxel in newly diagnosed HER2+ MBC.
- CDK 4/6 inhibitors (palbociclib, ribociclib, and abemaciclib) are being tested with various HER2-directed therapies.
- Other immunotherapy agents such as durvalumab and atezolizumab are being tested with HER2-directed therapy.

LIMITATIONS OF CURRENT STUDIES AND FUTURE DIRECTIONS

There is no doubt that the treatment of HER2+ MBC with targeted therapies has dramatically improved the outcomes for this patient population. Further, the introduction of these HER2-targeted agents into the adjuvant and neoadjuvant settings has been shown to reduce the number of women who develop metastatic disease. Despite these advances, the majority of patients with metastatic disease die from their cancer. Therefore, more work needs to be done.

A major unmet need in the treatment of HER2+ metastatic disease is metastases to the CNS. Breast cancer is the second most common source of brain metastases.[45] HER2+ patients tend to have an increased risk of developing CNS involvement. Brain metastases have become a challenge in the treatment of HER2+ breast cancer, especially as targeted therapies are allowing for excellent systemic control and prolonged survival. These new therapies have limited efficacy in treating brain metastases. Often, patients will develop brain metastases even when their visceral disease is well controlled. Research is needed for systemic treatments that will treat CNS disease as well as reduce the chance of developing brain metastases.

Despite treatment with trastuzumab and pertuzumab in the first-line metastatic setting, patients go on to develop progressive disease. Biomarker-driven studies may help identify patients for whom dual therapy is most beneficial versus those patients who may be resistant and progress early.

Another question that remains to be answered is the duration of pertuzumab in the metastatic setting. In the trials described, pertuzumab was discontinued at progression. Historically, despite disease progression on prior trastuzumab-based therapy, trastuzumab was continued along with a change in chemotherapy agent. Clinical trials later confirmed that continuing trastuzumab was beneficial.[46] A more thoughtful approach involving clinical trials should be pursued to determine if continuing pertuzumab is effective beyond progression.

It is clear that some patients with HER2+ breast cancer can benefit from HER2-targeted therapy in the absence of chemotherapy. For example, in the NeoSphere neoadjuvant trial,[47] a pathologic complete response rate of 18% was seen in patients treated with trastuzumab and pertuzumab alone without chemotherapy. If biomarkers can be found to identify these patients, we may be able to find a group of HER2+ patients who could be spared the toxicities of chemotherapy.

A major limitation of front-line trastuzumab and pertuzumab trials was the prohibition of endocrine therapy during the maintenance HER2-targeted phase of the trials. It is likely that survival would have been even better if endocrine treatment were allowed during nonchemotherapy maintenance, as it is in HER2-negative, HR+ disease, yet recent reports from the SystHERs trial show that this is not standard practice in the real world. Forty-one percent of HR-positive HER2+ patients did not receive hormone therapy during first-line treatment.[48]

The treatment of elderly patients with metastatic disease presents a challenge. Elderly patients are clearly underrepresented in clinical trials.[49] In a retrospective analysis published by the US FDA,[50] data on over 28,000 cancer patients from 55 registration trials were analyzed. They noted an underrepresentation of the elderly, particularly patients aged 70 years and above, in registration trials for all cancer treatments except for breast cancer hormone therapy trials. This underrepresentation in clinical trials may lead to a lack of information regarding the efficacy and toxicity of specific treatments in these patients.

Clinical trials of shorter durations of chemotherapy when it is combined with targeted therapy could show that less is more. These trial designs are unlikely to be supported by pharma but are within the mandate of CTEP.

Enrollment to clinical trials is imperative. With the introduction of HER2-targeted therapies to the early-stage neoadjuvant and adjuvant settings, fewer patients are progressing to develop MBC. This encouraging progress has led to fewer patients being available for clinical trials in the metastatic setting. Further progress in this disease will only be made through the completion of clinical trials using new agents and new combinations. Therefore, it is crucial that all physicians consider enrolling their patients with HER2+ MBC on clinical trials.

REFERENCES

1. Slamon DJ, Clark GM, Wong SG, Levin WJ, Ullrich A, McGuire WL. Human breast cancer: correlation of relapse and survival with amplification of the Her-2/*neu* oncogene. *Science*. 1987;235(4785):177−182.
2. Slamon DJ, Leyland-Jones B, Shak S, et al. Use of chemotherapy plus a monoclonal antibody against HER2 for metastatic breast cancer that overexpresses HER2. *N Engl J Med*. 2001;344(11):783−792.
3. Mass RD, Press MF, Anderson S, et al. Evaluation of clinical outcomes according to HER2 detection by fluorescence in situ hybridization in women with metastatic breast cancer treated with trastuzumab. *Clin Breast Cancer*. 2005;6(3):240−246.
4. Marty M, Cognetti F, Maraninchi D, et al. Randomized phase II trial of the efficacy and safety of trastuzumab combined with docetaxel in patients with human epidermal growth factor receptor 2-positive metastatic breast cancer administered as first-line treatment: the M77001 study group. *J Clin Oncol*. 2005;23(19):4265−4274.
5. Dawood S, Broglio K, Buzdar AU, Hortobagyi GN, Giordano SH. Prognosis of women with metastatic breast cancer by HER2 status and trastuzumab treatment: an institutional-based review. *J Clin Oncol*. 2010;28(1): 92−98.
6. Robert N, Leyland-Jones B, Asmar L, et al. Randomized phase III study of trastuzumab, paclitaxel, and carboplatin compared with trastuzumab and paclitaxel in women with HER-2-overexpressing metastatic breast cancer. *J Clin Oncol*. 2006;24(18):2786−2792.
7. Valero V, Forbes J, Pegram MD, et al. Multicenter phase III randomized trial comparing docetaxel and trastuzumab with docetaxel, carboplatin, and trastuzumab as first-line chemotherapy for patients with HER2-gene-amplified metastatic breast cancer (BCIRG 007 study): two highly active therapeutic regimens. *J Clin Oncol*. 2011;29(2): 149−156.
8. Wardley AM, Pivot X, Morales-Vasquez F, et al. Randomized phase II trial of first-line trastuzumab plus docetaxel and capecitabine compared with trastuzumab plus docetaxel in HER2-positive metastatic breast cancer. *J Clin Oncol*. 2010;28(6):976−983.
9. Gianni L, Romieu GH, Lichinitser M, et al. AVEREL: a randomized phase III Trial evaluating bevacizumab in combination with docetaxel and trastuzumab as first-line therapy for HER2-positive locally recurrent/metastatic breast cancer. *J Clin Oncol*. 2013;31(14): 1719−1725.
10. Hurvitz SA, Andre F, Jiang Z, et al. Combination of everolimus with trastuzumab plus paclitaxel as first-line treatment for patients with HER2-positive advanced breast cancer (BOLERO-1): a phase 3, randomised, double-blind, multicentre trial. *Lancet Oncol*. 2015; 16(7):816−829.
11. Burstein HJ, Harris LN, Marcom PK, et al. Trastuzumab and vinorelbine as first-line therapy for HER2-overexpressing metastatic breast cancer: multicenter phase II trial with clinical outcomes, analysis of serum tumor markers as predictive factors, and cardiac surveillance algorithm. *J Clin Oncol*. 2003;21(15):2889−2895.
12. Burstein HJ, Keshaviah A, Baron AD, et al. Trastuzumab plus vinorelbine or taxane chemotherapy for HER2-overexpressing metastatic breast cancer: the trastuzumab and vinorelbine or taxane study. *Cancer*. 2007;110(5): 965−972.
13. Andersson M, Lidbrink E, Bjerre K, et al. Phase III randomized study comparing docetaxel plus trastuzumab with vinorelbine plus trastuzumab as first-line therapy of metastatic or locally advanced human epidermal growth factor receptor 2-positive breast cancer: the HERNATA study. *J Clin Oncol*. 2011;29(3):264−271.
14. Schaller G, Fuchs I, Gonsch T, et al. Phase II study of capecitabine plus trastuzumab in human epidermal growth factor receptor 2 overexpressing metastatic breast cancer pretreated with anthracyclines or taxanes. *J Clin Oncol*. 2007;25(22):3246−3250.
15. Yamamoto D, Iwase S, Kitamura K, Odagiri H, Yamamoto C, Nagumo Y. A phase II study of trastuzumab and capecitabine for patients with HER2-overexpressing metastatic breast cancer: Japan Breast Cancer Research Network (JBCRN) 00 Trial. *Cancer Chemother Pharmacol*. 2008;61(3):509−514.
16. Vogel CL, Cobleigh MA, Tripathy D, et al. Efficacy and safety of trastuzumab as a single agent in first-line treatment of HER2-overexpressing metastatic breast cancer. *J Clin Oncol*. 2002;20(3):719−726.
17. Inoue K, Nakagami K, Mizutani M, et al. Randomized phase III trial of trastuzumab monotherapy followed by trastuzumab plus docetaxel versus trastuzumab plus docetaxel as first-line therapy in patients with HER2-positive metastatic breast cancer: the JO17360 Trial Group. *Breast Cancer Res Treat*. 2010;119(1):127−136.
18. Baselga J, Cortés J, Kim SB, et al. Pertuzumab plus trastuzumab plus docetaxel for metastatic breast cancer. *N Engl J Med*. 2012;366(2):109−119.
19. Swain SM, Baselga J, Kim SB, et al. Pertuzumab, trastuzumab, and docetaxel in HER2-positive metastatic breast cancer. *N Engl J Med*. 2015;372(8):724−734.

20. Smyth LM, Iyengar NM, Chen MF, et al. Weekly paclitaxel with trastuzumab and pertuzumab in patients with HER2-overexpressing metastatic breast cancer: overall survival and updated progression-free survival results from a phase II study. *Breast Cancer Res Treat.* 2016;158(1):91–97.
21. *NCCN Clinical Practice Guidelines in Oncology Breast Cancer Version 2.2017.* 2017. https://www.nccn.org/professionals/physician_gls/pdf/breast.pdf.
22. Perez EA, López-vega JM, Petit T, et al. Safety and efficacy of vinorelbine in combination with pertuzumab and trastuzumab for first-line treatment of patients with HER2-positive locally advanced or metastatic breast cancer: VELVET Cohort 1 final results. *Breast Cancer Res.* 2016;18(1):126.
23. Narui K, Yamashita T, Kitada M, et al. Eribulin in combination with pertuzumab plus trastuzumab for HER2-positive advanced or recurrent breast cancer (JBCRG-M03). *J Clin Oncol.* 2017;35(suppl):abstr 1025.
24. Lewis Phillips GD, Li G, Dugger DL, et al. Targeting HER2-positive breast cancer with trastuzumab-DM1, an antibody-cytotoxic drug conjugate. *Cancer Res.* 2008;68(22):9280–9290.
25. Verma S, Miles D, Gianni L, et al. Trastuzumab emtansine for HER2-positive advanced breast cancer. *N Engl J Med.* 2012;367(19):1783–1791.
26. Hurvitz SA, Dirix L, Kocsis J, et al. Phase II randomized study of trastuzumab emtansine versus trastuzumab plus docetaxel in patients with human epidermal growth factor receptor 2–positive metastatic breast cancer. *J Clin Oncol.* 2013;31(9):1157–1163.
27. Perez EA, Barrios C, Eiermann W, et al. Trastuzumab emtansine with or without pertuzumab versus trastuzumab plus taxane for human epidermal growth factor receptor 2-positive, advanced breast cancer: primary results from the phase III MARIANNE study. *J Clin Oncol.* 2017;35(2):141–148.
28. Gomez HL, Doval DC, Chavez MA, et al. Efficacy and safety of lapatinib as first-line therapy for ErbB2-amplified locally advanced or metastatic breast cancer. *J Clin Oncol.* 2008;26(18):2999–3005.
29. Di Leo A, Gomez HL, Aziz Z, et al. Phase III, double-blind, randomized study comparing lapatinib plus paclitaxel with placebo plus paclitaxel as first-line treatment for metastatic breast cancer. *J Clin Oncol.* 2008;26(34):5544–5552.
30. Sweetlove M. Phase III trial of lapatinib. *Pharm Med.* 2012;26(5):321–325.
31. Gelmon KA, Boyle FM, Kaufman B, et al. Lapatinib or trastuzumab plus taxane therapy for human epidermal growth factor receptor 2-positive advanced breast cancer: final results of NCIC CTG MA.31. *J Clin Oncol.* 2015;33(14):1574–1583.
32. Awada A, Colomer R, Inoue K, et al. Neratinib plus paclitaxel vs trastuzumab plus paclitaxel in previously untreated metastatic ERBB2-positive breast cancer: the NEfERT-T randomized clinical trial. *JAMA Oncol.* 2016;2(12):1557–1564.
33. Rugo HS, Barve A, Waller CF, et al. Effect of a proposed trastuzumab biosimilar compared with trastuzumab on overall response rate in patients with ERBB2 (HER2)-positive metastatic breast cancer: a randomized clinical trial. *JAMA.* 2017;317(1):37–47.
34. Untch M, Gelber RD, Jackisch C, et al. Estimating the magnitude of trastuzumab effects within patient subgroups in the HERA trial. *Ann Oncol.* 2008;19(6):1090–1096.
35. Perez EA, Romond EH, Suman VJ, et al. Updated results of the combined analysis of NCCTG N9831 and NSABP B-31 adjuvant chemotherapy with/without trastuzumab in patients with HER2-positive breast cancer. *J Clin Oncol.* 2007;25(18):abstr 512.
36. Brufsky A, Lembersky B, Schiffman K, Lieberman G, Paton VE. Hormone receptor status does not affect the clinical benefit of trastuzumab therapy for patients with metastatic breast cancer. *Clin Breast Cancer.* 2005;6(3):247–252.
37. Penault-Llorca F, Vincent-Salomon A, Mathieu MC, Trillet-Lenoir V, Khayat D, Marty M. Incidence and implications of HER2 and hormonal receptor overexpression in newly diagnosed metastatic breast cancer. *J Clin Oncol.* 2005;23(16):abstr 764.
38. Slamon D, Eiermann W, Robert N, et al. BCIRG 006: 2nd interim analysis phase III randomized trial comparing doxorubicin and cyclophosphamide followed by docetaxel with doxorubicin and cyclophosphamide followed by docetaxel and trastuzumab with docetaxel, carboplatin and trastuzumab (TCH) in Her2neu positive early breast cancer patients. In: *SABCS.* 2006. General Session 2: Abstract 52.
39. Kaufman B, Mackey JR, Clemens MR, et al. Trastuzumab plus anastrozole versus anastrozole alone for the treatment of postmenopausal women with human epidermal growth factor receptor 2-positive, hormone receptor-positive metastatic breast cancer: results from the randomized phase III TAnDEM study. *J Clin Oncol.* 2009;27(33):5529–5537.
40. Huober J, Fasching PA, Barsoum M, et al. Higher efficacy of letrozole in combination with trastuzumab compared to letrozole monotherapy as first-line treatment in patients with HER2-positive, hormone-receptor-positive metastatic breast cancer - results of the eLEcTRA trial. *Breast.* 2012;21(1):27–33.
41. Johnston S, Pippen Jr J, Pivot X, et al. Lapatinib combined with letrozole versus letrozole and placebo as first-line therapy for postmenopausal hormone receptor-positive metastatic breast cancer. *J Clin Oncol.* 2009;27(33):5538–5546.
42. Aprino G, Ferrero J-M, de la Haba-Rodriguez J, et al. Primary analysis of PERTAIN: a randomized, two-arm, open-label, multicenter phase II trial assessing the efficacy and safety of pertuzumab given in combination with trastuzumab plus an aromatase inhibitor in first-line patients with HER2-positive and hormone receptor-positive metastatic or locally advanced breast cancer. In: *Presented at: San Antonio Breast Cancer Symposium; December 6-10; San Antonio, TX.* 2016;Abstract S3–04.

43. Giordano SH, Temin S, Kirshner JJ, et al. Systemic therapy for patients with advanced human epidermal growth factor receptor 2-positive breast cancer: American Society of Clinical Oncology clinical practice guideline. *J Clin Oncol.* 2014;32(19):2078−2099.

44. Jain S, Santa-Maria CA, Rademaker A, Giles FJ, Cristofanilli M, Gradishar WJ. Phase I study of alpelisib (BYL-719) and T-DM1 in HER2-positive metastatic breast cancer after trastuzumab and taxane therapy. *J Clin Oncol.* 2017;35(15):abstr 1026.

45. Kamar FG, Posner JB. Brain metastases. *Semin Neurol.* 2010;30(3):217−235.

46. Blackwell KL, Burstein HJ, Storniolo AM, et al. Randomized study of Lapatinib alone or in combination with trastuzumab in women with ErbB2-positive, trastuzumab-refractory metastatic breast cancer. *J Clin Oncol.* 2010;28(7):1124−1130.

47. Gianni L, Pienkowski T, Im YH, et al. Efficacy and safety of neoadjuvant pertuzumab and trastuzumab in women with locally advanced, inflammatory, or early HER2-positive breast cancer (NeoSphere): a randomised multicentre, open-label, phase 2 trial. *Lancet Oncol.* 2012;13(1):25−32.

48. Cobleigh M, Yardley DA, Brufsky A, et al. Baseline (BL) characteristics, treatment (tx) patterns, and outcomes in patients with hormone receptor (HR)+ vs HR-HER2+ disease from the SystHERs registry. *Cancer Res.* 2017;77. https://doi.org/10.1158/1538-7445.SABCS16-P5-08-27. P5-08.

49. Murthy VH, Krumholz HM, Gross CP. Participation in cancer clinical trials: race-, sex-, and age-based disparities. *JAMA.* 2004;291(22):2720−2726.

50. Talarico L, Chen G, Pazdur R. Enrollment of elderly patients in clinical trials for cancer drug registration: a 7-year experience by the US Food and Drug Administration. *J Clin Oncol.* 2004;22(22):4626−4631.

CHAPTER 4

HER2-Positive Breast Cancer: Second Line and Beyond

SARAH SAMMONS, MD • KIMBERLY BLACKWELL, MD

INTRODUCTION

The treatment of HER2-positive (HER2+) metastatic breast cancer (mBC) has drastically evolved in the past two decades with the breakthrough clinical success of HER2-directed therapies. The discovery of trastuzumab has altered the clinical course of both early-stage and metastatic HER2+ breast cancer. As one of the largest victories in modern oncology, trastuzumab was approved in 1998 as a first-line treatment in combination with paclitaxel for HER2+ mBC.[1] Moving into the adjuvant setting in early-stage HER2+ breast cancer, the addition of trastuzumab to chemotherapy resulted in impressive improvements in both disease-free and overall survival (OS) and is now the standard of care.[2–4] Despite these major advances, up to 30% of patients with early-stage HER2+ breast cancer will develop metastatic recurrence.[2,5] Trastuzumab still plays a key role in the treatment of HER2+ mBC along with the newer HER2-directed monoclonal antibody pertuzumab, the small molecule inhibitor lapatinib, and the antibody-drug conjugate (ADC) trastuzumab emtansine.

For first-line treatment in HER2+ mBC, patients who have completed adjuvant trastuzumab-based treatment greater than 6 months before developing advanced disease are recommended by expert panels to receive combination therapy with pertuzumab, trastuzumab, and a taxane based on the results of the randomized phase III CLEOPATRA clinical trial.[6] The addition of pertuzumab to trastuzumab and docetaxel was associated with impressive improvements in both median progression-free survival (PFS) and OS with a median OS of 56.5 months.[7] Patients who progress on this regimen or patients who progressed within 6 months of adjuvant trastuzumab are recommended for second-line therapy.

The ADC, trastuzumab emtansine (T-DM1), is the most supported choice for second-line therapy in HER2+ mBC based on the results of the phase III EMILIA clinical trial, which showed improvements in PFS and OS over capecitabine and lapatinib.[8,9] Beyond second-line recommendations, there is little consensus or evidence for the sequence of agents; however, lapatinib combination therapies and trastuzumab/chemotherapy combinations have been well studied and are available. Clinical trials should always be considered in this patient population as well. Fig. 4.1 shows a schema for rational treatment options in the second line and beyond in HER2+ mBC.

Overall, HER2-directed therapies have drastically improved outcomes in HER2+ mBC in the second line and beyond. A recent analysis of 19 randomized controlled trials assessing changes in outcomes in HER2+ mBC in the last two decades confirmed these results.[10] In the second-line setting and beyond, OS has improved from 15.3 months[11] with lapatinib plus capecitabine[2] to 30 months[8] with trastuzumab emtansine.[8] In the third-line setting or beyond, the addition of lapatinib to trastuzumab has improved OS compared with lapatinib alone.[12] Similarly, in heavily pretreated populations after at least two HER2-directed therapies, T-DM1 improved OS versus treatment of physician's choice (PC) to a median of 22.7 months from 15.8 months.[13] A list of pivotal phase III clinical trials in metastatic HER2+ breast cancer treated in the second line and beyond can be seen in Table 4.1. For the purposes of this text, second line was defined as treatment after progression on trastuzumab and a taxane. These results confirm that HER2-directed therapies are drastically improving outcomes in an otherwise incurable disease.

This chapter will focus on established and approved treatment options in the second line and beyond, including the following:

- The principle of continuing HER2-directed therapy beyond progression on trastuzumab

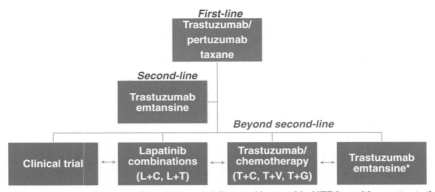

FIG. 4.1 **Schema for treatment options in second-line and beyond in HER2 positive metastatic breast cancer.** C, capecitabine; G, gemcitabine; L, lapatinib; T, trastuzumab; V, vinorelbine; *, Trastuzumab emtansine has shown efficacy in the third-line and beyond if not given in the second-line.

- The evidence and recommendations for the use of ADC trastuzumab emtansine in the second-line setting and beyond
- Lapatinib combinations in metastatic HER2+ breast cancer
- Chemotherapy/trastuzumab combinations in metastatic HER2+ breast cancer
- Hormone receptor positive, HER2+ mBC

CONTINUING HER2-DIRECTED THERAPY BEYOND PROGRESSION ON TRASTUZUMAB

Since the initial trials of trastuzumab, the issue of how to best manage patients whose tumors progress on trastuzumab-based therapy has emerged. For years, oncologists empirically practiced continuing HER2-directed therapy beyond progression on trastuzumab in patients with HER2+ mBC. Trastuzumab has synergistic effects with many cytotoxic chemotherapies[14]; therefore, theoretically, changing the chemotherapy backbone and keeping the targeted therapeutic could still provide benefit. Trastuzumab is extremely well tolerated with most agents other than anthracyclines, and continuing treatment causes little cumulative toxicity.

Several phase III clinical trials have demonstrated the benefit of continuing trastuzumab or HER2-directed therapy following disease progression on a trastuzumab-containing regimen. One phase III study investigated capecitabine with or without trastuzumab in patients who had progressed on trastuzumab.[15,16] The trial closed prematurely because of poor accrual, but data from the available 156 patients showed no significant difference in OS with capecitabine versus

capecitabine plus trastuzumab. However, median time to progression (TTP) favored the combination group (8.2 months vs. 5.6 months) (Table 4.1) with an unadjusted hazard ratio (HR) of 0.69 (95% CI 0.48–0.97; two-sided log-rank $P = .0338$).[16] In a post hoc analysis of the study, patients who continued or restarted treatment with trastuzumab or lapatinib after second progression (n = 52) had a postprogression survival of 18.8 months compared with 13.3 months for those who did not receive third-line treatment with anti-HER2 agents (n = 88) (HR 0.63; $P = .02$).[15] Continuation of trastuzumab was not associated with increased toxicity. Another phase III randomized clinical trial examined the role of lapatinib with capecitabine versus capecitabine alone in patients who had experienced progression after receiving (at minimum) trastuzumab, an anthracycline, and a taxane.[17] With 324 eligible patients, the trial met its primary endpoint of median time to disease progression in favor of lapatinib and capecitabine (8.4 months vs. 4.4 months; $P < .0019$) (Table 4.1).

These data together support the use of HER2-targeted therapy beyond progression of disease on a trastuzumab-containing regimen. The question of how long to continue HER2-directed therapy in the metastatic setting is unclear, and there are no randomized trials to guide us. Most experts would agree that after progression beyond trastuzumab/pertuzumab-taxane and trastuzumab emtansine, lapatinib-based combinations or trastuzumab/chemotherapy combinations should be considered if not limited by toxicity. The choice of how long to continue HER2-directed therapy at this time remains a highly individualized decision considering previous regimens, response to previous regimens, toxicity, and overall clinical status.

TABLE 4.1
Pivotal Phase III Clinical Trials in Metastatic HER2+ Breast Cancer Treated in the Second-line and Beyond. Second-line was defined as progression after trastuzumab containing regimen.

Trial Identifier	Patients	Regimen	Population	Median TTP or PFS (Months)	Median OS (Months)	ORR
TH3RESA (Krop et al., 2017)[13]	602	T-DM1 versus physician's choice	HER2+ mBC progression on two or more HER2-targeted regimens	6.2 vs. 3.3 (P < 0.0001)	22.7 vs. 15.8($P = 0\cdot0007$)	NR
EMILIA[8]	991	T-DM1 versus capecitabine and lapatinib	HER2+ mBC progression on trastuzumab and a taxane	9.6 vs. 6.4 (P < .001)	30.9 vs. 25.1 (P < .001)	44 (P < .001)
EGF104900[34]	296	Lapatinib with or without trastuzumab	HER2+ mBC progression on anthracycline, taxane, trastuzumab	11.1 vs. 8.1 (weeks) (P = 0.011)	14.0 vs. 9.5 (P = .026)	10 (P = .46)
von Minckwitz et al.[16]	156	Capecitabine with or without trastuzumab	HER2+ mBC progression on trastuzumab and up to one chemotherapy	8.2 vs. 5.6 (P = .034)	24.9 vs. 20.6 (P = .73)	48 (P = .012)
EGF100151[17]	324	Capecitabine with or without lapatinib	HER2+ mBC progression on anthracycline, a taxane, and trastuzumab	8.4 vs. 4.4 (P < .001)	75 vs. 64.7 (weeks) (P = .21)	22 (P = .09)

mBC, metastatic breast cancer; ORR, overall response rate; OS, overall survival; PFS, progression-free survival; TTP, time to progression.

TRASTUZUMAB EMTANSINE IN HER2-POSITIVE METASTATIC BREAST CANCER

Trastuzumab emtansine or ado-trastuzumab emtansine (T-DM1) is an ADC with the HER2-targeted antitumor properties of trastuzumab and the cytotoxic activity of the microtubule-inhibitory agent DM1 attached via a stable thioethel linker.[18] DM1, also called emtansine, is a thiol-containing maytansinoid that interferes with microtubule function. This ADC allows cytotoxic intracellular drug delivery to HER2-overexpressing cells while sparing normal tissues. The safety and recommended dosing of T-DM1 (3.6 mg/kg every 3 weeks) were first established in a phase 1 clinical trial.[19] The clinical benefit of T-DM1 for HER2+ mBC was first observed in phase II clinical trials in populations that were heavily pretreated with trastuzumab, lapatinib, anthracycline, taxane, and capecitabine.[20,21] T-DM1 is the most supported choice for second-line therapy after progression on trastuzumab and a taxane, showing superiority over lapatinib and capecitabine.[22,23] If not given in this setting, it has also shown efficacy beyond second line compared with physicians' choice therapies.[13]

Trastuzumab Emtansine for Second-Line Therapy

The efficacy of T-DM1 in the second line leading to regulatory approval was confirmed in the phase III EMILIA trial in which T-DM1 was compared with lapatinib plus capecitabine in patients with HER2+ mBC previously treated with trastuzumab and a taxane (Table 4.1). Most patients had visceral disease and half were also hormone receptor positive. The trial met both coprimary endpoints. T-DM1 improved PFS 9.6 months versus 6.4 months (HR 0.65; 95% CI 0.55–0.77; $P < .001$).[8] At second interim analysis, median OS was superior with T-DM1 at 30.9 months versus 25.1 months (HR 0.68; 95% CI 0.5–0.85; $P < .001$). OS was confirmed and was similar (29.9 months vs. 25.9 months) in the final analysis (HR 0.75; 95% CI 0.64–0.88).[22] Importantly, grade 3 or 4 toxicity was higher with lapatinib/capecitabine over T-DM1 (57.0% vs. 40.8%). T-DM1 is very well tolerated with the most frequent serious adverse events remaining thrombocytopenia and elevated liver enzymes. Of the 481 patients in the T-DM1 group, 1.7% developed left ventricular ejection fraction <50% versus 1.6% in the combination group. These results led to the FDA approval of T-DM1 in taxane- and trastuzumab-refractory HER2+ mBC in 2013.

EMILIA was conducted before the era of dual anti-HER2 therapy with trastuzumab and pertuzumab with a taxane as the standard of care for first-line HER2+ mBC. It remains unclear if pertuzumab-pretreated patients will achieve the same benefits from T-DM1. A recent retrospective, observational study involving 23 cancer centers and 250 patients addressed T-DM1 efficacy in HER2+ mBC patients treated in real-world practice and its activity in pertuzumab-pretreated patients.[24] In the overall population, PFS and OS in T-DM1 treated patients was similar in pertuzumab-pretreated and naïve patients. However, pertuzumab pretreatment did seem to negatively influence second-line T-DM1 efficacy. Pertuzumab pretreated patients who received T-DM1 as second-line treatment showed a mPFS of 3 months, whereas patients who did not receive previous pertuzumab had a mPFS of 8 months (p=0.0001). Further large-scale studies are necessary to determine T-DM1 efficacy when given as second-line treatment after pertuzumab.

Trastuzumab Emtansine Beyond Second Line

If T-DM1 is not given in the second line, it has still shown efficacy in the later setting. The phase III TH3RESA clinical trial showed that T-DM1 is effective over physicians' choice beyond second line in patients with HER2+ mBC who progressed on two or more HER2-targeted regimens (Table 4.1).[13] Eligible patients had HER2+ mBC and previously received two or more HER2-directed regimens in the advanced setting including trastuzumab, lapatinib, and taxane. Patients were randomly assigned to receive T-DM1 or PC. The majority of PC regimens were either trastuzumab plus single-agent chemotherapy or trastuzumab plus lapatinib. In this setting, T-DM1 provided a significant improvement in PFS compared with PC (6.2 months vs. 3.3 months; HR 0.528; 95% CI 0.422–0.661; $P < .0001$). OS was significantly longer with T-DM1 versus PC as well (22.7 months vs. 15.8 months; HR 0.68; 95% CI 0.54–0.85; $P = .0007$). The safety profile was also better with T-DM1.

Taken together, EMILIA and TH3RESA demonstrate improved outcomes and survival with T-DM1 over chemotherapy-based anti-HER2 regimens and provide strong support to incorporate T-DM1 routinely as second- or third-line therapy.

LAPATINIB COMBINATIONS IN HER2-POSITIVE METASTATIC BREAST CANCER

Upon disease progression following a first-line regimen of pertuzumab, trastuzumab, and taxane and second-line T-DM1, there is no consensus or evidence for the sequence of agents in HER2+ mBC. Several trials have investigated the efficacy and safety of lapatinib alone and in conjunction with other agents in the treatment of HER2+ mBC. Lapatinib-based regimens (lapatinib/ capecitabine or lapatinib/trastuzumab) have shown great clinical success in heavily pretreated populations and are a logical next choice (Fig. 4.1). It is important to note that neither of these regimens have efficacy data available in the setting of prior progression after multiple HER2-directed antibody-based strategies such as pertuzumab and T-DM1.

Lapatinib is an orally bioavailable small molecule that binds and reversibly inhibits the adenosine triphosphate binding site of the intracellular kinase domains of EGFR (epidermal growth factor receptor, also known as HER1) and HER2, blocking receptor phosphorylation and activation of downstream signaling pathways, including the MAPK/ERK (mitogen-activated protein kinase; extracellular signal–related kinase 1/2) and PI3K/Akt (phosphatidylinositol 3′ kinase; protein kinase B) pathways.[25,26] Lapatinib has mechanisms of action distinct from trastuzumab; therefore, in preclinical studies, lapatinib was not cross-resistant with trastuzumab, demonstrating significant activity in trastuzumab-resistant cell lines.[25,27]

Lapatinib has been studied as monotherapy in several phase II clinical trials, showing limited efficacy but tolerable safety.[28,29] The most common treatment-related adverse events were rash (47%), diarrhea (46%), nausea (31%), and fatigue (18%),[29] which were mild and manageable. Lapatinib in combination with either capecitabine or trastuzumab has shown better clinical efficacy in heavily pretreated populations,[12,17] leading to regulatory approvals. In 2007, lapatinib in combination with capecitabine was approved in the United States for patients with HER2+ mBC who had received prior therapies, including anthracycline, taxane, and trastuzumab, based on results from a phase III randomized study.[17]

Lapatinib Plus Capecitabine
The pivotal phase III clinical trial demonstrating lapatinib efficacy was a randomized study comparing lapatinib plus capecitabine with capecitabine alone in women with advanced, progressive HER2+ mBC following prior treatment with anthracyclines, taxanes, and trastuzumab[17] (Table 4.1). Taxanes could have been given in the adjuvant or metastatic setting. Nearly all patients had received trastuzumab in the first-line metastatic setting. The interim analysis showed that the addition of lapatinib to capecitabine was associated with a 51% reduction in the risk of disease progression. The median TTP was 8.4 months in the combination group versus 4.4 months with capecitabine alone

(HR 0.47; 95% CI 0.32−0.68; $P < .001$).[17] Toxicity was similar to either agent alone and was not cumulative. This regimen is no longer recommended in the second-line setting because of inferior efficacy to T-DM1.[22] Its clinical activity allows it to remain as an option after pertuzumab- and T-DM1-based regimens.

HER2+ mBC is associated with a higher prevalence of brain metastases when compared with other subtypes. Lapatinib alone and in combination with capecitabine has shown efficacy in the treatment of HER2+ brain metastases. A recent pooled analysis reviewed 12 studies in 799 patients with HER2+ brain metastases treated with lapatinib alone or lapatinib plus capecitabine.[30] The pooled overall response rate (ORR) was 21.4% for lapatinib alone (95% CI 11.7−35.9) and 29.2% (95% CI 18.5−42.7) for lapatinib plus capecitabine. The pooled median PFS and OS were 4.1 (95% CI 3.1−6.7) and 11.2 (95% CI 8.9−14.1) months, respectively.

The combination of lapatinib and capecitabine has also shown activity in untreated brain metastases in a single-arm phase II clinical trial of 45 HER2+ mBC patients (LANDSCAPE).[31] The primary endpoint was the proportion of patients with an objective central nervous system (CNS) response (decrease in volume of CNS lesions by 50% or more) and was found to be 65.9% (95% CI 50.1−79.5); all were partial responses. Owing to its activity, lapatinib plus capecitabine combination may be considered for HER2+ mBC with untreated or treatment-refractory brain metastases in conjunction with standard CNS treatment. Other small molecule inhibitors, such as neratinib, have also demonstrated activity in the CNS, either as single agents or in combination with capecitabine.[32]

Lapatinib Plus Trastuzumab
Synergistic activity for the combination of dual HER2-directed therapy with lapatinib and trastuzumab was first demonstrated in HER2-overexpressing cell lines, suggesting a potential for clinical activity with combination of HER2-targeted regimens.[25] A phase I study to evaluate the safety, feasibility, and dosing of trastuzumab combined with lapatinib in 54 patients with HER2+ advanced breast cancer revealed the optimal regimen was lapatinib 1000 mg daily with standard weekly trastuzumab.[33] There were no pharmacokinetic interactions between the two drugs.

Clinical efficacy was confirmed in the phase III clinical trial EGF104900 (Table 4.1), which compared lapatinib alone or in combination with trastuzumab in patients with HER2+ trastuzumab-refractory mBC.[12,34] Patients had received a median of three prior trastuzumab-containing regimens. PFS for the combination was superior to lapatinib alone at 11.1 weeks versus 8.1 weeks (HR 0.74; 95% CI 0.58–0.94; $P = .011$). In the updated final analysis of 291 patients, median OS was superior for lapatinib plus trastuzumab, offering a benefit of 4.5 months (HR 0.74; 95% CI 0.57–0.97; $P = .026$). Median OS was 14 months for the combination therapy versus 9.5 months for lapatinib alone. The proportion of patients experiencing adverse events was similar in both treatments. Diarrhea was higher in patients receiving the combination therapy compared with those receiving monotherapy (62% vs. 48%, respectively), but the incidence of grade ≥3 diarrhea was similar between the two treatment arms.

Lapatinib Plus Vinorelbine

The safety and efficacy of lapatinib plus vinorelbine was established in the open-label, multicenter, phase II VITAL study for patients with HER2+ mBC. In total, 112 patients were randomized 2:1 to treatment with lapatinib plus vinorelbine (n = 75) or the established regimen lapatinib plus capecitabine (n = 37). Results showed that the median PFS (primary endpoint) and OS (secondary endpoint) postrandomization were comparable between treatment arms with no new safety signals detected. Median OS in the lapatinib plus vinorelbine arm was 23.3 months (95% CI 18.5–31.1) compared with 20.3 months (95% CI 16.4–31.8) in the lapatinib plus capecitabine arm.[35] This regimen appears safe. There is no evidence of the CNS benefits achieved with lapatinib and capecitabine.

In conclusion, lapatinib combinations remain valuable treatment options beyond second line in HER2+ mBC. Lapatinib/capecitabine has shown efficacy in terms of PFS in taxane- and trastuzumab-refractory mBC and may be a particular attraction option in patients with brain metastases. Lapatinib/trastuzumab has shown efficacy in terms of OS and PFS in heavily pretreated patients with a median of three prior trastuzumab-containing regimens. Neither lapatinib/capecitabine nor lapatinib/trastuzumab has been evaluated in pertuzumab- or T-DM1-pretreated populations.

TRASTUZUMAB AND CHEMOTHERAPY COMBINATIONS IN HER2-POSITIVE METASTATIC BREAST CANCER

Preclinically, trastuzumab has shown synergistic or additive effects when used in combination with several different chemotherapeutic agents.[14,36] Trastuzumab in combination with paclitaxel for first-line treatment of HER2+ mBC was approved in 1998 based on the

results of a randomized phase III clinical trial showing that this combination produced higher response rates and had longer survival than treatment with chemotherapy alone.[1] This led to the standard-of-care treatment of a taxane plus trastuzumab for first-line HER2+ mBC for over a decade. Several later trials have shown safety and efficacy in combination with other cytotoxic chemotherapy agents, including vinorelbine, gemcitabine, capecitabine, and platinum agents.

In later lines of treatment, beyond pertuzumab-/trastuzumab-containing regimens and T-DM1, clinicians regularly default to sequential salvage chemotherapeutics given in combination with trastuzumab. As previously discussed, several trials have demonstrated benefit with continuing trastuzumab-based therapy following disease progression on a trastuzumab-containing regimen.[15] This approach is reasonable assuming trastuzumab toxicity has not occurred, although evidence to continue trastuzumab after more than two trastuzumab-containing regimens is lacking. We would recommend trastuzumab in combination with single-agent chemotherapy in the metastatic setting. Although combination chemotherapy with trastuzumab might improve response rates, these gains are associated with an excess risk for toxicity. Furthermore, no trials have demonstrated that this approach improves OS.[37,38] According to national guidelines,[9] patients not previously treated with pertuzumab in the first line can be considered for a combination regimen of pertuzumab, trastuzumab, and chemotherapy (vinorelbine, taxane, capecitabine) in later lines as well.[39–42] Continuing pertuzumab after progression on a pertuzumab- and/or trastuzumab-containing regimen has never shown a significant PFS or OS benefit.

There are several effective chemotherapy agents with safety data in combination with trastuzumab. National guidelines mention that trastuzumab can be given with any recommended single-agent chemotherapy used in the treatment of mBC with the exception of anthracyclines[9] because of additive cardiotoxicity. We will discuss the evidence for several well-studied and commonly used regimens, including vinorelbine plus trastuzumab, capecitabine plus trastuzumab, and gemcitabine plus trastuzumab, for the treatment of HER2+ mBC. Early-second line and beyond phase II clinical trials in patients treated with commonly used trastuzumab and chemotherapy regimens are listed in Table 4.2. Second line and beyond for these trials were defined as progression after at least one chemotherapy, as trastuzumab-pretreated populations were rarely included in early trials. Outcomes of these trials are

TABLE 4.2
Phase II clinical trials including chemotherapy-refractory patients treated with commonly used trastuzumab/chemotherapy-based regimens.

Trial Identifier	Regimen	Patients	Population	Prior T	Median TTP or PFS	RR
Burstein et al.[47]	T + vinorelbine (25 mg/m² weekly)	40	≥1 prior chemotherapy regimen (82%)	No	34 weeks first line 16 weeks second line	84% first line 60% second/third line
Papaldo et al.[52]	T + vinorelbine (25 mg/m² weekly)	35	≥1 prior chemotherapy regimen	No (9%)	9 months	51.4%
Bayo-Calero et al.[48]	T + vinorelbine (25 mg/m² weekly)	52	≥1 prior chemotherapy regimen (58%)	No	7 months	58%
Lee et al.[51]	T+ vinorelbine (25 mg/m² D1, 8 of 21 day cycle)	33	Previously treated taxane and anthracycline	No	6.8 months	30.3%
Schaller el al.[53]	T + capecitabine (1250 mg/m² bid for 14 days, 7 days off)	27	Previously treated taxane and anthracycline	No	6.7 months	45%
Bartsch et al.[54]	T + capecitabine (1250 mg/m² bid for 14 days, 7 days off)	40	Previously treated with taxane and anthracycline or vinorelbine; prior T	Yes (100%)	8 months	20%
O'Shaughnessy et al.[56]	T + gemcitabine (1200 mg/m² D1, 8 of 21-day cycle)	64	Previously treated taxane and anthracycline	No	5.8 months	44%
Bartsch et al.[58]	T + gemcitabine (1250 mg/m² D1, 8 of 21-day cycle)	29	Previously treated anthracyclines, docetaxel, and/or vinorelbine, and trastuzumab	Yes (100%)	3 months	19.2%

PFS, progression-free survival; *RR*, response rate; *T*, trastuzumab; *TTP*, time to progression.

likely not applicable to present-day HER2+ mBC patients, who are heavily pretreated with multiple HER2-directed therapies. We will not discuss taxanes and trastuzumab, as it is assumed that this regimen would have been given in the first-line metastatic setting as standard of care.

Trastuzumab Plus Vinorelbine

Vinorelbine is a vinca alkaloid that has demonstrated great antitumor synergy with trastuzumab in preclinical models.[14] Several phase II trials have been conducted with vinorelbine and trastuzumab as first-line therapy or in pretreated patients with HER2+ mBC, consistently demonstrating high efficacy with response rates in the range of 43%−85%.[43−52] In a single-center feasibility study, vinorelbine plus trastuzumab showed an 84% ORR and 34 week TTP in the first line and a 67% ORR and 16 week TTP in the second or third line.[46,47] These early studies do not include patient populations pretreated with trastuzumab or several HER2-directed therapies. Table 4.2 includes phase II clinical trials of trastuzumab and vinorelbine in patients treated beyond the first line in the metastatic setting.

In most trials, vinorelbine was administered weekly at 25−35 mg/m^2 with weekly trastuzumab until disease progression. Adverse events were primarily grade 3/4 neutropenia, which is manageable with dose reductions or delays. The dose of 35 mg/mg^2 leads to more dose reductions and delays than 30 mg/m^2.[45] The regimen appears to be safe and overall well tolerated. Vinorelbine is more tolerable than docetaxel as well. The HER-NATA trial compared docetaxel plus trastuzumab with vinorelbine plus trastuzumab in 284 first-line HER2+ mBC patients. There was no difference in ORR (59.3% in both groups); however, more patients in the docetaxel arm discontinued therapy because of toxicity ($P < .001$).[45]

Vinorelbine plus trastuzumab is a well-studied, safe, and effective regimen in HER2+ mBC. Most trials included first-line metastatic populations or patients previously treated with anthracyclines and taxanes; trastuzumab-pretreated populations were rarely included.

Trastuzumab Plus Capecitabine

Capecitabine (N^4-pentyloxycarbonyl-5′deoxy-5-fluorocytidine) is an orally administered prodrug of fluorouracil that is a valuable treatment option in advanced breast cancer. In patients treated previously with anthracyclines and taxanes, capecitabine is an approved single-agent therapy. Capecitabine has shown efficacy and safety when given with trastuzumab in the metastatic setting.[53,54] In a phase II clinical trial including 40 patients with HER2+ mBC treated with prior anthracycline, taxane, or vinorelbine and at least one line of trastuzumab-containing therapy for metastatic disease, capecitabine was administered at a dose of 1250 mg/m^2 twice a day for 14 consecutive days in 21-day cycles with standard dose trastuzumab.[54] TTP was a median of 8 months and OS was 24 months. There was no significant difference found for second-line and beyond second-line treatments. Diarrhea (5%) and hand-foot syndrome (15%) were the only grade 3 or 4 treatment-related adverse events.

Von Minckowitz et al. published a phase III study investigating capecitabine with or without trastuzumab in patients who had progressed on trastuzumab.[15] Median TTP favored the combination group at 8.2 months versus 5.6 months with an unadjusted hazard ratio of 0.69 (95% CI 0.48−0.97; two-sided log-rank $P = .0338$). In a post hoc analysis of the study, patients who received third-line HER2-directed therapy experienced longer median OS than those who did not (18.8 months vs. 13.3 months, respectively; $P = .02$).[15]

Trastuzumab and capecitabine appear to be effective and well-tolerated regimens in heavily pretreated, trastuzumab-pretreated patient populations.

Trastuzumab/Pertuzumab Plus Capecitabine

The addition of pertuzumab to trastuzumab and chemotherapy had not been previously studied in trastuzumab-resistant second-line populations until the recently published randomized phase III PHEREXA clinical trial. This study assessed the efficacy and safety of trastuzumab plus capecitabine with or without pertuzumab in patients with HER2+ mBC and disease progression during or after trastuzumab-based therapy and a taxane. Patients were randomly assigned to trastuzumab plus capecitabine (1250 mg/m^2 twice a day, 2 weeks on, 1 week off, every 3 weeks) or pertuzumab plus trastuzumab plus capecitabine (1000 mg/m^2).[42] The primary endpoint of median PFS was 9.0 months versus 11.1 months (HR 0.82; 95% CI 0.65−1.02; $P = .0731$) which was not statistically significant. The interim OS analysis showed an 8-month increase with the addition of pertuzumab from 28.1 to 36.1 months (HR 0.68; 95% CI 0.51− 0.90) which was not statistically significant. The regimen was overall safe. Adverse events of grade ≥3 were similar in both groups, although pertuzumab-treated patients had more grade 3 diarrhea and left ventricular systolic dysfunction. The addition of pertuzumab to chemotherapy/

trastuzumab in trastuzumab-refractory populations in the second-line setting has shown a nonsignificant OS benefit and cannot be routinely recommended at this time.

Trastuzumab Plus Gemcitabine

The combination of trastuzumab with gemcitabine in patients with HER2+ mBC has been reported as safe and effective in heavily pretreated populations. In a phase II study of trastuzumab plus gemcitabine (1200 mg/m^2 on days 1 and 8 every 3 weeks) in HER2+ mBC patients who had previously received a taxane and/or anthracycline, the ORR (n = 61) was 38%, the median OS time was 14.7 months, and the median TTP was 5.8 months.[55,56] The response rate of single-agent gemcitabine in mBC is 29%.[57]

Another phase II clinical trial evaluated the efficacy and safety of gemcitabine/trastuzumab after progression on anthracyclines, docetaxel and/or vinorelbine, and trastuzumab. Twenty-nine patients received gemcitabine at a dose of 1250 mg/m^2 on days 1 and 8 of a 21-day cycle with trastuzumab given every 21 days.[58] Patients were heavily pretreated and had received prior trastuzumab (100%), anthracycline (100%), vinorelbine (96.6%), docetaxel (72.4%), and capecitabine (72.4%). Partial response was seen in 19.2% patients, and clinical benefit rate (CBR) (complete response + partial response + stable disease > 6 months) was 46.2%. TTP was a median of 3 months and OS was 17 months. Neutropenia (20.7%), thrombocytopenia (13.8%), and nausea (3.4%) were the only treatment-related adverse events that occurred with grade 3 or 4 intensity. Phase II clinical trials of gemcitabine and trastuzumab in the second line and beyond are summarized in Table 4.2.

Gemcitabine plus trastuzumab is a safe and effective regimen in trastuzumab-pretreated patient populations and a viable therapy beyond second line.

HORMONE RECEPTOR POSITIVE, HER2-POSITIVE METASTATIC BREAST CANCER

In the first line, most patients with metastatic HER2+, hormone receptor positive (HR+) breast cancer receive dual HER2 blockade with trastuzumab, pertuzumab, and a taxane with or without the addition of endocrine therapy (ET). ET added to trastuzumab plus pertuzumab in the first-line metastatic setting has shown significant benefits over ET plus trastuzumab alone.[59] Two previous studies [60,61] have demonstrated the benefit of combining single-agent HER2 blockade plus ET (without chemotherapy) in the first line setting

compared with ET alone in HER2+ HR+ mBC. There is a paucity of data on ET plus HER2 blocking regimens in the second line and beyond.

ALTERNATIVE (EGF114299) evaluated the efficacy of dual HER2 blockade with lapatinib and trastuzumab plus aromatase inhibitor (AI) compared with trastuzumab plus AI or lapatinib plus AI in patients with HER2+ HR+ mBC who experienced disease progression after prior trastuzumab plus chemotherapy in the neoadjuvant, adjuvant, or first-line metastatic setting.[62] In this phase III study, 355 eligible patients were randomly assigned to receive either lapatinib + trastuzumab + AI, trastuzumab + AI, or lapatinib + AI. AI therapy was investigator's choice (exemestane, anastrozole, or letrozole). In the lapatinib + trastuzumab + AI, trastuzumab + AI, and lapatinib + AI arms, 68%, 57%, and 65% of patients received study treatment in the first-line metastatic setting and 32%, 41%, and 35% in the second-line setting or later, respectively. The primary endpoint was PFS of lapatinib + trastuzumab + AI versus trastuzumab + AI; secondary endpoints were PFS of all arms, OS, ORR, CBR, and safety. Nearly all patients had previously received at least one line of chemotherapy, trastuzumab, and ET. Superior PFS was observed with lapatinib + trastuzumab + AI versus trastuzumab + AI (median PFS 11 months vs. 5.7 months; HR 0.62; 95% CI 0.45−0.88; $P = .0064$). Median PFS of lapatinib + AI was 8.3 months (HR 0.71; 95% CI 0.51−0.98; $P = .0361$). The ORR with lapatinib + trastuzumab + AI, trastuzumab + AI, and lapatinib + AI was 31.7%, 13.7%, and 18.6%, respectively. The CBR was 41%, 31%, and 33%, respectively. OS data was immature at the time of this analysis but favored dual HER2 blockade. Diarrhea and rash were more common in lapatinib arms. The study was not powered for comparison between lapatinib + AI versus trastuzumab + AI; however, the results showed that lapatinib + AI (median PFS 8.3 months) was superior to trastuzumab + AI (median PFS 5.7 months) in patients with HER2+ HR+ mBC previously treated with trastuzumab and ET. Further studies are warranted to determine if lapatinib plus AI is superior to trastuzumab plus AI in this specific patient population.

This is the first large randomized controlled trial to show the benefit of dual HER2 blockade plus an AI in patients with HER2+ HR+ mBC after previous treatment with trastuzumab and ET. However, only 1/3 of the treatment population received previous trastuzumab in the metastatic setting. Lapatinib + trastuzumab + AI is a reasonable regimen to consider in patients with HER2+ HR+ mBC with progression after trastuzumab and ET.

CONCLUSIONS

Standard-of-care first-line therapy for HER2+ mBC is the combination regimen of pertuzumab, trastuzumab, and a taxane.[9] After progression, trastuzumab emtansine is the most evidence-based choice for second-line therapy and shows a survival advantage over lapatinib and capecitabine. After the second-line setting, there is little evidence for the optimal sequence of agents or the duration that patients derive benefit from continued HER2-directed therapy. However, we offer the following for consideration:

- It is highly recommended that patients be considered for a clinical trial.
- All patients should be offered therapy with pertuzumab and T-DM1 at some point in their metastatic treatment journey.
- Continuing HER2-directed therapy following progression on trastuzumab has shown benefit and is recommended.
- Lapatinib combination therapies with either capecitabine/lapatinib or trastuzumab/lapatinib are clinically efficacious in heavily pretreated populations.
- Capecitabine/lapatinib has shown efficacy in the treatment of HER2+ brain metastases.
- Trastuzumab/lapatinib has shown efficacy in patient populations heavily pretreated with several HER2-directed therapies.
- Trastuzumab plus lapatinib with an AI is a reasonable choice for HER2+ HR+ patients after progression on trastuzumab and ET.
- Sequential single-agent chemotherapy given in combination with trastuzumab is a reasonable approach in later lines of therapy with well-studied regimens including trastuzumab with vinorelbine, capecitabine, or gemcitabine.

There is a paucity of data in HER2+ mBC for regimens in pertuzumab- and T-DM1-pretreated populations; future research is needed in this space. The choice of how long to continue HER2-directed therapy remains a highly individualized decision with consideration of previous regimens, response to previous regimens, toxicity, and overall clinical status.

REFERENCES

1. Slamon DJ, Leyland-Jones B, Shak S, et al. Use of chemotherapy plus a monoclonal antibody against HER2 for metastatic breast cancer that overexpresses HER2. *N Engl J Med.* 2001;344(11):783−792.
2. Romond EH, Perez EA, Bryant J, et al. Trastuzumab plus adjuvant chemotherapy for operable HER2-positive breast cancer. *N Engl J Med.* 2005;353(16):1673−1684.
3. Joensuu H, Kellokumpu-Lehtinen PL, Bono P, et al. Adjuvant docetaxel or vinorelbine with or without trastuzumab for breast cancer. *N Engl J Med.* 2006;354(8):809−820.
4. Piccart-Gebhart MJ, Procter M, Leyland-Jones B, et al. Trastuzumab after adjuvant chemotherapy in HER2-positive breast cancer. *N Engl J Med.* 2005;353(16):1659−1672.
5. Cameron D, Piccart-Gebhart MJ, Gelber RD, et al. 11 years' follow-up of trastuzumab after adjuvant chemotherapy in HER2-positive early breast cancer: final analysis of the HERceptin Adjuvant (HERA) trial. *Lancet.* 2017;389(10075):1195−1205.
6. Giordano SH, Temin S, Kirshner JJ, et al. Systemic therapy for patients with advanced human epidermal growth factor receptor 2-positive breast cancer: American Society of Clinical Oncology clinical practice guideline. *J Clin Oncol.* 2014;32(19):2078−2099.
7. Swain SM, Ewer MS, Cortes J, et al. Cardiac tolerability of pertuzumab plus trastuzumab plus docetaxel in patients with HER2-positive metastatic breast cancer in CLEOPATRA: a randomized, double-blind, placebo-controlled phase III study. *Oncologist.* 2013;18(3):257−264.
8. Verma S, Miles D, Gianni L, et al. Trastuzumab emtansine for HER2-positive advanced breast cancer. *N Engl J Med.* 2012;367(19):1783−1791.
9. *Members NGVP. NCCN Clinical Practice Guidelines in Oncology- Breast Cancer. Version 2-2017.* 2017.
10. Mendes D, Alves C, Afonso N, et al. The benefit of HER2-targeted therapies on overall survival of patients with metastatic HER2-positive breast cancer—a systematic review. *Breast Cancer Res.* 2015;17:140.
11. Cameron D, Casey M, Press M, et al. A phase III randomized comparison of lapatinib plus capecitabine versus capecitabine alone in women with advanced breast cancer that has progressed on trastuzumab: updated efficacy and biomarker analyses. *Breast Cancer Res Treat.* 2008;112(3):533−543.
12. Blackwell KL, Burstein HJ, Storniolo AM, et al. Overall survival benefit with lapatinib in combination with trastuzumab for patients with human epidermal growth factor receptor 2-positive metastatic breast cancer: final results from the EGF104900 Study. *J Clin Oncol.* 2012;30(21):2585−2592.
13. Krop IE, Kim SB, Martin AG, et al. Trastuzumab emtansine versus treatment of physician's choice in patients with previously treated HER2-positive metastatic breast cancer (TH3RESA): final overall survival results from a randomised open-label phase 3 trial. *Lancet Oncol.* 2017;18(6):743−754.
14. Pegram M, Hsu S, Lewis G, et al. Inhibitory effects of combinations of HER-2/neu antibody and chemotherapeutic agents used for treatment of human breast cancers. *Oncogene.* 1999;18(13):2241−2251.
15. von Minckwitz G, Schwedler K, Schmidt M, et al. Trastuzumab beyond progression: overall survival analysis of the GBG 26/BIG 3-05 phase III study in HER2-positive breast cancer. *Eur J Cancer.* 2011;47(15):2273−2281.

16. von Minckwitz G, du Bois A, Schmidt M, et al. Trastuzumab beyond progression in human epidermal growth factor receptor 2-positive advanced breast cancer: a German breast group 26/breast international group 03-05 study. *J Clin Oncol.* 2009;27(12):1999−2006.

17. Geyer CE, Forster J, Lindquist D, et al. Lapatinib plus capecitabine for HER2-positive advanced breast cancer. *N Engl J Med.* 2006;355(26):2733−2743.

18. Lewis Phillips GD, Li G, Dugger DL, et al. Targeting HER2-positive breast cancer with trastuzumab-DM1, an antibody-cytotoxic drug conjugate. *Cancer Res.* 2008; 68(22):9280−9290.

19. Krop IE, Beeram M, Modi S, et al. Phase I study of trastuzumab-DM1, an HER2 antibody-drug conjugate, given every 3 weeks to patients with HER2-positive metastatic breast cancer. *J Clin Oncol.* 2010;28(16): 2698−2704.

20. Krop IE, LoRusso P, Miller KD, et al. A phase II study of trastuzumab emtansine in patients with human epidermal growth factor receptor 2-positive metastatic breast cancer who were previously treated with trastuzumab, lapatinib, an anthracycline, a taxane, and capecitabine. *J Clin Oncol.* 2012;30(26):3234−3241.

21. Burris HA 3rd, Rugo HS, Vukelja SJ, et al. Phase II study of the antibody drug conjugate trastuzumab-DM1 for the treatment of human epidermal growth factor receptor 2 (HER2)-positive breast cancer after prior HER2-directed therapy. *J Clin Oncol.* 2011;29(4):398−405.

22. Dieras V, Miles D, Verma S, et al. Trastuzumab emtansine versus capecitabine plus lapatinib in patients with previously treated HER2-positive advanced breast cancer (EMILIA): a descriptive analysis of final overall survival results from a randomised, open-label, phase 3 trial. *Lancet Oncol.* 2017;18(6):732−742.

23. Krop IE, Lin NU, Blackwell K, et al. Trastuzumab emtansine (T-DM1) versus lapatinib plus capecitabine in patients with HER2-positive metastatic breast cancer and central nervous system metastases: a retrospective, exploratory analysis in EMILIA. *Ann Oncol.* 2015;26(1): 113−119.

24. Vici P, Pizzuti L, Michelotti A, et al. A retrospective multicentric observational study of trastuzumab emtansine in HER2 positive metastatic breast cancer: a real-world experience. *Oncotarget.* 2017;8(34):56921−56931.

25. Konecny GE, Pegram MD, Venkatesan N, et al. Activity of the dual kinase inhibitor lapatinib (GW572016) against HER-2-overexpressing and trastuzumab-treated breast cancer cells. *Cancer Res.* 2006;66(3):1630−1639.

26. Rusnak DW, Lackey K, Affleck K, et al. The effects of the novel, reversible epidermal growth factor receptor/ErbB-2 tyrosine kinase inhibitor, GW2016, on the growth of human normal and tumor-derived cell lines in vitro and in vivo. *Mol Cancer Ther.* 2001;1(2):85−94.

27. Nahta R, Yuan LX, Du Y, Esteva FJ. Lapatinib induces apoptosis in trastuzumab-resistant breast cancer cells: effects on insulin-like growth factor I signaling. *Mol Cancer Ther.* 2007;6(2):667−674.

28. Burstein HJ, Storniolo AM, Franco S, et al. A phase II study of lapatinib monotherapy in chemotherapy-refractory HER2-positive and HER2-negative advanced or metastatic breast cancer. *Ann Oncol.* 2008;19(6):1068−1074.

29. Blackwell KL, Pegram MD, Tan-Chiu E, et al. Single-agent lapatinib for HER2-overexpressing advanced or metastatic breast cancer that progressed on first- or second-line trastuzumab-containing regimens. *Ann Oncol.* 2009; 20(6):1026−1031.

30. Petrelli F, Ghidini M, Lonati V, et al. The efficacy of lapatinib and capecitabine in HER-2 positive breast cancer with brain metastases: a systematic review and pooled analysis. *Eur J Cancer.* 2017;84:141−148.

31. Bachelot T, Romieu G, Campone M, et al. Lapatinib plus capecitabine in patients with previously untreated brain metastases from HER2-positive metastatic breast cancer (LANDSCAPE): a single-group phase 2 study. *Lancet Oncol.* 2013;14(1):64−71.

32. Awada A, Colomer R, Inoue K, et al. Neratinib plus paclitaxel vs trastuzumab plus paclitaxel in previously untreated metastatic ERBB2-positive breast cancer: the NEfERT-T randomized clinical trial. *JAMA Oncol.* 2016; 2(12):1557−1564.

33. Storniolo AM, Pegram MD, Overmoyer B, et al. Phase I dose escalation and pharmacokinetic study of lapatinib in combination with trastuzumab in patients with advanced ErbB2-positive breast cancer. *J Clin Oncol.* 2008;26(20):3317−3323.

34. Blackwell KL, Burstein HJ, Storniolo AM, et al. Randomized study of Lapatinib alone or in combination with trastuzumab in women with ErbB2-positive, trastuzumab-refractory metastatic breast cancer. *J Clin Oncol.* 2010;28(7):1124−1130.

35. Janni W, Sarosiek T, Karaszewska B, et al. Final overall survival analysis of a phase II trial evaluating vinorelbine and lapatinib in women with ErbB2 overexpressing metastatic breast cancer. *Breast.* 2015;24(6):769−773.

36. Pegram MD, Slamon DJ. Combination therapy with trastuzumab (Herceptin) and cisplatin for chemoresistant metastatic breast cancer: evidence for receptor-enhanced chemosensitivity. *Semin Oncol.* 1999;26(4 suppl 12):89−95.

37. Robert N, Leyland-Jones B, Asmar L, et al. Randomized phase III study of trastuzumab, paclitaxel, and carboplatin compared with trastuzumab and paclitaxel in women with HER-2-overexpressing metastatic breast cancer. *J Clin Oncol.* 2006;24(18):2786−2792.

38. Valero V, Forbes J, Pegram MD, et al. Multicenter phase III randomized trial comparing docetaxel and trastuzumab with docetaxel, carboplatin, and trastuzumab as first-line chemotherapy for patients with HER2-gene-amplified metastatic breast cancer (BCIRG 007 study): two highly active therapeutic regimens. *J Clin Oncol.* 2011;29(2):149−156.

39. Perez EA, Lopez-Vega JM, Petit T, et al. Safety and efficacy of vinorelbine in combination with pertuzumab and trastuzumab for first-line treatment of patients with HER2-positive locally advanced or metastatic breast cancer: VELVET Cohort 1 final results. *Breast Cancer Res.* 2016;18(1):126.

40. Swain SM, Kim SB, Cortes J, et al. Pertuzumab, trastuzumab, and docetaxel for HER2-positive metastatic breast cancer (CLEOPATRA study): overall survival results from a randomised, double-blind, placebo-controlled, phase 3 study. *Lancet Oncol.* 2013;14(6):461–471.

41. Andersson M, Lopez-Vega JM, Petit T, et al. Efficacy and safety of pertuzumab and trastuzumab administered in a single infusion bag, followed by vinorelbine: VELVET Cohort 2 final results. *Oncologist.* 2017;22(10):1160–1168.

42. Urruticoechea A, Rizwanullah M, Im SA, et al. Randomized phase III trial of trastuzumab plus capecitabine with or without pertuzumab in patients with human epidermal growth factor receptor 2-positive metastatic breast cancer who experienced disease progression during or after trastuzumab-based therapy. *J Clin Oncol.* 2017;35(26):3030–3038.

43. Jahanzeb M, Mortimer JE, Yunus F, et al. Phase II trial of weekly vinorelbine and trastuzumab as first-line therapy in patients with HER2(+) metastatic breast cancer. *Oncologist.* 2002;7(5):410–417.

44. Chan A, Martin M, Untch M, et al. Vinorelbine plus trastuzumab combination as first-line therapy for HER 2-positive metastatic breast cancer patients: an international phase II trial. *Br J Cancer.* 2006;95(7):788–793.

45. Andersson M, Lidbrink E, Bjerre K, et al. Phase III randomized study comparing docetaxel plus trastuzumab with vinorelbine plus trastuzumab as first-line therapy of metastatic or locally advanced human epidermal growth factor receptor 2-positive breast cancer: the HERNATA study. *J Clin Oncol.* 2011;29(3):264–271.

46. Burstein HJ, Harris LN, Marcom PK, et al. Trastuzumab and vinorelbine as first-line therapy for HER2-overexpressing metastatic breast cancer: multicenter phase II trial with clinical outcomes, analysis of serum tumor markers as predictive factors, and cardiac surveillance algorithm. *J Clin Oncol.* 2003;21(15):2889–2895.

47. Burstein HJ, Kuter I, Campos SM, et al. Clinical activity of trastuzumab and vinorelbine in women with HER2-overexpressing metastatic breast cancer. *J Clin Oncol.* 2001;19(10):2722–2730.

48. Bayo-Calero JL, Mayordomo JI, Sanchez-Rovira P, et al. A phase II study of weekly vinorelbine and trastuzumab in patients with HER2-positive metastatic breast cancer. *Clin Breast Cancer.* 2008;8(3):264–268.

49. De Maio E, Pacilio C, Gravina A, et al. Vinorelbine plus 3-weekly trastuzumab in metastatic breast cancer: a single-centre phase 2 trial. *BMC Cancer.* 2007;7:50.

50. Schilling G, Bruweleit M, Harbeck N, et al. Phase II trial of vinorelbine and trastuzumab in patients with HER2-positive metastatic breast cancer. A prospective, open label, non-controlled, multicenter phase II trial (to investigate efficacy and safety of this combination chemotherapy). *Investig New Drugs.* 2009;27(2):166–172.

51. Lee YR, Huh SJ, Lee DH, et al. Phase II study of vinorelbine plus trastuzumab in HER2 overexpressing metastatic breast cancer pretreated with anthracyclines and taxanes. *J Breast Cancer.* 2011;14(2):140–146.

52. Papaldo P, Fabi A, Ferretti G, et al. A phase II study on metastatic breast cancer patients treated with weekly vinorelbine with or without trastuzumab according to HER2 expression: changing the natural history of HER2-positive disease. *Ann Oncol.* 2006;17(4):630–636.

53. Schaller G, Fuchs I, Gonsch T, et al. Phase II study of capecitabine plus trastuzumab in human epidermal growth factor receptor 2 overexpressing metastatic breast cancer pretreated with anthracyclines or taxanes. *J Clin Oncol.* 2007;25(22):3246–3250.

54. Bartsch R, Wenzel C, Altorjai G, et al. Capecitabine and trastuzumab in heavily pretreated metastatic breast cancer. *J Clin Oncol.* 2007;25(25):3853–3858.

55. O'Shaughnessy J. Gemcitabine and trastuzumab in metastatic breast cancer. *Semin Oncol.* 2003;30(2 suppl 3):22–26.

56. O'Shaughnessy JA, Vukelja S, Marsland T, Kimmel G, Ratnam S, Pippen JE. Phase II study of trastuzumab plus gemcitabine in chemotherapy-pretreated patients with metastatic breast cancer. *Clin Breast Cancer.* 2004;5(2):142–147.

57. Spielmann M, Llombart-Cussac A, Kalla S, et al. Single-agent gemcitabine is active in previously treated metastatic breast cancer. *Oncology.* 2001;60(4):303–307.

58. Bartsch R, Wenzel C, Gampenrieder SP, et al. Trastuzumab and gemcitabine as salvage therapy in heavily pre-treated patients with metastatic breast cancer. *Cancer Chemother Pharmacol.* 2008;62(5):903–910.

59. Arpino G, Ferrero J-M, de la Haba-Rodriguez J, et al. Abstract S3-04: primary analysis of PERTAIN: a randomized, two-arm, open-label, multicenter phase II trial assessing the efficacy and safety of pertuzumab given in combination with trastuzumab plus an aromatase inhibitor in first-line patients with HER2-positive and hormone receptor-positive metastatic or locally advanced breast cancer. *Cancer Res.* 2017;77(suppl 4):S3–04-S03-04.

60. Kaufman B, Mackey JR, Clemens MR, et al. Trastuzumab plus anastrozole versus anastrozole alone for the treatment of postmenopausal women with human epidermal growth factor receptor 2-positive, hormone receptor-positive metastatic breast cancer: results from the randomized phase III TAnDEM study. *J Clin Oncol.* 2009;27(33):5529–5537.

61. Johnston S, Pippen Jr J, Pivot X, et al. Lapatinib combined with letrozole versus letrozole and placebo as first-line therapy for postmenopausal hormone receptor-positive metastatic breast cancer. *J Clin Oncol.* 2009;27(33):5538–5546.

62. Johnston SRD, Hegg R, Im SA, et al. Phase III, randomized study of dual human epidermal growth factor receptor 2 (HER2) blockade with lapatinib plus trastuzumab in combination with an aromatase inhibitor in postmenopausal women with HER2-positive, hormone receptor-positive metastatic breast cancer: ALTERNATIVE. *J Clin Oncol.* 2017. JCO2017747824.

CHAPTER 5

Central Nervous System Metastases in HER2-Positive Breast Cancer

JOSÉ PABLO LEONE, MD[a] • AYAL A. AIZER, MD, MHS[a] • NANCY U. LIN, MD

BACKGROUND

One of the most feared complications in patients with breast cancer is the development of metastases to the central nervous system (CNS). Historically, brain metastases have been described in 10%–16% of patients with metastatic breast cancer (MBC) overall;[1] however, data over the past decade has illuminated a particularly high frequency in patients with metastatic human epidermal growth factor receptor 2 (HER2)-positive breast cancer, in which CNS involvement can be seen in up to 50% of patients by the end of their lives.[2]

The pathophysiology of CNS metastases involves a highly complex process that consists of breast cancer cell invasion into the connective tissue and blood vessels, travel through the bloodstream, disruption of the blood-brain barrier (BBB), and colonization and growth in the CNS parenchyma.[3,4] The median time from initial breast cancer diagnosis until CNS metastasis has been reported as approximately 32 months[5] but varies according to the tumor subtype and stage at diagnosis. Patients with triple-negative and with HER2-positive (HER2+) breast cancer generally experience shorter intervals to the development of CNS metastases, whereas those with estrogen receptor (ER)-positive tumors tend to have longer intervals.[6]

The development of CNS metastases in breast cancer patients continues to represent a very challenging clinical problem. Despite treatment, the prognosis is generally poor, with median survival in the range of 2–25.3 months.[7–9] Moreover, CNS metastases can cause progressive neurologic deficits leading to increased morbidity and reduced quality of life.[10] In more recent years, the incidence of CNS metastases appears to have increased secondary to the improved survival of patients with effective systemic therapy, as well as the use of more sensitive diagnostic studies for detection of CNS disease. The efficacy of current systemic therapies is of particular relevance in patients with HER2+ disease, in whom CNS relapses can occur in the setting of well-controlled extracranial metastases.[11]

Treatment options for HER2+ breast cancer patients with CNS metastases include the use of surgery with resection of the metastatic disease, stereotactic radiosurgery (SRS), whole-brain radiation therapy (WBRT), systemic chemotherapy, and targeted agents.[12] This chapter will describe key issues in the diagnosis, clinical management, and future perspectives for patients with HER2+ CNS metastases from breast cancer.

DIAGNOSIS

The radiologic diagnosis of CNS metastases is most commonly confirmed by using magnetic resonance imaging (MRI) with and without gadolinium contrast, which has higher sensitivity and specificity than contrast-enhanced computed tomography scans.[13] For most patients, imaging alone is sufficient for diagnosis in the appropriate clinical scenario (i.e., HER2-positive breast cancer with biopsy-proven systemic metastatic disease). However, in cases such as an isolated CNS lesion, pathologic analysis of metastatic tissue is necessary to confirm the presumed diagnosis of CNS involvement originating from breast cancer and to obtain tumor biomarkers that may help guide therapy selection. HER2 may be a target that is particularly enriched in the CNS. Although data is conflicting, some recent studies have suggested that 16%–23% of HER2-negative breast cancers may develop HER2+ CNS metastases, and such patients may be candidates for anti-HER2 therapy.[14–16]

Although CNS metastases are not uncommon in those with HER2+ breast cancer, imaging studies to detect the presence of CNS metastases should be triggered when patients present with neurologic symptoms

---

[a]Contributed equally to this work.

or signs rather than as part of an initial staging strategy or in routine surveillance of asymptomatic patients after treatment with curative intent. The estimated incidence of CNS metastases in patients with early-stage HER2+ breast cancer is between 2% and 3.7%,[17,18] and CNS involvement can occur in up to 50% of patients with metastatic HER2+ breast cancer.[2] However, in the absence of data showing any meaningful clinical benefit for early detection of CNS relapse, CNS screening is not currently endorsed by the American Society of Clinical Oncology (ASCO) HER2 guidelines[19] nor by the European School of Oncology-MBC guidelines[20] outside of the context of prospective studies. Further studies evaluating both the positive and negative impacts of screening may shed additional light on this important issue.

PROGNOSTIC FACTORS

There are several important factors to be considered when assessing prognosis in patients with CNS metastases, including tumor biology, the overall health of the patient, and treatment modalities.[21,22] Patients with triple-negative breast cancer tend to have the worst prognosis with median overall survival (OS) between 3 and 6 months.[23–25] Conversely, although the rates of CNS metastases are higher, patients with HER2+ tumors tend to have the best OS with median of 21–23 months,[24–26] likely due to better control of extracranial disease.

Performance status is strongly associated with survival. A number of studies have shown that OS is longer among patients with Karnofsky Performance Status (KPS) score ≥70 of 100, reasonably defined as those who are able to perform their own self-care without assistance.[8,9] Age at the time of diagnosis of CNS metastases is another factor to consider, with older age being associated with shorter OS in adjusted models.[24,26] Some, but not all, studies have demonstrated a relationship between OS and the number of brain metastases or the presence of extracranial disease that is refractory to systemic therapy.[26,27]

The graded prognostic assessment (GPA) is a commonly used, retrospectively validated clinical tool in the prognostic assessment of patients with brain metastases.[28] When initially published in 2008, this index included patient age, KPS score, number of brain metastases, and the presence of extracranial disease as predictive factors.[29] Subsequently, the dataset was expanded, and tumor subtypes were incorporated to create a breast cancer–specific GPA model with consideration given to age and KPS score.[9] This breast cancer–specific GPA was recently validated and refined with the inclusion of the number of brain metastases.[30] This is a valuable index to consider for patient selection in clinical trials and for risk stratification.

TREATMENT

The treatment of CNS metastases from breast cancer can be considered in terms of localized therapy modalities and systemic therapies. Localized therapy modalities are targeted to the disease confined to the CNS and include surgical resection of metastatic disease and radiation therapy. Systemic therapies consist of systemic chemotherapy and targeted agents. Unfortunately, with rare exceptions, CNS metastases represent incurable disease. Because of the multiple potential treatment modalities, treatment should ideally be planned in the context of a multidisciplinary team that may include some combination of neurosurgeons, radiation oncologists, medical oncologists, neuro-oncologists, palliative care providers, and rehabilitation specialists.

SURGICAL RESECTION

Patients who present with a single or very few (≤3) CNS metastases may be considered as candidates for surgical resection. The case for surgical management is particularly compelling in the setting of symptomatic CNS involvement in patients with otherwise good performance status and well-controlled extracranial disease. Treatment with surgical resection has a number of advantages over radiation or medical management, such as the potential for immediate improvement of neurologic deficits, management of intracranial hypertension, and the possibility of obtaining tissue diagnosis in patients with disease limited to the CNS. Disadvantages include the invasiveness of the procedure, limitations inherent to the anatomic location of the metastases, the potential need for prolonged rehabilitation, and delays in systemic therapy as the patient heals. Craniotomy for brain metastasectomy is generally a safe intervention in appropriate candidates at high-volume centers, with mortality rates declining to <5% in the past few decades in correlation with an increase in caseload.[31]

The role of surgical resection versus radiation therapy was evaluated in a study by Patchell et al., in which 48 patients with solitary brain metastases from any primary tumor were randomized to surgical resection followed by WBRT or needle biopsy followed by WBRT.[32] The rate of brain recurrence was lower in the surgery group compared with the control group

(20% vs. 52%, respectively; $P < .02$). Median OS was superior in the surgery group compared with the control group (40 weeks vs. 15 weeks, respectively; $P < .01$). Patients treated with surgery were also able to remain functionally independent for a longer period of time (median of 38 weeks vs. 8 weeks; $P < .005$).

Similarly, a study by Vecht et al. evaluated 63 patients with systemic cancer and solitary brain metastasis with randomization to surgical resection plus WBRT or WBRT alone.[33] There was a preplanned stratification by status of extracranial disease (progressive vs. stable). In patients with stable extracranial disease, the combination arm resulted in longer OS ($P = .04$) and functionally independent survival (FIS) ($P = .06$) compared with WBRT alone with median OS (mOS) 12 months versus 7 months, respectively, and median FIS (mFIS) 9 months versus 4 months, respectively. Conversely, patients with progressive extracranial disease had a mOS of 5 months and a mFIS of 2.5 months irrespective of treatment arm, a finding that was also confirmed by another randomized study.[34] This study in particular highlights the importance of extracranial disease control in the survival and functional status of patients with CNS metastases. Three other studies, albeit nonrandomized, have also shown improvements in overall survival, brain recurrences, and neurologic outcomes with surgical resection in addition to WBRT.[35–37]

RADIATION THERAPY

Radiation therapy represents an important component of management for most patients with brain metastases. In patients with HER2+ breast cancer, although systemic options for intracranial control exist, most patients with brain metastases will generally receive recommendations for brain-directed radiation therapy. However, although radiation is commonly used to manage patients with brain metastases, caution should be exerted not to overutilize this approach given the potential toxicity of both stereotactic and WBRT. Accordingly, patients with a large systemic disease burden and few remaining options for systemic control who present with modest intracranial disease burden may benefit from observation rather than up-front radiation, a concept illustrated in the QUARTZ study, as discussed in the following section.[38]

Whole Brain Radiation

Whole-brain radiation remains the standard radiotherapeutic option for patients with a large number of brain metastases (>3) or when radiation must be started immediately. The latter scenario is relatively rare given that most patients who need immediate therapy for brain metastases due to a large, symptomatic lesion typically benefit from up-front surgery. Whole-brain radiation is typically given in 5–15 daily fractions over 1–3 weeks, with longer courses utilizing a lower radiation dose per day. Most randomized trials comparing different dose per fractionation schemes for WBRT have not yielded meaningful differences in outcome.[39–41] In the United States, the most commonly used regimens are administered over 10–15 fractions.[38,42] The primary adverse effects associated with WBRT include fatigue, nausea, headache, anorexia, skin irritation, and alopecia in the short to intermediate term, of which fatigue tends to be the most bothersome to patients,[43] and ototoxicity and neurocognitive decline in the longer term.[44] Short-term side effects typically abate with time, whereas long-term toxicities are often permanent.

A number of strategies have been used to minimize long-term neurocognitive dysfunction associated with WBRT. Memantine is an N-methyl-D-aspartate receptor antagonist used in the management of patients with primary neurocognitive disorders.[45] In a study evaluating a potential role for memantine for the prevention of neurocognitive decline secondary to WBRT, Brown et al. randomized patients receiving WBRT to memantine versus placebo for 6 months with initiation of treatment within the first 3 days of radiation therapy and with titration from 5 mg daily to 20 mg daily over a 4 week lead-in period.[45] The investigators found that memantine generally reduced the likelihood of cognitive decline as assessed by a battery of neuropsychologic tests, although the primary endpoint (Hopkins Verbal Learning Test–Revised for delayed recall) only showed a trend to improvement with memantine ($P = .059$). Donepezil, a neurocognitive-protecting agent with a different mechanism of action, has also shown promising neurocognitive benefits in randomized studies of patients receiving radiation for a variety of indications.[43,46] Given that the data for memantine stem from a study of patients receiving WBRT for brain metastases (as opposed to data supporting donepezil, which is derived from patients with a variety of tumors who receive radiation in one of several forms), most providers have chosen memantine over donepezil to try to preserve neurocognitive function in patients receiving WBRT.

Another strategy to reduce the neurocognitive impact of WBRT focuses on sparing the hippocampi

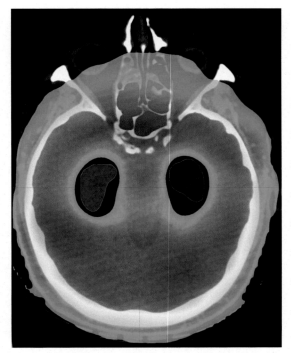

FIG. 5.1 Radiation Dose Distribution in a Patient Receiving Hippocampal-Sparing Whole-Brain Radiation Therapy for Brain Metastases. *Shaded (green-yellow-red) regions* depict areas of higher radiation dose. Note the sparing of the blue/red contoured structures (hippocampi).

from receiving the full dose of radiation, a technique called hippocampal-sparing or hippocampal-avoidance WBRT. The hippocampi are integral to learning and memory, but whether excluding them from the target of the radiation field improves outcomes is uncertain. When hippocampal-sparing WBRT is used, the hippocampi receive approximately 47%–70% of the prescribed radiation dose, although biologically, given the nonlinear impact of dose received in a single day, such sparing may translate to a reduction in biologic dose of approximately 62%–83%.[47] A radiation plan for a patient treated with hippocampal-sparing WBRT is presented in Fig. 5.1.

Although hippocampal-sparing WBRT has theoretical appeal, definitive evidence showing its superiority over conventional WBRT is lacking. Prospective evidence supporting the use of hippocampal-sparing WBRT stems from RTOG 0933. In this single arm, phase II trial of hippocampal-sparing WBRT in patients with brain metastases (patients with metastases near the hippocampi excluded), the investigators observed a reduced rate of decline in recall than in historic controls managed with conventional WBRT.[48] However, the historic controls had a poorer median survival than patients in RTOG 0933, thereby confounding the interpretation of this study. Randomized phase II–III studies comparing WBRT and hippocampal-sparing WBRT are now under way (NCT02147028, NCT02360215).

Although conducted in patients with non–small cell lung cancer, the QUARTZ study likely illustrates the limited benefit of WBRT in patients with brain metastases of any underlying histology with a limited life expectancy, particularly if the prognosis is driven by progressive systemic disease.[38] The QUARTZ study randomized 538 patients with non–small cell lung cancer and brain metastases to receive WBRT versus supportive care; patients were only enrolled on the study if they were "unsuitable for either surgery or stereotactic radiotherapy." It is of interest to note that the majority of patients had a modest burden of intracranial disease with only 1–4 brain metastases; in the modern era, there are few situations whereby such patients would be candidates for WBRT but unsuitable for stereotactic radiation. Subgroup analyses suggested that patients less than 70 years of age, with a KPS ≥70 (capable of self-care), and with controlled systemic disease displayed a trend to improved survival with WBRT, but the median overall survival was approximately 2 months in both cohorts, suggesting that the majority of enrolled patients had an extremely poor prognosis. Approximately 10% of patients assigned to the WBRT arm died before WBRT could be initiated or declined to the point that WBRT could not be used. QUARTZ could be considered to validate withholding of brain-directed radiation in lieu of best supportive care in patients with a very poor prognosis limited by systemic disease.

In general practice, brain-directed radiation treatment is commonly recommended to those patients whose lives are not imminently threatened by the burden of metastatic disease, but most patients with a limited number of brain metastases benefit from stereotactic radiation as opposed to WBRT.

Brain-Directed Stereotactic Radiation

Stereotactic radiation involves delivery of focused radiation to each brain metastasis with relative sparing of the nondiseased brain tissue. Because the whole brain is not targeted in the radiation fields, radiation doses can be higher with a corresponding increase in CNS tumor control. Stereotactic radiation, when given in a

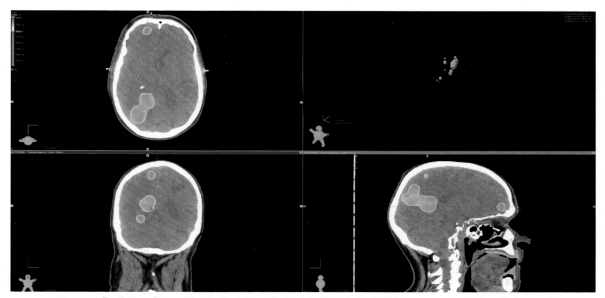

FIG. 5.2 Radiation Dose Distribution in a Patient With 11 Brain Metastases Receiving Stereotactic Radiotherapy, 30 Gy in Five Fractions. *Shaded regions* represent regions receiving the prescription dose.

single fraction in 1 day, is termed SRS, with doses ranging from 15 to 24 Gy in most series.[49] When lesions exceed the maximal size that can safely be treated in a single day,[50,51] smaller doses (fractions) of targeted radiation is given over 2−5 days (typically to 20−30 Gy in total), a technique termed stereotactic radiotherapy (SRT). An example of an SRT plan is presented in Fig. 5.2.

RTOG 9508 established the survival benefit associated with stereotactic radiation in the management of a single brain metastasis. In this study, patients with 1−3 brain metastases were randomized to receive WBRT alone or WBRT in combination with a stereotactic radiation boost. The study was powered a priori to analyze this relationship in patients with a single brain metastasis; in this population, stereotactic radiation improved overall survival of patients with an mOS of 4.9 in patients receiving WBRT alone versus 6.5 months in those receiving WBRT + stereotactic radiation (P = .04), establishing stereotactic radiation as a beneficial option in patients with a single brain metastasis.

Acute side effects associated with stereotactic radiation are typically of a lesser magnitude then those associated with WBRT, although seizures and intracranial bleeding may be more common given the higher radiation doses used.[52,53] Whereas the most dreaded long-term complication of WBRT is dementia, the primary long-term adverse effect associated with stereotactic radiation for brain metastases is radiation

necrosis—uncontrolled tissue death in the irradiated area that usually occurs within the first 1 or 2 years after radiation.[50] Radiation necrosis is common and always occurs in the original location of the tumor that was treated.[51] Conventional MRI shows enhancing lesions in both tumor recurrence and radiation necrosis, making discernment of radiation necrosis from tumor recurrence or progression difficult. Other imaging studies, such as perfusion-weighted MRI,[54,55] diffusion-weighted MRI,[56,57] MRI spectroscopy,[58−60] positron emission tomography,[61,62] and single photon emission computer tomography[63,64] can be used to attempt to distinguish radiation necrosis from tumor recurrence, but the sensitivity and specificity of these tests are limited; as a result, neurosurgical resection remains the standard for distinguishing these entities.[65] However, neurosurgical resection is associated with morbidity, quality of life decrement, and delay in resumption of systemic therapy.[66,67]

The ability to reliably distinguish tumor recurrence from radiation necrosis after stereotactic radiation is of great clinical significance, as it may reduce the need for neurosurgical resection for diagnostic purposes. In addition, it would allow for noninvasive, targeted treatment, such as repeat radiation for recurrent tumors[68] and bevacizumab for radiation necrosis, to be used.[69] Such therapies cannot be given without an accurate and reliable diagnostic test to distinguish tumor recurrence from progression given the potential

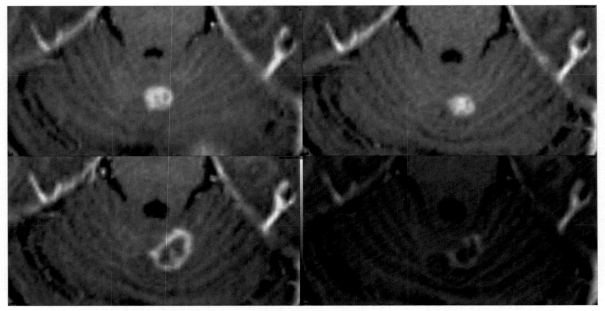

FIG. 5.3 Radiation Necrosis in a Patient With a Brain Metastasis in the Vermis Who Received Stereotactic Radiation. Top left: preradiation. Top right: 3 months postradiation. Bottom left: 12 months postradiation with enlargement of the treated lesion. Bottom right: 18 months postradiation with a decrease in the size of the treated lesion in the absence of systemic therapy, consistent with radiation necrosis.

for additional radiation to exacerbate necrosis and the possibility of intracranial hemorrhage with bevacizumab use in patients with progressive brain metastases.[70,71] The lack of sustained growth on MRI in the absence of systemic therapy with intracranial penetration is perhaps the most useful differentiator. An example of a patient with radiation necrosis is presented in Fig. 5.3.

WBRT Versus Stereotactic Radiation

No studies have compared WBRT alone versus stereotactic radiation alone as sole management for brain metastases, although a number of prior studies have examined local therapy (herein defined as surgery and/or stereotactic radiation) alone versus local therapy followed by WBRT in patients with ≤4 brain metastases.[44,72,73] In all studies, intracranial tumor control was better with the addition of WBRT, but in no study was overall survival improved, likely due to the competing risks of systemic disease progression and lack of salvage options for intracranial progression.

More modern studies have generally shown that WBRT may diminish quality of life and neurocognition relative to local therapy alone.[42,44,74,75] As a result, stereotactic radiation is generally preferred to WBRT in patients with 1−4 brain metastases, particularly if none have been resected surgically.[42,74,75]

Among patients with 1−4 brain metastases who have undergone resection of one or more brain metastases, whether to pursue adjuvant WBRT or stereotactic radiation is less clear. A large multicenter study in the United States found less of a detriment in neurocognitive function in patients who underwent SRS following surgery than those who received adjuvant SRS + WBRT, although without a definitive improvement in overall quality of life, whereas a very small Polish study found that longer-term quality of life may be better in patients receiving adjuvant WBRT versus stereotactic radiation after resection of a single brain metastasis.[75−77]

In the modern era, combining WBRT and stereotactic radiation as a joint, upfront therapy is discouraged; rather, most patients should be managed with a single modality of radiotherapeutic care with additional radiation reserved for salvage purposes. Table 5.1 summarizes the trials that compared local therapy alone versus local therapy followed by WBRT.

Stereotactic Radiation in Patients With More Than Four Brain Metastases

Although stereotactic radiation has been shown in most studies to yield improved quality of life and to have less neurocognitive dysfunction relative to WBRT in patients with ≤4 brain metastases, no randomized studies have

TABLE 5.1
Randomized Trials of WBRT in Patients With 1—4 CNS Metastases

Study	No. of Breast Cancer Patients	CNS Lesions	Arms	Intracranial Recurrence With WBRT	OS With WBRT
Patchell[78]	95	1	1. Resection 2. Resection + WBRT	Lower	No difference
JROSG 99-1[72]	132	1—4	1. SRS 2. SRS + WBRT	Lower	No difference
MDACC[44]	58	1—3	1. SRS 2. SRS + WBRT	Lower	Worse
EORTC 22952[73]	359	1—3	1. Local therapy 2. Local therapy + WBRT	Lower	No difference
NCCTG N0574[42]	213	1—3	1. SRS 2. SRS + WBRT	Lower	No difference
JCOG0504[79]	271	1—4	1. Resection + SRS 2. Resection + WBRT	Lower	No difference
Polish[77]	59	1	1. Resection + SRS 2. Resection + WBRT	Trend toward lower	Improved
NCCTG 107C[75]	194	1—4	1. Resection + SRS 2. Resection + SRS + WBRT	Lower	No difference

CNS, central nervous system; OS, overall survival; SRS, stereotactic radiosurgery; WBRT, whole-brain radiation therapy.

compared stereotactic radiation with WBRT in patients with >4 brain metastases. Because the risks of WBRT generally remain static as lesion number increases, but the risks of stereotactic radiation (bleeding, seizure, necrosis) increase with the number of lesions treated, caution should be exerted before employing stereotactic radiation regardless of the number of lesions present. The whole brain dose received as scatter radiation while giving stereotactic radiation to many brain metastases can be significant, resulting in whole brain toxicities despite intentions to the contrary. It is also worth considering that high numbers of gross brain metastases could signal widespread microscopic involvement with a higher likelihood of intracranial progression if the entire brain is not treated.

A nonrandomized, prospective Japanese study evaluated the viability of stereotactic radiation for up to 10 brain metastases. The authors found no significant difference in outcomes (overall survival, deterioration of neurologic function, local recurrence, new lesions, use of salvage radiation or surgery, or use of systemic anticancer agents) between patients with 2—4 brain metastases versus 5—10 brain metastases;[80] however, the study is limited given that patients could

only be enrolled if the total intracranial disease burden was <15 cc, thereby excluding patients with larger numbers of bulky metastases. In addition, the authors suspected that they would accrue patients with 2—4 and 5—10 brain metastases in a 1:1 ratio, but the final cohort contained a >2:1 ratio between these respective cohorts. Randomized studies of stereotactic radiation versus WBRT are needed before the optimal radiotherapeutic modality for patients with >4 brain metastases can be determined. One such study is ongoing at our institution (NCT03075072; Fig. 5.4).

To summarize, brain-directed radiation is an important modality of care for patients with HER2+ breast cancer with brain metastases but should be used judiciously, particularly in patients with limited life expectancies that are driven by systemic disease. The optimal modality of radiation for patients with 1—4 brain metastases is stereotactic radiation, although in patients who have undergone resection of one or more brain metastases, this assertion may be more doubtful. Further evaluation of stereotactic radiation versus WBRT in patients with >4 brain metastases is warranted.

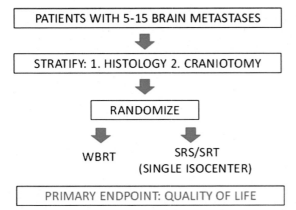

FIG. 5.4 Phase III Randomized Study of WBRT Versus Stereotactic Radiation in Patients With 5–15 Brain Metastases Being Conducted at Brigham and Women's Hospital/Dana-Farber Cancer Institute. *SRS*, stereotactic radiosurgery; *SRT*, stereotactic radiotherapy, *WBRT*, whole-brain radiation therapy.

SYSTEMIC THERAPIES

The use of systemic therapies in patients with HER2+ CNS metastases is critical, not only with the goal of obtaining responses in the CNS but also to control the extracranial disease which can be responsible for the clinical deterioration of the patient. The optimal utilization of anti-HER2 agents in patients with metastatic breast cancer has resulted in a dramatic improvement in overall survival over the years.[81] However, these patients are unfortunately at an increased risk for the development of relapses in the CNS, which represents a significant challenge.[2]

The activity of HER2-directed treatments to provide longer duration of responses in patients with MBC has uncovered the ability of HER2+ cancer cells to avidly colonize the CNS and prosper despite the use of highly effective systemic therapies. One possible contributing factor to this is that most drugs used in the management of these patients either do not cross the intact BBB or can be pumped out of the CNS through P-glycoproteins present in the BBB. As a result, standard systemic treatments for HER2+ disease may not achieve sufficient therapeutic concentrations in the CNS for the treatment of micrometastatic deposits.

Subtherapeutic CNS penetration may contribute to the development of drug resistance in the CNS by placing a degree of selective pressure on cancer cells while failing to reach cytotoxic levels.[1] Although the blood-tumor barrier is significantly more permissive than the intact BBB, it is only heterogeneously permissive, which can also contribute to variations in drug levels within and between brain metastases, and may also be associated with therapeutic resistance.[82,83]

The brain microenvironment may also be a relatively advantageous milieu for HER2+ cancer cells to grow. Recent data suggest that despite appropriate drug accumulation in the CNS lesions, HER2-amplified tumors are resistant to phosphatidylinositide 3-kinase (PI3K) inhibition through increased HER3 expression. This mechanism was not observed in extracranial sites and may provide a basis for therapeutic resistance specific to the brain microenvironment.[84]

Finally, because brain metastases appear to occur somewhat stochastically over time, the tumor cells seeding the CNS may have been exposed to a variety of prior systemic therapies and the development of therapeutic resistance before residence in the CNS. Radiation therapy may provoke additional alterations directly in the tumor and/or microenvironment that contribute to a resistant phenotype.[85]

Trastuzumab

Trastuzumab has historically been thought to not cross the BBB. This was demonstrated in the study of a patient with meningeal carcinomatosis, in which the ratio of trastuzumab in plasma to trastuzumab in the cerebrospinal fluid was >300:1.[86] However, the use of cranial surgery and radiation therapy may disrupt the BBB, allowing drug penetration into the CNS. In addition, the vasculature can be quite disordered within brain metastases, which can contribute to a leaky blood-tumor barrier. HER2+ CNS metastasis uptake has been observed in imaging studies using trastuzumab labeled with the radioisotopes zirconium 89 or copper 64.[87–89]

Whether or not trastuzumab crosses the BBB, treatment remains of value in patients with CNS metastases. A number of clinical studies have shown that the use of trastuzumab with chemotherapy results in survival improvements in breast cancer patients with HER2+ CNS metastases,[90,91] although this is difficult to separate from the survival benefit attributed to improved control of extracranial disease.[92]

Pertuzumab

In the first line setting, the addition of pertuzumab to a trastuzumab-taxane backbone results in an absolute improvement in median overall survival of 15.7 months compared with placebo plus trastuzumab plus docetaxel.[81] An exploratory analysis of CLEOPATRA showed that although the incidence of CNS metastases as first site of disease progression was similar between groups (13.7% in the pertuzumab arm compared with 12.6% in the placebo arm), the time to CNS progression was somewhat longer in the pertuzumab-containing arm (15 months vs. 11.9 months, $P = .0049$).[93] Whether this observation simply stems from better systemic tumor control (and hence less seeding to the CNS) or a true antitumor effect in the CNS is unknown at this time, particularly given that neither baseline nor follow-up CNS imaging were mandated per protocol.

Trastuzumab Emtansine

Trastuzumab emtansine (T-DM1) is an antibody-drug conjugate indicated for the treatment of trastuzumab and pretreated HER2+ MBC. In the EMILIA trial, T-DM1 demonstrated overall superior survival and a more favorable toxicity profile compared with lapatinib plus capecitabine.[94] Like nearly all prospective trials in HER2+ breast cancer, the EMILIA trial excluded patients with active brain metastases at the time of study entry. However, 95 patients were enrolled who had stable/treated brain metastases at baseline. A retrospective exploratory analysis of this subset of patients demonstrated similar rates of CNS progression between arms; however, median overall survival was significantly improved with T-DM1 compared with lapatinib plus trastuzumab (26.8 months vs. 12.9 months, respectively; $P = .008$).[95]

Unfortunately, none of the early-phase or registration trials evaluating T-DM1 allowed patients with active/progressive brain metastases at study entry, but since its approval, several groups have reported on the activity of T-DM1 in the CNS in case series. A study of 10 patients treated in Austria reported three patients with partial response and four patients with stable disease.[96] A larger study from France included 39 patients and documented a clinical benefit rate of 59% (44% partial response and 15% stable disease) and a median progression-free survival of 6.1 months.[97]

Lapatinib

Lapatinib, a tyrosine-kinase inhibitor (TKI) of epidermal growth factor receptor (EGFR) and HER2, is approved in combination with capecitabine for the treatment of HER2+ MBC previously treated with trastuzumab. Because of its small size, it was hypothesized to cross a leaky blood-tumor barrier, and has been studied in several nonrandomized prospective trials.

Despite the initial excitement, clinical trials evaluating lapatinib as a single agent in heavily pretreated populations described only modest response rates in the CNS of between 2.6% and 6%.[98,99] However, response rates increased to 20%–38% when capecitabine was added to lapatinib.[99–103] Previously untreated patients derived the most benefit from this combination, with objective response rate of 65.9%, median time to progression of 5.5 months, and 1-year survival rates >70%.[104] An ad hoc analysis of the pivotal trial showed that the combination of lapatinib plus capecitabine was also noted to decrease the frequency of CNS involvement at first progression when compared with capecitabine alone (6% vs. 2%, $P = .045$).[105] To build on this observation, the CEREBEL trial was designed to test whether lapatinib has a role in the prevention of CNS metastases. Patients with HER2+ MBC were screened with brain MRI, and those without CNS metastases were randomized to lapatinib plus capecitabine or trastuzumab plus capecitabine. There was no significant difference in the primary endpoint of incidence of CNS metastases between arms (3% for lapatinib vs. 5% for trastuzumab, $P = .36$). Furthermore, progression-free survival and overall survival favored the trastuzumab arm.[106] Thus, there is no data at present to support transitioning patients with stable, treated CNS metastases to lapatinib-capecitabine for the purpose of prevention of subsequent CNS events.

Cytotoxic Chemotherapy

Traditional cytotoxic chemotherapy agents have also been evaluated in the treatment of CNS metastases. Initial studies with combined drugs reported response rates of around 50%.[107,108] Temozolomide, a drug commonly used in the treatment of primary CNS tumors, has not induced meaningful responses as a single agent.[109] However, temozolomide in combination with cisplatin or capecitabine resulted in response rates of 40% and 18%, respectively, although these responses most likely demonstrated an effect of the chemotherapy partner rather than the temozolomide itself.[110,111] Capecitabine, which is commonly used in combination with other targeted agents as noted earlier, has limited retrospective data to support its use as a single agent.[112] Platinum-containing regimens have shown significant activity in CNS metastases from breast cancer with response rates between 37.5% and 55%.[110,113,114] Anthracyclines have also been reported to have CNS activity. The activities of several different cytotoxic agents are summarized in Table 5.2.

INVESTIGATIONAL APPROACHES AND FUTURE DIRECTIONS

Although great strides have been made in cancer therapy, CNS metastases portend a poor prognosis with current treatment options. For patients with HER2+ CNS metastases, there are a number of ongoing

TABLE 5.2
Overall CNS Response Rates in Select Trials of Cytotoxic Chemotherapy Agents

Agent	Type of Study	Regimen	No. of Breast Cancer Patients	CNS ORR Among Breast Cancer (%)
Anthracyclines	Phase II[115]	Pegylated liposomal doxorubicin	8	62
	Retrospective[116]	Liposomal doxorubicin + cyclophosphamide	29	41
	Case series[107]	Doxorubicin + cyclophosphamide	6	17
Capecitabine	Phase I[111]	Capecitabine + temozolomide	24	18
	Case series[112]	Capecitabine	7	43
Cisplatin	Prospective[113]	Cisplatin + etoposide	56	37.5
	Case series[114]	Cisplatin + etoposide	22	55
	Phase II[110]	Cisplatin + temozolomide	15	40
Irinotecan	Phase II[117]	Irinotecan + iniparib	37	12
Temozolomide	Phase II[118]	Temozolomide	51	4
	Phase II[109]	Temozolomide	19	0
	Phase II[119]	Temozolomide	10	0
	Phase II[120]	Temozolomide	4	0
	Phase II[121]	Temozolomide + vinorelbine	11	0

CNS, central nervous system; *ORR*, overall response rate (complete and partial responses).

trials evaluating novel targets as well as cytotoxic agents, a few of which are highlighted in the following section.

HER2-Targeted Tyrosine-Kinase Inhibitors

Lapatinib, neratinib, afatinib, and tucatinib are among the TKIs which have been studied in HER2+ breast cancer. Neratinib, an irreversible TKI of EGFR and HER2, is being evaluated in multiple cohorts of patients with CNS metastases in an ongoing phase II study. The first cohort (n = 40) was treated with single agent neratinib with a reported CNS response rate of 8%.[122] The second cohort (n = 37) received neratinib plus capecitabine with a CNS response rate of 49% but increased toxicity with a 32% rate of grade 3 diarrhea.[123]

Afatinib, also an irreversible TKI of both EGFR and HER2, has been approved for the treatment of patients with non–small cell lung cancers characterized by particular activating EGFR mutations.[124] In patients with HER2+ breast cancer brain metastases, afatinib showed no additional benefits in a phase II study comparing single agent afatinib or afatinib plus vinorelbine versus treatment of investigator's choice.[65] Because of these results, along with results from a similarly designed trial enrolling patients without brain

metastases,[125] no further studies are planned for this drug in breast cancer.

Unlike neratinib and afatinib, tucatinib is a more selective inhibitor of HER2 with less anti-EGFR activity, resulting in less diarrhea and rash. In a phase I study testing, the combination of tucatinib and trastuzumab without chemotherapy, the CNS response rate was 12%, and prolonged stable disease was also observed.[126] In a phase Ib study combining tucatinib with trastuzumab and capecitabine, 42% of patients with CNS metastases achieved a CNS objective response.[127] These results have led to an ongoing, randomized trial testing trastuzumab-capecitabine versus the triplet of trastuzumab-capecitabine-tucatinib (NCT02614794). An innovative feature of this study is the inclusion of patients with or without brain metastases, and even the inclusion of patients with active (i.e., untreated with surgical resection or radiation) brain metastases at study baseline.

Cell Cycle Inhibitors

The cyclin D1-CDK4/6 pathway involved in cell cycle progression has gained significant interest as a target in breast cancer, particularly for hormone receptor–positive breast cancers. The CDK4/6 and cyclin D1 complex phosphorylate the tumor suppressor retinoblastoma protein, which releases the transcription factor E2F, leading to cell proliferation and transition from the G1 phase to the S phase of the cell cycle. There are currently three drugs that inhibit CDK4/6— palbociclib, ribociclib, and abemaciclib—all of which have FDA approval for use in hormone receptor–positive/HER2-negative MBC.[128–130] The role of CDK4/6 inhibitors are being evaluated in two phase II trials that include patients with HER2+ CNS metastases (NCT02774681, NCT02308020).

Immunotherapy-Based Approaches

Recent data have shown that tumor infiltration by immune cells has prognostic value in HER2+ MBC,[131] and expression of the T-cell inhibitory transmembrane molecule programmed death-ligand 1 has been reported in 53% of brain metastases.[132] Immune checkpoint inhibitors have become an important treatment option for metastatic melanoma and lung cancer, particularly in the setting of CNS metastases.[133] The combination of nivolumab and ipilimumab has resulted in CNS response rates of 42%–44% in two recent melanoma trials.[134,135] Studies evaluating immune checkpoint inhibitors for CNS metastases in patients with HER2+ breast cancer are ongoing (NCT02886585, NCT02669914).

Targeting of the PI3K/Mammalian Target of Rapamycin Pathway

Alterations in the phosphatidylinositol 3-kinase (PI3K) pathway are one of the most frequent changes in breast cancer cells with constitutive activation of the class IA PI3K pathway resulting from mutational activation of the PIK3CA gene or loss of phosphatase and tensin homolog (PTEN).[136–139] PI3K is such a central conduit of HER2 signaling that HER2 is unable to transform mouse embryonic fibroblasts lacking a functional p110α subunit of PI3K.[140]

Previous studies have suggested an important role for signaling down the PI3K pathway, and particularly, for PTEN loss, in the development of brain metastases from breast cancer. Adamo et al. analyzed phosphorylation levels of protein kinase B (p-AKT), phosphorylation of protein S6 (p-S6), and expression of PTEN by immunohistochemistry in 52 brain metastases samples and found that p-AKT and p-S6 were common, indicating signaling through the PI3K pathway.[141] PTEN loss was noted in 25% of samples and was correlated with shorter time to distant and brain recurrence. Wikman et al. performed array comparative genetic

hybridization on matched primary tumors and breast cancer brain metastases and also found PTEN allelic imbalance more frequently in brain metastases (52%) and primary tumors with CNS relapse (59%) compared with primary tumors from patients without relapse (18%, $P = .003$) or relapse in other sites (12%, $P = .006$).[142] PTEN mRNA expression was also downregulated in brain metastases compared with primary tumors. Finally, in patient-derived xenograft models using human breast cancer brain metastases, the combination of PI3K and mammalian target of rapamycin (mTOR) inhibition led to dramatic intracranial tumor regressions.[143]

In the clinic, a phase II trial combining everolimus with vinorelbine and trastuzumab for patients with HER2+ breast cancer brain metastases has recently been completed. While the response rate (4%) was somewhat disappointing, the CNS clinical benefit rate (which includes stable disease) at 6 months was 27%.[144] Everolimus is also being evaluated in combination with capecitabine and lapatinib (NCT01783756). Trials testing combinations of PI3K inhibitors and mTOR inhibitors in patients with HER2+ brain metastases are being actively planned.

Cytotoxic Agents

Two chemotherapeutic agents of particular interest due to their CNS penetration are ANG1005 and etirinotecan pegol. ANG1005 is a novel peptide-drug conjugate of angiopep-2 and paclitaxel, which can cross the BBB through the lipoprotein receptor–related protein 1.[145] Early-phase studies have shown promising responses in the CNS with additional studies ongoing (NCT02048059).[146,147] Etirinotecan pegol is an extended-release formulation of irinotecan, a topoisomerase-I inhibitor. This drug showed improved overall survival in a preplanned analysis of a subset of patients with stable CNS metastases treated under a larger phase III trial,[148] which prompted the conduction of an ongoing confirmatory phase III trial focusing on CNS metastases from breast cancer, including HER2+ subtypes (NCT02915744).

Alternative Dosing Schedules

Because of the concerns about the CNS penetration of anti-HER2 agents, a number of studies are evaluating alternative doses or routes of administration of these drugs including a phase II study evaluating a higher dose of trastuzumab (6 mg/kg IV weekly) with pertuzumab standard dose (NCT02536339). A planned interim analysis after enrollment of the first 15 patients showed a CNS response rate of 20%, which met prespecified criteria; full enrollment (n = 40) is ongoing.[149] Another trial is testing intermittent higher doses of lapatinib with capecitabine (NCT02650752). Regarding drug delivery into the CNS, a phase I trial is exploring a dose escalation of intrathecal pertuzumab plus intrathecal trastuzumab 80 mg (NCT02598427).

TREATMENT APPROACH

The main factors to consider when deciding on treatment options for individual patients are the number of CNS metastases, the symptoms from CNS disease, the status of the systemic disease, and the prognosis of the patient. Specific considerations in patients with HER2+ disease have also been recently addressed by the ASCO in a clinical practice guideline.[19]

Initial Presentation

Fig. 5.5 illustrates an algorithm that may be considered at initial presentation. It is critical to highlight the role of multidisciplinary management for these patients, as

at each decision point, the positive and negative attributes of each treatment modality and their integration/sequencing should be weighed. In addition, given the limited standard options, clinical trials should always be a consideration when available.

Subsequent Central Nervous System Progression After Initial Local Therapy

CNS progression after initial local therapy is a common clinical problem. In this scenario, some of the most important factors to consider are the level of control of extracranial disease, the type(s) of local therapy on which the patient has progressed, performance status, and the availability and potential efficacy of systemic therapies and/or clinical trials. In patients with controlled extracranial disease and limited CNS progression (for example, a single enlarging lesion), attempting a new (or repeated) form of local therapy is usually favored when possible, and the systemic therapy can remain unchanged. On the other hand, if the CNS progression occurs as part of extracranial

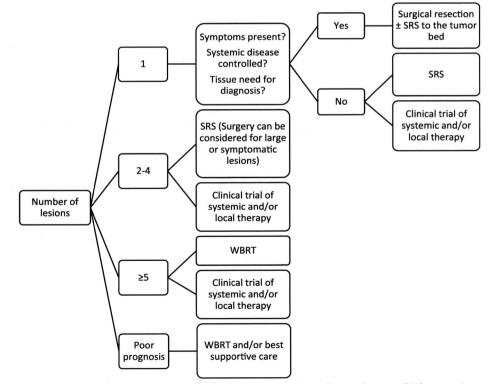

FIG. 5.5 Algorithm for the Management of CNS Metastases From Breast Cancer. *CNS*, central nervous system; *SRS*, stereotactic radiosurgery; *WBRT*, whole-brain radiation therapy.

progression, or if there are multiple new/worsening lesions (especially if prior WBRT has already been given), transitioning to a previously untired form of systemic therapy is preferred, and local therapy modalities to the CNS can be considered, especially to symptomatic lesions. Once again, multidisciplinary planning and clinical trial participation are highly encouraged. Fig. 5.6 shows a possible algorithm for patients who have disease progression in the CNS after initial local therapy.

Isolated Central Nervous System Progression in the Absence of Extracranial Disease

A small proportion of patients present with CNS-only recurrence without evidence of extracranial involvement. Initial management of these patients includes a form of local therapy such as surgery, radiation, or both. Surgery is of particular relevance in this situation because it can provide tissue diagnosis and analysis of receptor status in addition to prolonging survival of patients with single lesions. After local therapy, our practice has been to monitor patients with interval brain MRI every 2—4 months.

There are no prospective data to guide systemic therapy in patients with CNS-only relapse after completion of local therapy, but a recent retrospective study suggested an improved survival with the use of systemic therapy after local treatment in patients with CNS-only relapse.[150] Options include observation alone, endocrine therapy if estrogen receptor positive (ER+) and/or progesterone receptor positive (PR+), or some form of HER2-based therapy if HER2+. Some important factors to consider when deciding between these options include the patient's age, performance status, the duration of the disease-free interval, and the patient's preferences with regard to treatment. In older patients or those with prolonged disease-free interval, observation after local therapy may be appropriate. In younger patients, we consider trastuzumab alone,

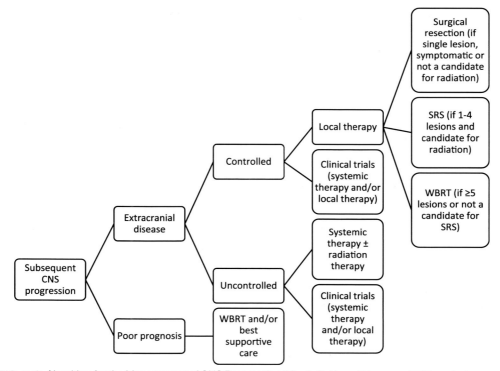

FIG. 5.6 Algorithm for the Management of CNS Progression After Initial Local Therapy. *CNS*, central nervous system; *SRS*, stereotactic radiosurgery; *WBRT*, whole-brain radiation therapy.

trastuzumab with pertuzumab, and/or endocrine therapy if ER+ and/or PR+ (particularly if the relapse is late). In the absence of prospective data demonstrating clinical benefit, we generally prefer to avoid combinations of chemotherapy with anti-HER2 therapy (e.g., such as lapatinib-capecitabine) in the frontline treatment of patients with locally treated, CNS-only relapses due to the toxicity profile.

CONCLUSIONS

Patients with HER2+ MBC have recently experienced significant gains in overall survival with an increasing number of efficacious treatment options. However, these patients have an increased risk of developing CNS metastases, which represent a significant clinical challenge. Although treatment options are somewhat limited, a multidisciplinary collaboration for individual patients is strongly advised. Appropriate selection of surgical candidates, the timing and modality of radiation therapy, and considerations for systemic therapy with targeted agents should all be discussed as part of the management plan. Ongoing clinical trials that include breast cancer patients with CNS metastases are a much-needed step toward improving treatment options for this poor-prognosis group of patients.

REFERENCES

1. Lin NU, Bellon JR, Winer EP. CNS metastases in breast cancer. *J Clin Oncol.* 2004;22(17):3608−3617.
2. Aversa C, Rossi V, Geuna E, et al. Metastatic breast cancer subtypes and central nervous system metastases. *Breast.* 2014;23(5):623−628.
3. Weil RJ, Palmieri DC, Bronder JL, Stark AM, Steeg PS. Breast cancer metastasis to the central nervous system. *Am J Pathol.* 2005;167(4):913−920.
4. Nguyen DX, Bos PD, Massague J. Metastasis: from dissemination to organ-specific colonization. *Nat Rev Cancer.* 2009;9(4):274−284.
5. Leone JP, Lee AV, Brufsky AM. Prognostic factors and survival of patients with brain metastasis from breast cancer who underwent craniotomy. *Cancer Med.* 2015;4(7):989−994.
6. Sperduto PW, Kased N, Roberge D, et al. The effect of tumor subtype on the time from primary diagnosis to development of brain metastases and survival in patients with breast cancer. *J Neurooncol.* 2013;112(3):467−472.
7. Lee SS, Ahn JH, Kim MK, et al. Brain metastases in breast cancer: prognostic factors and management. *Breast Cancer Res Treat.* 2008;111(3):523−530.
8. Ogawa K, Yoshii Y, Nishimaki T, et al. Treatment and prognosis of brain metastases from breast cancer. *J Neurooncol.* 2008;86(2):231−238.
9. Sperduto PW, Kased N, Roberge D, et al. Effect of tumor subtype on survival and the graded prognostic assessment for patients with breast cancer and brain metastases. *Int J Radiat Oncol Biol Phys.* 2012;82(5):2111−2117.
10. Klos KJ, O'Neill BP. Brain metastases. *Neurol.* 2004;10(1):31−46.
11. Dawood S, Broglio K, Esteva FJ, et al. Defining prognosis for women with breast cancer and CNS metastases by HER2 status. *Ann Oncol.* 2008;19(7):1242−1248.
12. Leone JP, Leone BA. Breast cancer brain metastases: the last frontier. *Exp Hematol Oncol.* 2015;4:33.
13. Barajas RF Jr, Cha S. Imaging diagnosis of brain metastasis. *Prog Neurol Surg.* 2012;25:55−73.
14. Duchnowska R, Dziadziuszko R, Trojanowski T, et al. Conversion of epidermal growth factor receptor 2 and hormone receptor expression in breast cancer metastases to the brain. *Breast Cancer Res.* 2012;14(4):R119.
15. Thomson AH, McGrane J, Mathew J, et al. Changing molecular profile of brain metastases compared with matched breast primary cancers and impact on clinical outcomes. *Br J Cancer.* 2016;114(7):793−800.
16. Priedigkeit N, Hartmaier RJ, Chen Y, et al. Intrinsic subtype switching and acquired ERBB2/HER2 amplifications and mutations in breast cancer brain metastases. *JAMA Oncol.* 2017;3(5):666−671.
17. Pestalozzi BC, Holmes E, de Azambuja E, et al. CNS relapses in patients with HER2-positive early breast cancer who have and have not received adjuvant trastuzumab: a retrospective substudy of the HERA trial (BIG 1-01). *Lancet Oncol.* 2013;14(3):244−248.
18. Arvold ND, Oh KS, Niemierko A, et al. Brain metastases after breast-conserving therapy and systemic therapy: incidence and characteristics by biologic subtype. *Breast Cancer Res Treat.* 2012;136(1):153−160.
19. Ramakrishna N, Temin S, Chandarlapaty S, et al. Recommendations on disease management for patients with advanced human epidermal growth factor receptor 2-positive breast cancer and brain metastases: American Society of Clinical Oncology clinical practice guideline. *J Clin Oncol.* 2014;32(19):2100−2108.
20. Lin NU, Thomssen C, Cardoso F, et al. International guidelines for management of metastatic breast cancer (MBC) from the European School of Oncology (ESO)-MBC Task Force: surveillance, staging, and evaluation of patients with early-stage and metastatic breast cancer. *Breast.* 2013;22(3):203−210.
21. Niwinska A, Murawska M, Pogoda K. Breast cancer brain metastases: differences in survival depending on biological subtype, RPA RTOG prognostic class and systemic treatment after whole-brain radiotherapy (WBRT). *Ann Oncol.* 2010;21(5):942−948.
22. Niikura N, Hayashi N, Masuda N, et al. Treatment outcomes and prognostic factors for patients with brain metastases from breast cancer of each subtype: a multicenter retrospective analysis. *Breast Cancer Res Treat.* 2014;147(1):103−112.

23. Anders CK, Deal AM, Miller CR, et al. The prognostic contribution of clinical breast cancer subtype, age, and race among patients with breast cancer brain metastases. *Cancer.* 2011;117(8):1602–1611.

24. Leone JP, Leone J, Zwenger AO, Iturbe J, Leone BA, Vallejo CT. Prognostic factors and survival according to tumour subtype in women presenting with breast cancer brain metastases at initial diagnosis. *Eur J Cancer.* 2017; 74:17–25.

25. Martin AM, Cagney DN, Catalano PJ, et al. Brain metastases in newly diagnosed breast cancer: a population-based study. *JAMA Oncol.* 2017;3(8):1069–1077.

26. Melisko ME, Moore DH, Sneed PK, De Franco J, Rugo HS. Brain metastases in breast cancer: clinical and pathologic characteristics associated with improvements in survival. *J Neurooncol.* 2008;88(3):359–365.

27. Lentzsch S, Reichardt P, Weber F, Budach V, Dorken B. Brain metastases in breast cancer: prognostic factors and management. *Eur J Cancer.* 1999;35(4):580–585.

28. Sperduto PW, Berkey B, Gaspar LE, Mehta M, Curran W. A new prognostic index and comparison to three other indices for patients with brain metastases: an analysis of 1,960 patients in the RTOG database. *Int J Radiat Oncol Biol Phys.* 2008;70(2):510–514.

29. Sperduto CM, Watanabe Y, Mullan J, et al. A validation study of a new prognostic index for patients with brain metastases: the graded prognostic assessment. *J Neurosurg.* 2008;109(suppl):87–89.

30. Subbiah IM, Lei X, Weinberg JS, et al. Validation and development of a modified breast graded prognostic assessment as a tool for survival in patients with breast cancer and brain metastases. *J Clin Oncol.* 2015;33(20): 2239–2245.

31. Barker FG 2nd. Craniotomy for the resection of metastatic brain tumors in the U.S., 1988-2000: decreasing mortality and the effect of provider caseload. *Cancer.* 2004; 100(5):999–1007.

32. Patchell RA, Tibbs PA, Walsh JW, et al. A randomized trial of surgery in the treatment of single metastases to the brain. *N Engl J Med.* 1990;322(8):494–500.

33. Vecht CJ, Haaxma-Reiche H, Noordijk EM, et al. Treatment of single brain metastasis: radiotherapy alone or combined with neurosurgery? *Ann Neurol.* 1993;33(6): 583–590.

34. Mintz AH, Kestle J, Rathbone MP, et al. A randomized trial to assess the efficacy of surgery in addition to radiotherapy in patients with a single cerebral metastasis. *Cancer.* 1996;78(7):1470–1476.

35. Sause WT, Crowley JJ, Morantz R, et al. Solitary brain metastasis: results of an RTOG/SWOG protocol evaluation surgery + RT versus RT alone. *Am J Clin Oncol.* 1990;13(5):427–432.

36. Ampil FL, Nanda A, Willis BK, Nandy I, Meehan R. Metastatic disease in the cerebellum. The LSU experience in 1981-1993. *Am J Clin Oncol.* 1996;19(5):509–511.

37. Rades D, Kieckebusch S, Haatanen T, Lohynska R, Dunst J, Schild SE. Surgical resection followed by whole brain radiotherapy versus whole brain radiotherapy alone for single brain metastasis. *Int J Radiat Oncol Biol Phys.* 2008;70(5):1319–1324.

38. Mulvenna P, Nankivell M, Barton R, et al. Dexamethasone and supportive care with or without whole brain radiotherapy in treating patients with non-small cell lung cancer with brain metastases unsuitable for resection or stereotactic radiotherapy (QUARTZ): results from a phase 3, non-inferiority, randomised trial. *Lancet.* 2016;388(10055):2004–2014.

39. Borgelt B, Gelber R, Kramer S, et al. The palliation of brain metastases: final results of the first two studies by the Radiation Therapy Oncology Group. *Int J Radiat Oncol Biol Phys.* 1980;6(1):1–9.

40. Gelber RD, Larson M, Borgelt BB, Kramer S. Equivalence of radiation schedules for the palliative treatment of brain metastases in patients with favorable prognosis. *Cancer.* 1981;48(8):1749–1753.

41. Kurtz JM, Gelber R, Brady LW, Carella RJ, Cooper JS. The palliation of brain metastases in a favorable patient population: a randomized clinical trial by the Radiation Therapy Oncology Group. *Int J Radiat Oncol Biol Phys.* 1981;7(7):891–895.

42. Brown PD, Jaeckle K, Ballman KV, et al. Effect of radiosurgery alone vs radiosurgery with whole brain radiation therapy on cognitive function in patients with 1 to 3 brain metastases: a randomized clinical trial. *JAMA.* 2016;316(4):401–409.

43. Page BR, Shaw EG, Lu L, et al. Phase II double-blind placebo-controlled randomized study of armodafinil for brain radiation-induced fatigue. *Neuro Oncol.* 2015; 17(10):1393–1401.

44. Chang EL, Wefel JS, Hess KR, et al. Neurocognition in patients with brain metastases treated with radiosurgery or radiosurgery plus whole-brain irradiation: a randomised controlled trial. *Lancet Oncol.* 2009;10(11):1037–1044.

45. Brown PD, Pugh S, Laack NN, et al. Memantine for the prevention of cognitive dysfunction in patients receiving whole-brain radiotherapy: a randomized, double-blind, placebo-controlled trial. *Neurooncol.* 2013;15(10): 1429–1437.

46. Shaw EG, Rosdhal R, D'Agostino Jr RB, et al. Phase II study of donepezil in irradiated brain tumor patients: effect on cognitive function, mood, and quality of life. *J Clin Oncol.* 2006;24(9):1415–1420.

47. Thames HD, Bentzen SM, Turesson I, Overgaard M, Van den Bogaert W. Time-dose factors in radiotherapy: a review of the human data. *Radiother Oncol.* 1990;19(3): 219–235.

48. Gondi V, Pugh SL, Tome WA, et al. Preservation of memory with conformal avoidance of the hippocampal neural stem-cell compartment during whole-brain radiotherapy for brain metastases (RTOG 0933): a phase II multi-institutional trial. *J Clin Oncol.* 2014;32(34):3810–3816.

49. Shaw E, Scott C, Souhami L, et al. Single dose radiosurgical treatment of recurrent previously irradiated primary brain tumors and brain metastases: final report of RTOG protocol 90-05. *Int J Radiat Oncol Biol Phys.* 2000;47(2):291–298.

50. Blonigen BJ, Steinmetz RD, Levin L, Lamba MA, Warnick RE, Breneman JC. Irradiated volume as a predictor of brain radionecrosis after linear accelerator stereotactic radiosurgery. *Int J Radiat Oncol Biol Phys.* 2010;77(4):996−1001.

51. Minniti G, Clarke E, Lanzetta G, et al. Stereotactic radiosurgery for brain metastases: analysis of outcome and risk of brain radionecrosis. *Radiat Oncol.* 2011;6:48.

52. Williams BJ, Suki D, Fox BD, et al. Stereotactic radiosurgery for metastatic brain tumors: a comprehensive review of complications. *J Neurosurg.* 2009;111(3):439−448.

53. Chen CC, Hsu PW, Erich Wu TW, et al. Stereotactic brain biopsy: single center retrospective analysis of complications. *Clin Neurol Neurosurg.* 2009;111(10): 835−839.

54. Sugahara T, Korogi Y, Tomiguchi S, et al. Posttherapeutic intraaxial brain tumor: the value of perfusion-sensitive contrast-enhanced MR imaging for differentiating tumor recurrence from nonneoplastic contrast-enhancing tissue. *Am J Neuroradiol.* 2000;21(5):901−909.

55. Mitsuya K, Nakasu Y, Horiguchi S, et al. Perfusion weighted magnetic resonance imaging to distinguish the recurrence of metastatic brain tumors from radiation necrosis after stereotactic radiosurgery. *J Neurooncol.* 2010;99(1):81−88.

56. Asao C, Korogi Y, Kitajima M, et al. Diffusion-weighted imaging of radiation-induced brain injury for differentiation from tumor recurrence. *Am J Neuroradiol.* 2005; 26(6):1455−1460.

57. Rock JP, Scarpace L, Hearshen D, et al. Associations among magnetic resonance spectroscopy, apparent diffusion coefficients, and image-guided histopathology with special attention to radiation necrosis. *Neurosurgery.* 2004;54(5):1111−1117, discussion 1117−1119.

58. Kimura T, Sako K, Tanaka K, et al. Evaluation of the response of metastatic brain tumors to stereotactic radiosurgery by proton magnetic resonance spectroscopy, 201TlCl single-photon emission computerized tomography, and gadolinium-enhanced magnetic resonance imaging. *J Neurosurg.* 2004;100(5):835−841.

59. Henry RG, Vigneron DB, Fischbein NJ, et al. Comparison of relative cerebral blood volume and proton spectroscopy in patients with treated gliomas. *Am J Neuroradiol.* 2000;21(2):357−366.

60. Davidson A, Tait DM, Payne GS, et al. Magnetic resonance spectroscopy in the evaluation of neurotoxicity following cranial irradiation for childhood cancer. *Br J Radiol.* 2000;73(868):421−424.

61. Horky LL, Hsiao EM, Weiss SE, Drappatz J, Gerbaudo VH. Dual phase FDG-PET imaging of brain metastases provides superior assessment of recurrence versus post-treatment necrosis. *J Neurooncol.* 2011;103(1):137−146.

62. Doyle WK, Budinger TF, Valk PE, Levin VA, Gutin PH. Differentiation of cerebral radiation necrosis from tumor recurrence by [18F]FDG and 82Rb positron emission tomography. *J Comput Assist Tomogr.* 1987;11(4): 563−570.

63. Buchpiguel CA, Alavi JB, Alavi A, Kenyon LC. PET versus SPECT in distinguishing radiation necrosis from tumor recurrence in the brain. *J Nucl Med.* 1995;36(1): 159−164.

64. Lai G, Mahadevan A, Hackney D, et al. Diagnostic accuracy of PET, SPECT, and arterial spin-labeling in differentiating tumor recurrence from necrosis in cerebral metastasis after stereotactic radiosurgery. *Am J Neuroradiol.* 2015;36(12):2250−2255.

65. Cortes J, Dieras V, Ro J, et al. Afatinib alone or afatinib plus vinorelbine versus investigator's choice of treatment for HER2-positive breast cancer with progressive brain metastases after trastuzumab, lapatinib, or both (LUX-Breast 3): a randomised, open-label, multicentre, phase 2 trial. *Lancet Oncol.* 2015;16(16):1700−1710.

66. Ferrara M, Bizzozzero L, Talamonti G, D'Angelo VA. Surgical treatment of 100 single brain metastases. Analysis of the results. *J Neurosurg Sci.* 1990;34(3−4): 303−308.

67. Patel AJ, Suki D, Hatiboglu MA, Rao VY, Fox BD, Sawaya R. Impact of surgical methodology on the complication rate and functional outcome of patients with a single brain metastasis. *J Neurosurg.* 2015;122(5): 1132−1143.

68. McKay WH, McTyre ER, Okoukoni C, et al. Repeat stereotactic radiosurgery as salvage therapy for locally recurrent brain metastases previously treated with radiosurgery. *J Neurosurg.* 2016:1−9.

69. Levin VA, Bidaut L, Hou P, et al. Randomized double-blind placebo-controlled trial of bevacizumab therapy for radiation necrosis of the central nervous system. *Int J Radiat Oncol Biol Phys.* 2011;79(5):1487−1495.

70. Seet RC, Rabinstein AA, Lindell PE, Uhm JH, Wijdicks EF. Cerebrovascular events after bevacizumab treatment: an early and severe complication. *Neurocrit Care.* 2011; 15(3):421−427.

71. Nishimura T, Furihata M, Kubo H, et al. Intracranial hemorrhage in patients treated with bevacizumab: report of two cases. *World J Gastroenterol.* 2011;17(39): 4440−4444.

72. Aoyama H, Shirato H, Tago M, et al. Stereotactic radiosurgery plus whole-brain radiation therapy vs stereotactic radiosurgery alone for treatment of brain metastases: a randomized controlled trial. *JAMA.* 2006;295(21): 2483−2491.

73. Kocher M, Soffietti R, Abacioglu U, et al. Adjuvant whole-brain radiotherapy versus observation after radiosurgery or surgical resection of one to three cerebral metastases: results of the EORTC 22952-26001 study. *J Clin Oncol.* 2011;29(2):134−141.

74. Soffietti R, Kocher M, Abacioglu UM, et al. A European Organisation for Research and Treatment of Cancer phase III trial of adjuvant whole-brain radiotherapy versus observation in patients with one to three brain metastases from solid tumors after surgical resection or radiosurgery: quality-of-life results. *J Clin Oncol.* 2013; 31(1):65−72.

75. Brown PD, Ballman KV, Cerhan JH, et al. Postoperative stereotactic radiosurgery compared with whole brain radiotherapy for resected metastatic brain disease (NCCTG N107C/CEC.3): a multicentre, randomised, controlled, phase 3 trial. *Lancet Oncol*. 2017;18(8):1049–1060.

76. Mahajan A, Ahmed S, McAleer MF, et al. Post-operative stereotactic radiosurgery versus observation for completely resected brain metastases: a single-centre, randomised, controlled, phase 3 trial. *Lancet Oncol*. 2017;18(8):1040–1048.

77. Kepka L, Tyc-Szczepaniak D, Osowiecka K, Sprawka A, Trabska-Kluch B, Czeremszynska B. Quality of life after whole brain radiotherapy compared with radiosurgery of the tumor bed: results from a randomized trial. *Clin Transl Oncol*. 2017;(2):150–159.

78. Patchell RA, Tibbs PA, Regine WF, et al. Postoperative radiotherapy in the treatment of single metastases to the brain: a randomized trial. *JAMA*. 1998;280(17):1485–1489.

79. Kayama T, Sato S, Sakurada K, et al. JCOG0504: a phase III randomized trial of surgery with whole brain radiation therapy versus surgery with salvage stereotactic radiosurgery in patients with 1 to 4 brain metastases. *J Clin Oncol*. 2016;34(15 suppl):2003.

80. Yamamoto M, Serizawa T, Shuto T, et al. Stereotactic radiosurgery for patients with multiple brain metastases (JLGK0901): a multi-institutional prospective observational study. *Lancet Oncol*. 2014;15(4):387–395.

81. Swain SM, Baselga J, Kim SB, et al. Pertuzumab, trastuzumab, and docetaxel in HER2-positive metastatic breast cancer. *N Engl J Med*. 2015;372(8):724–734.

82. Lockman PR, Mittapalli RK, Taskar KS, et al. Heterogeneous blood-tumor barrier permeability determines drug efficacy in experimental brain metastases of breast cancer. *Clin Cancer Res*. 2010;16(23):5664–5678.

83. Steeg PS, Camphausen KA, Smith QR. Brain metastases as preventive and therapeutic targets. *Nat Rev Cancer*. 2011;11(5):352–363.

84. Kodack DP, Askoxylakis V, Ferraro GB, et al. The brain microenvironment mediates resistance in luminal breast cancer to PI3K inhibition through HER3 activation. *Sci Transl Med*. 2017;9(391).

85. Barker HE, Paget JT, Khan AA, Harrington KJ. The tumour microenvironment after radiotherapy: mechanisms of resistance and recurrence. *Nat Rev Cancer*. 2015;15(7):409–425.

86. Pestalozzi BC, Brignoli S. Trastuzumab in CSF. *J Clin Oncol*. 2000;18(11):2349–2351.

87. Dijkers EC, Oude Munnink TH, Kosterink JG, et al. Biodistribution of 89Zr-trastuzumab and PET imaging of HER2-positive lesions in patients with metastatic breast cancer. *Clin Pharmacol Ther*. 2010;87(5):586–592.

88. Tamura K, Kurihara H, Yonemori K, et al. 64Cu-DOTA-trastuzumab PET imaging in patients with HER2-positive breast cancer. *J Nucl Med*. 2013;54(11):1869–1875.

89. Lewis Phillips GD, Nishimura MC, Lacap JA, et al. Trastuzumab uptake and its relation to efficacy in an animal model of HER2-positive breast cancer brain metastasis. *Breast Cancer Res Treat*. 2017;164(3):581–591.

90. Bartsch R, Rottenfusser A, Wenzel C, et al. Trastuzumab prolongs overall survival in patients with brain metastases from Her2 positive breast cancer. *J Neurooncol*. 2007;85(3):311–317.

91. Brufsky AM, Mayer M, Rugo HS, et al. Central nervous system metastases in patients with HER2-positive metastatic breast cancer: incidence, treatment, and survival in patients from registHER. *Clin Cancer Res*. 2011;17(14):4834–4843.

92. Park YH, Park MJ, Ji SH, et al. Trastuzumab treatment improves brain metastasis outcomes through control and durable prolongation of systemic extracranial disease in HER2-overexpressing breast cancer patients. *Br J Cancer*. 2009;100(6):894–900.

93. Swain SM, Baselga J, Miles D, et al. Incidence of central nervous system metastases in patients with HER2-positive metastatic breast cancer treated with pertuzumab, trastuzumab, and docetaxel: results from the randomized phase III study CLEOPATRA. *Ann Oncol*. 2014;25(6):1116–1121.

94. Verma S, Miles D, Gianni L, et al. Trastuzumab emtansine for HER2-positive advanced breast cancer. *N Engl J Med*. 2012;367(19):1783–1791.

95. Krop IE, Lin NU, Blackwell K, et al. Trastuzumab emtansine (T-DM1) versus lapatinib plus capecitabine in patients with HER2-positive metastatic breast cancer and central nervous system metastases: a retrospective, exploratory analysis in EMILIA. *Ann Oncol*. 2015;26(1):113–119.

96. Bartsch R, Berghoff AS, Vogl U, et al. Activity of T-DM1 in Her2-positive breast cancer brain metastases. *Clin Exp Metastasis*. 2015;32(7):729–737.

97. Jacot W, Pons E, Frenel JS, et al. Efficacy and safety of trastuzumab emtansine (T-DM1) in patients with HER2-positive breast cancer with brain metastases. *Breast Cancer Res Treat*. 2016;157(2):307–318.

98. Lin NU, Carey LA, Liu MC, et al. Phase II trial of lapatinib for brain metastases in patients with human epidermal growth factor receptor 2-positive breast cancer. *J Clin Oncol*. 2008;26(12):1993–1999.

99. Lin NU, Dieras V, Paul D, et al. Multicenter phase II study of lapatinib in patients with brain metastases from HER2-positive breast cancer. *Clin Cancer Res*. 2009;15(4):1452–1459.

100. Sutherland S, Ashley S, Miles D, et al. Treatment of HER2-positive metastatic breast cancer with lapatinib and capecitabine in the lapatinib expanded access programme, including efficacy in brain metastases—the UK experience. *Br J Cancer*. 2010;102(6):995–1002.

101. Metro G, Foglietta J, Russillo M, et al. Clinical outcome of patients with brain metastases from HER2-positive breast cancer treated with lapatinib and capecitabine. *Ann Oncol*. 2011;22(3):625–630.

102. Smith DC, McDermott DF, Powderly JD, et al. *N Engl J.* 2012:2443–2454.

103. Lin NU, Eierman W, Greil R, et al. Randomized phase II study of lapatinib plus capecitabine or lapatinib plus topotecan for patients with HER2-positive breast cancer brain metastases. *J Neurooncol.* 2011;105(3):613–620.

104. Bachelot T, Romieu G, Campone M, et al. Lapatinib plus capecitabine in patients with previously untreated brain metastases from HER2-positive metastatic breast cancer (LANDSCAPE): a single-group phase 2 study. *Lancet Oncol.* 2013;14(1):64–71.

105. Cameron D, Casey M, Press M, et al. A phase III randomized comparison of lapatinib plus capecitabine versus capecitabine alone in women with advanced breast cancer that has progressed on trastuzumab: updated efficacy and biomarker analyses. *Breast Cancer Res Treat.* 2008;112(3):533–543.

106. Pivot X, Manikhas A, Zurawski B, et al. CEREBEL (EGF111438): a phase III, randomized, open-label study of lapatinib plus capecitabine versus trastuzumab plus capecitabine in patients with human epidermal growth factor receptor 2-positive metastatic breast cancer. *J Clin Oncol.* 2015;33(14):1564–1573.

107. Rosner D, Nemoto T, Lane WW. Chemotherapy induces regression of brain metastases in breast carcinoma. *Cancer.* 1986;58(4):832–839.

108. Boogerd W, Dalesio O, Bais EM, van der Sande JJ. Response of brain metastases from breast cancer to systemic chemotherapy. *Cancer.* 1992;69(4):972–980.

109. Trudeau ME, Crump M, Charpentier D, et al. Temozolomide in metastatic breast cancer (MBC): a phase II trial of the National Cancer Institute of Canada - Clinical Trials Group (NCIC-CTG). *Ann Oncol.* 2006;17(6):952–956.

110. Christodoulou C, Bafaloukos D, Linardou H, et al. Temozolomide (TMZ) combined with cisplatin (CDDP) in patients with brain metastases from solid tumors: a Hellenic Cooperative Oncology Group (HeCOG) Phase II study. *J Neurooncol.* 2005;71(1):61–65.

111. Rivera E, Meyers C, Groves M, et al. Phase I study of capecitabine in combination with temozolomide in the treatment of patients with brain metastases from breast carcinoma. *Cancer.* 2006;107(6):1348–1354.

112. Ekenel M, Hormigo AM, Peak S, Deangelis LM, Abrey LE. Capecitabine therapy of central nervous system metastases from breast cancer. *J Neurooncol.* 2007;85(2):223–227.

113. Franciosi V, Cocconi G, Michiara M, et al. Front-line chemotherapy with cisplatin and etoposide for patients with brain metastases from breast carcinoma, nonsmall cell lung carcinoma, or malignant melanoma: a prospective study. *Cancer.* 1999;85(7):1599–1605.

114. Cocconi G, Lottici R, Bisagni G, et al. Combination therapy with platinum and etoposide of brain metastases from breast carcinoma. *Cancer Investig.* 1990;8(3–4):327–334.

115. Caraglia M, Addeo R, Costanzo R, et al. Phase II study of temozolomide plus pegylated liposomal doxorubicin in the treatment of brain metastases from solid tumours. *Cancer Chemother Pharmacol.* 2006;57(1):34–39.

116. Linot B, Campone M, Augereau P, et al. Use of liposomal doxorubicin-cyclophosphamide combination in breast cancer patients with brain metastases: a monocentric retrospective study. *J Neurooncol.* 2014;117(2):253–259.

117. Anders C, Deal AM, Abramson V, et al. TBCRC 018: phase II study of iniparib in combination with irinotecan to treat progressive triple negative breast cancer brain metastases. *Breast Cancer Res Treat.* 2014;146(3):557–566.

118. Siena S, Crino L, Danova M, et al. Dose-dense temozolomide regimen for the treatment of brain metastases from melanoma, breast cancer, or lung cancer not amenable to surgery or radiosurgery: a multicenter phase II study. *Ann Oncol.* 2010;21(3):655–661.

119. Abrey LE, Olson JD, Raizer JJ, et al. A phase II trial of temozolomide for patients with recurrent or progressive brain metastases. *J Neurooncol.* 2001;53(3):259–265.

120. Christodoulou C, Bafaloukos D, Kosmidis P, et al. Phase II study of temozolomide in heavily pretreated cancer patients with brain metastases. *Ann Oncol.* 2001;12(2):249–254.

121. Iwamoto FM, Omuro AM, Raizer JJ, et al. A phase II trial of vinorelbine and intensive temozolomide for patients with recurrent or progressive brain metastases. *J Neurooncol.* 2008;87(1):85–90.

122. Freedman RA, Gelman RS, Wefel JS, et al. Translational breast Cancer Research Consortium (TBCRC) 022: a phase II trial of neratinib for patients with human epidermal growth factor receptor 2-positive breast cancer and brain metastases. *J Clin Oncol.* 2016;34(9):945–952.

123. Freedman RA, Gelman RS, Melisko ME, et al. TBCRC 022: phase II trial of neratinib+ capecitabine for patients (Pts) with human epidermal growth factor receptor 2 (HER2+) breast cancer brain metastases (BCBM). *J Clin Oncol.* 2017;35(15 suppl):1005.

124. Sequist LV, Yang JC, Yamamoto N, et al. Phase III study of afatinib or cisplatin plus pemetrexed in patients with metastatic lung adenocarcinoma with EGFR mutations. *J Clin Oncol.* 2013;31(27):3327–3334.

125. Harbeck N, Huang CS, Hurvitz S, et al. Afatinib plus vinorelbine versus trastuzumab plus vinorelbine in patients with HER2-overexpressing metastatic breast cancer who had progressed on one previous trastuzumab treatment (LUX-Breast 1): an open-label, randomised, phase 3 trial. *Lancet Oncol.* 2016;17(3):357–366.

126. Metzger O, Barry W, Krop I, et al. *Abstract P1-12-04: Phase I Dose-Escalation Trial of ONT-380 in Combination with Trastuzumab in Patients (pts) with HER2+ Breast Cancer Brain Metastases.* AACR; 2017.

127. Hamilton E, Borges V, Conlin A, Walker L, Moulder S. *Abstract P4-21-01: Efficacy Results of a Phase 1b Study of ONT-380, an Oral HER2-Specific Inhibitor, in Combination with Capecitabine (C) and Trastuzumab (T) in HER2+ Metastatic Breast Cancer (MBC), Including Patients (pts) with Brain Metastases (mets).* AACR; 2017.

128. Hortobagyi GN, Stemmer SM, Burris HA, et al. Ribociclib as first-line therapy for HR-positive, advanced breast cancer. *N Engl J Med.* 2016;375(18):1738–1748.

129. Finn RS, Martin M, Rugo HS, et al. Palbociclib and Letrozole in advanced breast cancer. *N Engl J Med.* 2016; 375(20):1925–1936.
130. Sledge Jr GW, Toi M, Neven P, et al. MONARCH 2: abemaciclib in combination with fulvestrant in women with HR+/HER2- advanced breast cancer who had progressed while receiving endocrine therapy. *J Clin Oncol.* 2017;35(25):2875–2884.
131. Luen SJ, Salgado R, Fox S, et al. Tumour-infiltrating lymphocytes in advanced HER2-positive breast cancer treated with pertuzumab or placebo in addition to trastuzumab and docetaxel: a retrospective analysis of the CLEOPATRA study. *Lancet Oncol.* 2017;18(1):52–62.
132. Duchnowska R, Peksa R, Radecka B, et al. Immune response in breast cancer brain metastases and their microenvironment: the role of the PD-1/PD-L axis. *Breast Cancer Res.* 2016;18(1):43.
133. Goldberg SB, Gettinger SN, Mahajan A, et al. Pembrolizumab for patients with melanoma or non-small-cell lung cancer and untreated brain metastases: early analysis of a non-randomised, open-label, phase 2 trial. *Lancet Oncol.* 2016;17(7):976–983.
134. Tawbi HA-H, Forsyth PA, Algazi AP, et al. Efficacy and safety of nivolumab (NIVO) plus ipilimumab (IPI) in patients with melanoma (MEL) metastatic to the brain: results of the phase II study CheckMate 204. *J Clin Oncol.* 2017;35(15 suppl):9507.
135. Long GV, Atkinson V, Menzies AM, et al. A randomized phase II study of nivolumab or nivolumab combined with ipilimumab in patients (pts) with melanoma brain metastases (mets): the Anti-PD1 Brain Collaboration (ABC). *J Clin Oncol.* 2017;35(15 suppl):9508.
136. Samuels Y, Wang Z, Bardelli A, et al. High frequency of mutations of the PIK3CA gene in human cancers. *Science (New York NY).* 2004;304(5670):554.
137. Liu P, Cheng H, Roberts TM, Zhao JJ. Targeting the phosphoinositide 3-kinase pathway in cancer. *Nat Rev.* 2009;8(8):627–644.
138. Vogt PK, Kang S, Elsliger MA, Gymnopoulos M. Cancer-specific mutations in phosphatidylinositol 3-kinase. *Trends Biochem Sci.* 2007;32(7):342–349.
139. Yuan TL, Cantley LC. PI3K pathway alterations in cancer: variations on a theme. *Oncogene.* 2008;27(41):5497–5510.
140. Zhao JJ, Cheng H, Jia S, et al. The p110alpha isoform of PI3K is essential for proper growth factor signaling and oncogenic transformation. *Proc Natl Acad Sci USA.* 2006;103(44):16296–16300.
141. Adamo B, Deal AM, Burrows E, et al. Phosphatidylinositol 3-kinase pathway activation in breast cancer brain metastases. *Breast Cancer Res.* 2011;13(6):R125.
142. Wikman H, Lamszus K, Detels N, et al. Relevance of PTEN loss in brain metastasis formation in breast cancer patients. *Breast Cancer Res.* 2012;14(2):R49.
143. Ni J, Ramkissoon SH, Xie S, et al. Combination inhibition of PI3K and mTORC1 yields durable remissions in mice bearing orthotopic patient-derived xenografts of HER2-positive breast cancer brain metastases. *Nat Med.* 2016;22(7):723–726.
144. Anders CK, Deal AM, Van Swearingen AED, et al. LCCC 1025: phase II study of everolimus, trastuzumab, and vinorelbine for HER2+ breast cancer brain metastases (BCBM). *J Clin Oncol.* 2017;35(15 suppl):1011.
145. Thomas FC, Taskar K, Rudraraju V, et al. Uptake of ANG1005, a novel paclitaxel derivative, through the blood-brain barrier into brain and experimental brain metastases of breast cancer. *Pharm Res.* 2009;26(11):2486–2494.
146. O'Sullivan CC, Lindenberg M, Bryla C, et al. ANG1005 for breast cancer brain metastases: correlation between 18F-FLT-PET after first cycle and MRI in response assessment. *Breast Cancer Res Treat.* 2016;160(1):51–59.
147. Kumthekar P, Tang S-C, Brenner AJ, et al. ANG1005, a novel brain-penetrant taxane derivative, for the treatment of recurrent brain metastases and leptomeningeal carcinomatosis from breast cancer. *J Clin Oncol.* 2016;34(15 suppl):2004.
148. Cortes J, Rugo HS, Awada A, et al. Prolonged survival in patients with breast cancer and a history of brain metastases: results of a preplanned subgroup analysis from the randomized phase III BEACON trial. *Breast Cancer Res Treat.* 2017;165(2):329–341.
149. Lin NU, Stein A, Nicholas A, et al. Planned interim analysis of PATRICIA: an open-label, single-arm, phase II study of pertuzumab (P) with high-dose trastuzumab (H) for the treatment of central nervous system (CNS) progression post radiotherapy (RT) in patients (pts) with HER2-positive metastatic breast cancer (MBC). *J Clin Oncol.* 2017;35(15 suppl):2074.
150. Niwinska A. Brain metastases as site of first and isolated recurrence of breast cancer: the role of systemic therapy after local treatment. *Clin Exp Metastasis.* 2016;33(7):677–685.

CHAPTER 6

Neoadjuvant Treatment of HER2-Positive Breast Cancer—A Review

PETER A. FASCHING, MD • NAIBA NABIEVA, MD • FREDERIK STÜBS, MD • MICHAEL UNTCH, MD, PHD

INTRODUCTION AND RATIONALE FOR NEOADJUVANT THERAPY IN HER2-POSITIVE PATIENTS

Around 15%−25% of breast cancer (BC) patients have a tumor that overexpresses human epidermal growth factor receptor 2 (HER2) or has an amplification of the *HER2* gene.[1,2] Anti-HER2-directed therapy with the monoclonal antibody trastuzumab was first approved for metastatic BC on the basis of a significant improvement in progression-free survival (PFS) as well as overall survival (OS).[3] Further studies also demonstrated a significant benefit in disease-free survival (DFS) and OS when adding trastuzumab to adjuvant chemotherapy for HER2-positive (HER2+) BC. On this basis, trastuzumab became the standard of care in the adjuvant treatment setting of HER2+ BC patients.[4−6]

Several studies have shown that neoadjuvant treatment is equivalent to adjuvant treatment with regard to prognosis.[7−9] A recent metaanalysis of the Early Breast Cancer Trialists Collaborative Group confirmed that neoadjuvant therapy had no disadvantages with regard to distant recurrence and mortality, but tumors downsized by neoadjuvant chemotherapy may have higher local recurrence after breast-conserving therapy than tumors of similar size which were treated with primary surgery.[10]

Neoadjuvant treatment offers some advantages over adjuvant treatment. Neoadjuvant therapy not only results in a higher rate of breast-conserving surgeries because of a reduction in tumor size[10,11] but also yields important prognostic information.[9] A pathologic complete response (pCR) at surgery is associated with a better survival than is seen in patients who do not achieve a pCR.[8,9,12] This has been confirmed in pooled analyses that have found a strong association between pCR and DFS and OS in patients with triple-negative BC and HER2+ BC, especially hormone receptor-negative,

HER2+ BC.[13,14] In fact, to accelerate approval of new drugs, both the Food and Drug Administration (FDA) and the European Medicines Agency (EMA) allow pCR as a primary endpoint for neoadjuvant clinical trials as a surrogate marker for prognosis.[15−17]

CLINICAL STUDIES FOR NEOADJUVANT ANTI-HER2 TREATMENT

A series of studies in the neoadjuvant setting have been conducted with primary HER2+ BC patients. Table 6.1 shows a summary of the relevant trials, trial designs, and results.

Introduction of Trastuzumab Into the Neoadjuvant Therapy Setting

The TECHNO trial was one of the first trials to analyze the frequency of pCR with neoadjuvant chemotherapy combined with trastuzumab and its effect on prognosis. A total of 39% of patients achieved a pCR, proving the high efficacy of this therapy in the neoadjuvant setting. Those who attained pCR had a 3-year OS of 96.3% compared with 85.0% in those without pCR ($P = .007$). pCR was the only significant prognostic factor for patient survival (DFS hazard ratio [HR] 2.49, 95% CI 1.22−5.09, $P = .013$; OS HR 4.91, 95% CI 1.42−17.00, $P = .012$).[18]

In the NOAH trial, chemotherapy was given in the neoadjuvant setting with or without trastuzumab (neoadjuvantly in combination with chemotherapy followed by adjuvant monotherapy to complete a year of therapy) in patients with locally advanced BC. Thirty-eight percent of HER2+ patients in the trastuzumab arm achieved a pCR versus only 19% in the control arm ($P = .001$). The 3-year DFS was 71% (95% CI 61−78) and OS 87% (95% CI 79−92) with trastuzumab compared with 56% (95% CI 46−65) and 79% (95% CI 70−86), respectively, with chemotherapy

TABLE 6.1
Differently Defined pCR Across the Studies

Study	Year	Country	Number of Patients (n)	Phase	Randomization	Neoadjuvant Treatment Arms	pCR	p
BERENICE[49]	2017	International	400	II	Yes	A: Doxorubicin plus cyclophosphamide, followed by paclitaxel plus trastuzumab plus pertuzumab B: Fluorouracil plus epirubicin plus cyclophosphamide, followed by docetaxel plus trastuzumab plus pertuzumab	A: 61.8% (95% CI 54.7–68.6) B: 60.7% (95% CI 53.6–67.5)	NA
CALGB 40601[26]	2016	USA	295	III	Yes	A: Taxane plus trastuzumab B: Taxane plus lapatinib C: Taxane plus trastuzumab plus lapatinib	A: 44% (95% CI 35%–53%) B: 27% (95% CI 18%–40%) C: 52% (95% CI 43%–61%)	NA
CHER-LOB[50]	2012	Italy	121	II	Yes	A: Paclitaxel plus trastuzumab, followed by fluorouracil plus epirubicin plus cyclophosphamide plus trastuzumab B: Paclitaxel plus lapatinib, followed by fluorouracil plus epirubicin plus cyclophosphamide plus lapatinib C: Paclitaxel plus trastuzumab plus lapatinib, followed by fluorouracil plus epirubicin plus cyclophosphamide plus trastuzumab plus lapatinib	A: 25% (90% CI 13.1%–36.9%) B: 26.3% (90% CI 14.5%–38.1%) C: 46.7% (90% CI 34.4%–58.9%)	C versus A and B: 0.019
GEICAM/ 2006–14[51]	2014	Spain	99	II	Yes	A: Epirubicin plus cyclophosphamide, followed by docetaxel plus trastuzumab B. Epirubicin plus cyclophosphamide, followed by docetaxel plus lapatinib	A: 47.9% (95% CI 33.8%–62.0%) B: 23.5% (95% CI 11.9%–35.1%)	0.0112

Study	Year	Country	Phase	Randomized	Treatment	pCR	p-value
GeparQuattro[21]	2010	Germany	III	Yes	A: Epirubicin plus cyclophosphamide plus trastuzumab, followed by docetaxel plus trastuzumab B: Epirubicin plus cyclophosphamide plus trastuzumab, followed by docetaxel plus trastuzumab plus capecitabine C: Epirubicin plus cyclophosphamide plus trastuzumab, followed by docetaxel plus trastuzumab, followed by capecitabine plus trastuzumab	A: 32.9% (no CI available) B: 31.3% (no CI available) C: 34.6% (no CI available)	NA
GeparQuinto[23]	2012	Germany Switzerland	III	Yes	A: Epirubicin plus cyclophosphamide plus trastuzumab, followed by docetaxel plus trastuzumab B: Epirubicin plus cyclophosphamide plus lapatinib, followed by docetaxel plus lapatinib	A: 30.3% (no CI available) B: 22.7% (no CI available)	0.04
GeparSixto[52]	2014	Germany	II	Yes	A: Paclitaxel plus nonpegylated liposomal doxorubicin plus trastuzumab plus lapatinib plus carboplatin B: Paclitaxel plus nonpegylated liposomal doxorubicin plus trastuzumab plus lapatinib	A: 32.8% (95% CI 25.0–40.7) B: 36.8% (95% CI 28.7–44.9)	0.581
GeparSepto[36]	2016	Germany	III	Yes	A: Nab-paclitaxel plus trastuzumab plus pertuzumab, followed by epirubicin plus cyclophosphamide plus trastuzumab plus pertuzumab B: Paclitaxel plus trastuzumab plus pertuzumab, followed by epirubicin plus cyclophosphamide plus trastuzumab plus pertuzumab	A: 62% (no CI available) B: 54% (no CI available)	0.13
HannaH[53]	2012	International	III	Yes	A: Docetaxel plus trastuzumab intravenous, followed by fluorouracil plus epirubicin plus cyclophosphamide plus trastuzumab intravenous B: Docetaxel plus trastuzumab subcutaneous, followed by fluorouracil plus epirubicin plus cyclophosphamide plus trastuzumab subcutaneous	A: 34.2% (95% CI 28.5–40.3) B: 39.2% (95% CI 33.3–45.5)	NA

Continued

TABLE 6.1
Differently Defined pCR Across the Studies—cont'd

Study	Year	Country	Number of Patients (n)	Phase	Randomization	Neoadjuvant Treatment Arms	pCR	p
KRISTINE[33]	2018	International	444	III	Yes	A: Trastuzumab emtansine plus pertuzumab B: Docetaxel plus carboplatin plus trastuzumab plus pertuzumab	A: 44.4% (no CI available) B: 55.7% (no CI available)	0.016
NeoALTTO[24]	2012	International	440	III	Yes	A: Lapatinib, followed by paclitaxel plus lapatinib B: Trastuzumab, followed by paclitaxel plus trastuzumab C: Lapatinib plus trastuzumab, followed by paclitaxel plus lapatinib plus trastuzumab	A: 20.0% (97.5% CI 13.9–27.3) B: 27.6% (97.5% CI 20.5–36.2) C: 46.8% (no CI available)	B versus C: 0.13 C versus B: 0.0007
NeoSphere[29]	2012	International	417	II	Yes	A: Trastuzumab plus docetaxel B: Trastuzumab plus pertuzumab plus docetaxel C: Trastuzumab plus pertuzumab D: Pertuzumab plus docetaxel	A: 21.5% (95% CI 14.1–30.5) B: 39.3% (95% CI 30.0–49.2) C: 11.2% (95% CI 5.9–18.8) D: 17.7% (95% CI 10.7–26.8)	NA
NOAH[19]	2010	International	235	III	Yes	A: Doxorubicin plus paclitaxel, followed by paclitaxel, followed by cyclophosphamide plus methotrexate plus fluorouracil B: Doxorubicin plus paclitaxel, followed by paclitaxel, followed by cyclophosphamide plus methotrexate plus fluorouracil plus trastuzumab	A: 19% (no CI available) B: 38% (no CI available)	0.001
NSABP B41[27]	2013	USA	518	III	Yes	A: Doxorubicin plus cyclophosphamide, followed by paclitaxel plus trastuzumab B: Doxorubicin plus cyclophosphamide, followed by paclitaxel plus lapatinib C: Doxorubicin plus cyclophosphamide, followed by paclitaxel plus trastuzumab plus lapatinib	A: 49.4% (95% CI 41.8–56.5) B: 47.4% (95% CI 39.8–54.6) C: 60.2% (95% CI 52.5–67.1)	C versus A: 0.056 B versus A: 0.78

Study	Year	Country	N	Phase	Randomized	Treatment	pCR	p
TECHNO[18]	2011	Germany	217	II	No	Epirubicin plus cyclophosphamide, followed by paclitaxel plus trastuzumab	pCR: 22.6% (no CI available)	NA
TRYPHAENA[54]	2013	International	225	II	Yes	A: Fluorouracil plus epirubicin plus cyclophosphamide plus trastuzumab plus pertuzumab, followed by docetaxel plus trastuzumab plus pertuzumab B: Fluorouracil plus epirubicin plus cyclophosphamide, followed by docetaxel plus trastuzumab plus pertuzumab C: Docetaxel plus carboplatin plus trastuzumab plus pertuzumab	A: 50.7% (no CI available) B: 45.3% (no CI available) C: 51.9% (no CI available)	NA
WSG-ADAPT HER2+/HR-[55]	2017	Germany	132	II	Yes	A: Trastuzumab plus pertuzumab B: Trastuzumab plus pertuzumab plus paclitaxel	A: 24.4% (no CI available) B: 78.6% (no CI available)	NA
WSG-ADAPT HER2+/HR+[32]	2016	Germany	376	II	Yes	A: T-DM1 B: T-DM1 plus endocrine treatment C: Trastuzumab plus endocrine treatment	A: 40.5% (no CI available) B: 45.8% (no CI available) C: 6.7% (no CI available)	A and B versus C: 0.001

NA, not assessed. If ypT0 ypN0 and ypT0/is ypN0 were both reported in an analysis, then the results on ypT0 ypN0 are reported here. If pCR results were demonstrated for breast and for breast with lymph nodes separately, then results on breast with lymph nodes are reported here. If there were only results on ypT0/is ypN0 or only on pCR of the breast, these results are listed as pCR in the present work.

alone.[19] With longer follow-up, the survival benefit in the trastuzumab group was maintained. Patients who achieved a pCR under treatment with trastuzumab had a significantly improved DFS (HR 0.29, 95% CI 0.11–0.78) and OS (HR 0.27, 95% CI 0.09–0.83), again demonstrating that pCR is associated with a better prognosis in HER2+ BC patients receiving anti-HER2 therapy with trastuzumab.[20] A beneficial impact on pCR with the addition of trastuzumab to neoadjuvant chemotherapy with anthracyclines was also demonstrated in GeparQuattro.[21]

Lapatinib and Trastuzumab in the Neoadjuvant Treatment

Lapatinib, a small molecule dual tyrosine kinase inhibitor, was first approved for the therapy of HER2+ metastatic BC.[22] GeparQuinto investigated whether neoadjuvant lapatinib is equivalent to trastuzumab when combined with chemotherapy. 30.3% of the patients in the trastuzumab arm and only 22.7% of the patients in the lapatinib arm had a pCR (OR 0.68, 95% CI 0.47%–0.97%, P = .04).[23] In the NeoALLTO trial, lapatinib, trastuzumab, and lapatinib plus trastuzumab were analyzed in combination with neoadjuvant chemotherapy. Patients given lapatinib achieved a pCR of 20.0% versus 27.6% with trastuzumab (P = .13). The combination of lapatinib and trastuzumab, however, resulted in a significantly higher pCR rate of 46.8% compared with trastuzumab alone (OR 2.39; 97.5% CI 1.36–4.26; P = .0007). Lapatinib was associated with more adverse events than trastuzumab.[24] Later analyses showed a 3-year event-free survival (EFS) of 78% (95% CI 70%–84%) and OS of 93% (95% CI 87%–96%) with lapatinib, 76% (95% CI 68%–82%) and 90% (95% CI 84%–94%) with trastuzumab, and 84% (95% CI 77%–89%) and 95% (95% CI 90%–98%) with the combination. Neither EFS nor OS differed significantly between the three arms. However, women who achieved a pCR had a significant improvement in 3-year EFS (HR 0.38, 95% CI 0.22–0.63, P = .0003) and OS (HR 0.35, 95% CI 0.15–0.70, P = .005), confirming again the importance of pCR with neoadjuvant treatment.[25] In contrast, the NSABP B41 and CALGB 40601 did not demonstrate superiority of the substitution of trastuzumab with lapatinib or a combination of both drugs compared with trastuzumab alone with regard to pCR[26,27]. Therefore, lapatinib has not been recommended for neoadjuvant use.

Pertuzumab and Trastuzumab

The safety and efficacy of dual HER2 blockade was also investigated with the anti-HER2 antibody pertuzumab, also first approved for metastatic BC[28] combined with trastuzumab. In the 4-arm, phase II NeoSphere trial, patients received neoadjuvant therapy with either docetaxel plus trastuzumab (TH), docetaxel plus pertuzumab (TP), docetaxel plus trastuzumab and pertuzumab (THP), or trastuzumab plus pertuzumab without chemotherapy (HP). All patients received FEC chemotherapy in the adjuvant setting. The highest pCR rate was observed in the THP arm (45.8%; 95% CI 36.1–55.7). In contrast, TH was associated with a pCR of 29.0% (95% CI 20.6–38.5), TP with a pCR of 24.0% (95% CI 15.8–33.7), and HP with a pCR of only 16.8% (95% CI 10.3–25.3). The high pCR rate associated with the THP regimen (without a significant increase in the occurrence of severe adverse events) led to the approval of this neoadjuvant regimen by the FDA in 2013.[29] The 5-year PFS and DFS in patients who received docetaxel in combination with trastuzumab and pertuzumab were 86% (95% CI 77–91) and 84% (95% CI 72–91), respectively. Women across all groups who achieved pCR benefitted from a longer PFS than those without pCR (85% vs. 76%; HR 0.54; 95% CI 0.29–1.00).[30]

The 3-arm phase II TRYPHAENA trial also evaluated dual HER2-targeting with pertuzumab plus trastuzumab in the neoadjuvant setting. Because the combination of anthracyclines with concurrent trastuzumab is associated with cardiotoxicity,[3,31] one arm of this study evaluated a nonanthracycline-based regimen (docetaxel, carboplatin, trastuzumab [TCH]) which demonstrated similar efficacy and improved toxicity compared with an anthracycline-based regimen in the adjuvant setting.[6] Patients assigned to this arm received six cycles of TCHP before surgery. The other two arms evaluated the safety and pCR rates for anthracycline-based regimens: three cycles of FEC given concurrently with HP followed by three cycles of THP (FECHP-THP) or three cycles of FEC followed by three cycles of THP (FEC-THP). High pCR rates were observed for all three regimens with the highest pCR rates in the nonanthracycline TCHP arm. pCR (ypT0/is) for TCHP was 66.2% (n = 76), 61.6% for FECHP-THP (n = 72), and 57.3% for FEC-THP (n = 75). The results from this study led to the FDA approval of the TCHP and FEC-THP regimens as neoadjuvant therapy in 2013. The arm with concurrent anthracyclines and HP (FECHP-THP) has not received FDA approval because of the lack of established cardiac safety.

Trastuzumab Emtansine (T-DM1)

Given the activity and excellent tolerability of the antibody drug conjugate T-DM1 in the metastatic setting, studies have been designed to evaluate whether this molecule could replace traditional cytotoxic chemotherapy in the early stage setting. In the ADAPT trial for patients with HER2+, hormone receptor-positive BC compared T-DM1 (alone or with an aromatase inhibitor [AI]) with trastuzumab plus an aromatase inhibitor in the neoadjuvant setting. The interim analysis showed meaningful pCR rates of greater than 40% after treatment with T-DM1 for 12 weeks,[32] which was statistically significantly higher than that achieved with trastuzumab plus AI. Interestingly, addition of an AI to T-DM1 did not improve pCR rates. While these data are intriguing and support the further evaluation of a deescalation strategy in some patients with hormone receptor coexpressing tumors, the phase III KRISTINE (TRIO-021) study demonstrated a clear superiority of neoadjuvant TCHP over T-DM1 combined with pertuzumab in terms of pCR (55.7% vs. 44.4%, $P = .016$).[33] For now, T-DM1 remains investigational in the early stage setting. Ongoing studies such as ATEMPT (NCT01853748) will further define whether T-DM1 has a role in the curative setting for lower risk patients.

CDK4/6 Inhibitors

Given their efficacy in hormone receptor-positive, HER2-negative BCs, CDK4/6 inhibitors are being investigated in combination with anti-HER2 therapy in the hormone receptor-positive, HER2+ setting.[34] Patients with hormone receptor-positive, HER2+ BC were given neoadjuvant treatment with trastuzumab, pertuzumab, selective estrogen receptor antagonist fulvestrant, and CDK4/6 inhibitor palbociclib in the NA-PHER2 study. At the time of surgery, Ki-67 expression was significantly reduced compared with baseline expression before therapy ($P = .013$), indicating that CDK4/6 inhibition might be a reasonable combination therapy in this patient group.[35]

Optimizing Neoadjuvant Chemotherapy

The neoadjuvant setting has also been used to evaluate a number of chemotherapies for HER2+ disease. For example, the GeparSepto trial compared the efficacy of the addition of nab-paclitaxel versus paclitaxel to neoadjuvant chemotherapy with epirubicin and cyclophosphamide in patients with hormonally driven, HER2+, or triple-negative BCs. Patients with HER2+ disease received concurrent pertuzumab and trastuzumab. There was no significant difference in pCR with nab-paclitaxel compared with solvent-based paclitaxel (62% vs. 54%; $P = .13$), and there was also no significant difference in pCR in patients with hormone receptor-negative, HER2+ disease versus hormone receptor-positive, HER2+ BC ($P = .49$ and $P = .30$,

respectively).[36] The total study population showed a clear benefit from nab-paclitaxel with regard to disease-free survival (HR = 0.69; 95% CI 0.54–0.89). Although there was no statistically significant benefit in the HER2+ subpopulation, patients with hormone receptor-negative, HER2+ disease showed the lowest HR (0.50; 95% CI: 0.18–1.41).

pCR AND PROGNOSIS: IMPLICATIONS FOR CLINICAL USE

National and international therapy guidelines have included therapeutic options for the neoadjuvant treatment of HER2+ BC for several years. Given that pCR may be a surrogate marker for long-term prognosis[13,14] of HER2+ disease, both the FDA and the EMA consider pCR rate an acceptable endpoint in the neoadjuvant setting.[15,16] In fact, pCR was sufficient for the approval of pertuzumab for neoadjuvant treatment of primary BC.[37,38]

While there seems to be a consistent positive correlation between increases in pCR rates and better prognosis in anti-HER2 clinical trials,[17,30] the large benefit in pCR rates with the addition of pertuzumab to standard trastuzumab-based chemotherapy did not translate into a correspondingly large improvement in DFS in the adjuvant APHINITY trial. That said, several trials in the neoadjuvant setting comparing either trastuzumab and chemotherapy with chemotherapy alone or comparing two anti-HER2-directed therapies seemed to demonstrate a reasonable correlation between odds ratios and HRs (Fig. 6.1). The higher the improvement of pCRs in those trials, the more patients benefited with regard to prognosis.

EVALUATION OF MOLECULAR PREDICTORS OF RESPONSE

One advantage of the neoadjuvant study design is that serial tumor biopsies can be taken before, during, and after treatment with systemic therapy, which allows scientists to evaluate various mechanisms of resistance and to explore for biomarkers that are predictive of response to therapy.

Genomic Instability

Genomic analysis of tumor samples collected during the NeoALTTO trial suggests that higher pCR rate may be associated with higher genomic instability ($P = .03$) as measured by copy number alterations. This effect seemed stronger in patients with hormone receptor-positive, HER2+ BC. While a gene or region that predicts EFS could not be found, the amplification

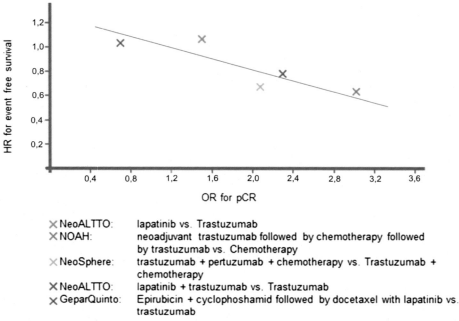

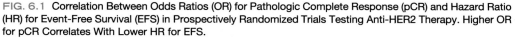

✕ NeoALTTO:	lapatinib vs. Trastuzumab
✕ NOAH:	neoadjuvant trastuzumab followed by chemotherapy followed by trastuzumab vs. Chemotherapy
✕ NeoSphere:	trastuzumab + pertuzumab + chemotherapy vs. Trastuzumab + chemotherapy
✕ NeoALTTO:	lapatinib + trastuzumab vs. Trastuzumab
✕ GeparQuinto:	Epirubicin + cyclophoshamid followed by docetaxel with lapatinib vs. trastuzumab

FIG. 6.1 Correlation Between Odds Ratios (OR) for Pathologic Complete Response (pCR) and Hazard Ratio (HR) for Event-Free Survival (EFS) in Prospectively Randomized Trials Testing Anti-HER2 Therapy. Higher OR for pCR Correlates With Lower HR for EFS.

of two regions on chromosome 6 was identified to be significantly associated with higher pCR ($P = .00005$ and $P = .00087$).[39]

Gene Expression

In CALBG 40601 study, genomic signatures were also investigated. Higher *HER2* expression was considered an independent factor associated with higher pCR rates, while estrogen receptor 1 (*ESR1*) expression seemed to be linked to lower pCR rates. Multivariable analysis demonstrated a significant association between pCR and *ESR1* (OR 0.71; 95% CI 0.54–0.93; $P = .0139$), *HER2* (OR 1.68; CI 95% 1.25–2.28; $P < .001$), and *TP53* (OR 2.33; 95% CI 1.18–4.71; $P = .014$) signatures.[26]

The role of phosphatase and tensin homologue (*PTEN*) has also been investigated. High *PTEN*-expressing tumors were associated with higher pCR rates compared with those with low *PTEN*-expressing tumors (57.1% vs. 27.6%; $P = .010$). This analysis also showed a potential interaction between *PTEN* and phosphatidylinositol 3-kinase (*PI3KCA*) mutations, which needs further investigation.[40]

Activating Mutations in Phosphatidylinositol 3-Kinase

PI3KCA mutation has been shown to be significantly associated with a lower pCR in HER2+ BC ($P < .001$), especially in patients with hormone receptor coexpression (7.6% vs. 24.2% in the wild-type group; $P < .001$). Those patients with hormone receptor-positive disease seemed also to have a significantly worse DFS (HR 1.56; 95% CI 1.00–2.45; $P = .050$), indicating that there might be an interaction between hormone receptor and *PI3KCA* mutation status that leads to resistance mechanisms for anti-HER2 treatment.[41] Further studies show similar results.[42,43] Based on the understanding that activating *PI3KCA* mutations can contribute to tumor resistance to HER2-directed therapy, the neoPHOEBE trial was designed to assess the efficacy of the PI3K inhibitor buparlisib to trastuzumab and chemotherapy in the neoadjuvant setting. Because of a high proportion of patients suffering from liver toxicity, enrollment was stopped and the study could not be completed.[44] The PI3K inhibitor alpelisib seems to be less toxic than buparlisib and effective in hormone receptor-positive/HER2-negative metastatic BC patients with a *PI3KCA* mutation.[45] PI3K inhibition could further improve patients' outcomes in HER2-positive BC.

Immune Responsiveness

Immune responsiveness may also be prognostic or predictive of outcomes for HER2+ BC. Analysis of RNA-based gene expression signatures from the neoadjuvant CALGB 40601 showed that immune activation, as measured by an IgG signature, was significantly associated with longer DFS (HR = 0.69; P = .05), suggesting this signature could be of possible prognostic value.[46] Moreover, data indicate that patients who achieve pCR seem to have an activated immune response.[47] Margetuximab, a HER2-targeted antibody designed with an Fc portion that has high affinity to Fc-γ receptor IIIA, seems to enhance antibody-dependent cellular cytotoxicity (ADCC) and to be well-tolerated.[48] It is currently being investigated in HER2+ metastatic BC in the phase III SOPHIA trial.

CONCLUSIONS

Many open questions regarding the optimal neoadjuvant treatment of HER2+ BC remain. Novel treatment combinations and sequences are being investigated in current trials. De novo resistance mechanisms and predictive factors for response are not fully understood. The implementation of therapies from the metastatic setting into neoadjuvant treatment algorithms requires significant improvement in patient outcomes and tolerability. Further analyses are necessary to answer these questions.

REFERENCES

1. Wolff AC, Hammond ME, Hicks DG, et al. Recommendations for human epidermal growth factor receptor 2 testing in breast cancer: American Society of Clinical Oncology/College of American Pathologists clinical practice guideline update. *J Clin Oncol.* 2013;31:3997—4013.
2. Hartkopf AD, Huober J, Volz B, et al. Treatment landscape of advanced breast cancer patients with hormone receptor positive HER2 negative tumors - data from the German PRAEGNANT breast cancer registry. *Breast.* 2018;37:42—51.
3. Slamon DJ, Leyland-Jones B, Shak S, et al. Use of chemotherapy plus a monoclonal antibody against HER2 for metastatic breast cancer that overexpresses HER2. *N Engl J Med.* 2001;344:783—792.
4. Piccart-Gebhart MJ, Procter M, Leyland-Jones B, et al. Trastuzumab after adjuvant chemotherapy in HER2-positive breast cancer. *N Engl J Med.* 2005;353:1659—1672.
5. Perez EA, Romond EH, Suman VJ, et al. Trastuzumab plus adjuvant chemotherapy for human epidermal growth factor receptor 2-positive breast cancer: planned joint analysis of overall survival from NSABP B-31 and NCCTG N9831. *J Clin Oncol.* 2014;32:3744—3752.
6. Slamon D, Eiermann W, Robert N, et al. Adjuvant trastuzumab in HER2-positive breast cancer. *N Engl J Med.* 2011;365:1273—1283.
7. Mauri D, Pavlidis N, Ioannidis JP. Neoadjuvant versus adjuvant systemic treatment in breast cancer: a meta-analysis. *J Natl Cancer Inst.* 2005;97:188—194.
8. Mieog JS, van der Hage JA, van de Velde CJ. Preoperative chemotherapy for women with operable breast cancer. *Cochrane Database Syst Rev.* 2007:CD005002.
9. Fisher B, Bryant J, Wolmark N, et al. Effect of preoperative chemotherapy on the outcome of women with operable breast cancer. *J Clin Oncol.* 1998;16:2672—2685.
10. Early Breast Cancer Trialists' Collaborative G. Long-term outcomes for neoadjuvant versus adjuvant chemotherapy in early breast cancer: meta-analysis of individual patient data from ten randomised trials. *Lancet Oncol.* 2018;19:27—39.
11. Fisher B, Brown A, Mamounas E, et al. Effect of preoperative chemotherapy on local-regional disease in women with operable breast cancer: findings from National Surgical Adjuvant Breast and Bowel Project B-18. *J Clin Oncol.* 1997;15:2483—2493.
12. Esserman LJ, Berry DA, DeMichele A, et al. Pathologic complete response predicts recurrence-free survival more effectively by cancer subset: results from the I-SPY 1 TRIAL—CALGB 150007/150012, ACRIN 6657. *J Clin Oncol.* 2012;30:3242—3249.
13. Cortazar P, Zhang L, Untch M, et al. Pathological complete response and long-term clinical benefit in breast cancer: the CTNeoBC pooled analysis. *Lancet.* 2014;384:164—172.
14. von Minckwitz G, Untch M, Blohmer JU, et al. Definition and impact of pathologic complete response on prognosis after neoadjuvant chemotherapy in various intrinsic breast cancer subtypes. *J Clin Oncol.* 2012;30:1796—1804.
15. European Medicines Agency. *The Role of the Pathological Complete Response as an Endpoint in Neoadjuvant Breast Cancer Studies*; 2014. http://www.ema.europa.eu/docs/en_GB/document_library/Scientific_guideline/2014/04/WC500165781.pdf.
16. US Department of Health and Human Services. *Guidance for Industry Pathological Complete Response in Neoadjuvant Treatment of High-risk Early-stage Breast Cancer: Use as an Endpoint to Support Accelerated Approval*. Food and Drug Administration Center for Drug Evaluation and Research; 2014. https://www.fda.gov/downloads/drugs/guidances/ucm305501.pdf 2014.
17. Cortazar P, Geyer Jr CE. Pathological complete response in neoadjuvant treatment of breast cancer. *Ann Surg Oncol.* 2015;22:1441—1446.

18. Untch M, Fasching PA, Konecny GE, et al. Pathologic complete response after neoadjuvant chemotherapy plus trastuzumab predicts favorable survival in human epidermal growth factor receptor 2-overexpressing breast cancer: results from the TECHNO trial of the AGO and GBG study groups. *J Clin Oncol.* 2011;29:3351−3357.

19. Gianni L, Eiermann W, Semiglazov V, et al. Neoadjuvant chemotherapy with trastuzumab followed by adjuvant trastuzumab versus neoadjuvant chemotherapy alone, in patients with HER2-positive locally advanced breast cancer (the NOAH trial): a randomised controlled superiority trial with a parallel HER2-negative cohort. *Lancet.* 2010; 375:377−384.

20. Gianni L, Eiermann W, Semiglazov V, et al. Neoadjuvant and adjuvant trastuzumab in patients with HER2-positive locally advanced breast cancer (NOAH): follow-up of a randomised controlled superiority trial with a parallel HER2-negative cohort. *Lancet Oncol.* 2014;15:640−647.

21. Untch M, Rezai M, Loibl S, et al. Neoadjuvant treatment with trastuzumab in HER2-positive breast cancer: results from the GeparQuattro study. *J Clin Oncol.* 2010;28: 2024−2031.

22. Cameron D, Casey M, Press M, et al. A phase III randomized comparison of lapatinib plus capecitabine versus capecitabine alone in women with advanced breast cancer that has progressed on trastuzumab: updated efficacy and biomarker analyses. *Breast Cancer Res Treat.* 2008;112: 533−543.

23. Untch M, Loibl S, Bischoff J, et al. Lapatinib versus trastuzumab in combination with neoadjuvant anthracycline-taxane-based chemotherapy (GeparQuinto, GBG 44): a randomised phase 3 trial. *Lancet Oncol.* 2012;13:135−144.

24. Baselga J, Bradbury I, Eidtmann H, et al. Lapatinib with trastuzumab for HER2-positive early breast cancer (NeoALTTO): a randomised, open-label, multicentre, phase 3 trial. *Lancet.* 2012;379:633−640.

25. de Azambuja E, Holmes AP, Piccart-Gebhart M, et al. Lapatinib with trastuzumab for HER2-positive early breast cancer (NeoALTTO): survival outcomes of a randomised, open-label, multicentre, phase 3 trial and their association with pathological complete response. *Lancet Oncol.* 2014; 15:1137−1146.

26. Carey LA, Berry DA, Cirrincione CT, et al. Molecular heterogeneity and response to neoadjuvant human epidermal growth factor receptor 2 targeting in CALGB 40601, a randomized phase III trial of paclitaxel plus trastuzumab with or without lapatinib. *J Clin Oncol.* 2016;34:542−549.

27. Robidoux A, Tang G, Rastogi P, et al. Lapatinib as a component of neoadjuvant therapy for HER2-positive operable breast cancer (NSABP protocol B-41): an open-label, randomised phase 3 trial. *Lancet Oncol.* 2013;14: 1183−1192.

28. Swain SM, Kim SB, Cortes J, et al. Pertuzumab, trastuzumab, and docetaxel for HER2-positive metastatic breast cancer (CLEOPATRA study): overall survival results from a randomised, double-blind, placebo-controlled, phase 3 study. *Lancet Oncol.* 2013;14:461−471.

29. Gianni L, Pienkowski T, Im YH, et al. Efficacy and safety of neoadjuvant pertuzumab and trastuzumab in women with locally advanced, inflammatory, or early HER2-positive breast cancer (NeoSphere): a randomised multicentre, open-label, phase 2 trial. *Lancet Oncol.* 2012;13: 25−32.

30. Gianni L, Pienkowski T, Im YH, et al. 5-year analysis of neoadjuvant pertuzumab and trastuzumab in patients with locally advanced, inflammatory, or early-stage HER2-positive breast cancer (NeoSphere): a multicentre, open-label, phase 2 randomised trial. *Lancet Oncol.* 2016; 17:791−800.

31. Romond EH, Perez EA, Bryant J, et al. Trastuzumab plus adjuvant chemotherapy for operable HER2-positive breast cancer. *N Engl J Med.* 2005;353:1673−1684.

32. Harbeck N, Gluz O, Christgen M, et al. Abstract S5−03: final analysis of WSG-ADAPT HER2+/HR+ phase II trial: efficacy, safety, and predictive markers for 12-weeks of neoadjuvant TDM1 with or without endocrine therapy versus trastuzumab+endocrine therapy in HER2-positive hormone-receptor-positive early breast cancer. *Cancer Res.* 2016;76:S5-03-S05-03.

33. Hurvitz SA, Martin M, Symmans WF, et al. Neoadjuvant trastuzumab, pertuzumab, and chemotherapy versus trastuzumab emtansine plus pertuzumab in patients with HER2-positive breast cancer (KRISTINE): a randomised, open-label, multicentre, phase 3 trial. *Lancet Oncol.* 2018; 19:115−126.

34. Corona SP, Ravelli A, Cretella D, et al. CDK4/6 inhibitors in HER2-positive breast cancer. *Crit Rev Oncol Hematol.* 2017;112:208−214.

35. Gianni L, Bisagni G, Colleoni M, et al. Neoadjuvant treatment with trastuzumab and pertuzumab plus palbociclib and fulvestrant in HER2-positive, ER-positive breast cancer (NA-PHER2): an exploratory, open-label, phase 2 study. *Lancet Oncol.* 2018;19:249−256.

36. Untch M, Jackisch C, Schneeweiss A, et al. Nab-paclitaxel versus solvent-based paclitaxel in neoadjuvant chemotherapy for early breast cancer (GeparSepto-GBG 69): a randomised, phase 3 trial. *Lancet Oncol.* 2016;17: 345−356.

37. Food and Drug Administration U.S. Perjeta, Highlights of Prescribing Information https://www.accessdata.fda.gov/drugsatfda_docs/label/2013/125409s051lbl.pdf.

38. European Medicines Agency. Perjeta Product Information, Annex I. http://www.ema.europa.eu/docs/en_GB/document_library/EPAR_-_Product_Information/human/002547/WC500140980.pdf.

39. Sotiriou C, Rothé F, Maetens M, et al. Abstract GS1−04: copy number aberration analysis to predict response to neoadjuvant anti-HER2 therapy: results from the NeoALTTO phase III trial. *Cancer Res.* 2018;78:GS1-04-GS01-04.

40. Loibl S, Darb-Esfahani S, Huober J, et al. Integrated analysis of PTEN and p4EBP1 protein expression as predictors for pCR in HER2-positive breast cancer. *Clin Cancer Res.* 2016;22:2675−2683.

41. Loibl S, Majewski I, Guarneri V, et al. PIK3CA mutations are associated with reduced pathological complete response rates in primary HER2-positive breast cancer: pooled analysis of 967 patients from five prospective trials investigating lapatinib and trastuzumab. *Ann Oncol.* 2016; 27:1519−1525.

42. Majewski IJ, Nuciforo P, Mittempergher L, et al. PIK3CA mutations are associated with decreased benefit to neoadjuvant human epidermal growth factor receptor 2-targeted therapies in breast cancer. *J Clin Oncol.* 2015;33: 1334−1339.

43. Loibl S, von Minckwitz G, Schneeweiss A, et al. PIK3CA mutations are associated with lower rates of pathologic complete response to anti-human epidermal growth factor receptor 2 (her2) therapy in primary HER2-overexpressing breast cancer. *J Clin Oncol.* 2014;32:3212−3220.

44. Loibl S, de la Pena L, Nekljudova V, et al. Neoadjuvant buparlisib plus trastuzumab and paclitaxel for women with HER2+ primary breast cancer: a randomised, double-blind, placebo-controlled phase II trial (NeoPHOEBE). *Eur J Cancer.* 2017;85:133−145.

45. Mayer IA, Abramson VG, Formisano L, et al. A phase Ib study of alpelisib (BYL719), a PI3Kalpha-specific inhibitor, with Letrozole in ER+/HER2- metastatic breast cancer. *Clin Cancer Res.* 2017;23:26−34.

46. Krop I, Hillman D, Polley M-Y, et al. Abstract GS3−02: invasive disease-free survival and gene expression signatures in CALGB (Alliance) 40601, a randomized phase III neoadjuvant trial of dual HER2-targeting with lapatinib added to chemotherapy plus trastuzumab. *Cancer Res.* 2018;78:GS3-02-GS03-02.

47. Lesurf R, Griffith OL, Griffith M, et al. Genomic characterization of HER2-positive breast cancer and response to neoadjuvant trastuzumab and chemotherapy-results from the ACOSOG Z1041 (Alliance) trial. *Ann Oncol.* 2017;28:1070−1077.

48. Bang YJ, Giaccone G, Im SA, et al. First-in-human phase 1 study of margetuximab (MGAH22), an Fc-modified chimeric monoclonal antibody, in patients with HER2-positive advanced solid tumors. *Ann Oncol.* 2017;28: 855−861.

49. Swain SM, Ewer MS, Viale G, et al. Pertuzumab, trastuzumab, and standard anthracycline- and taxane-based chemotherapy for the neoadjuvant treatment of patients with HER2-positive localized breast cancer (BERENICE): a phase II, open-label, multicenter, multinational cardiac safety study. *Ann Oncol.* 2017.

50. Guarneri V, Frassoldati A, Bottini A, et al. Preoperative chemotherapy plus trastuzumab, lapatinib, or both in human epidermal growth factor receptor 2-positive operable breast cancer: results of the randomized phase II CHER-LOB study. *J Clin Oncol.* 2012;30:1989−1995.

51. Alba E, Albanell J, de la Haba J, et al. Trastuzumab or lapatinib with standard chemotherapy for HER2-positive breast cancer: results from the GEICAM/2006-14 trial. *Br J Cancer.* 2014;110:1139−1147.

52. von Minckwitz G, Schneeweiss A, Loibl S, et al. Neoadjuvant carboplatin in patients with triple-negative and HER2-positive early breast cancer (GeparSixto; GBG 66): a randomised phase 2 trial. *Lancet Oncol.* 2014;15: 747−756.

53. Ismael G, Hegg R, Muehlbauer S, et al. Subcutaneous versus intravenous administration of (neo)adjuvant trastuzumab in patients with HER2-positive, clinical stage I-III breast cancer (HannaH study): a phase 3, open-label, multicentre, randomised trial. *Lancet Oncol.* 2012;13: 869−878.

54. Schneeweiss A, Chia S, Hickish T, et al. Pertuzumab plus trastuzumab in combination with standard neoadjuvant anthracycline-containing and anthracycline-free chemotherapy regimens in patients with HER2-positive early breast cancer: a randomized phase II cardiac safety study (TRYPHAENA). *Ann Oncol.* 2013;24:2278−2284.

55. Nitz UA, Gluz O, Christgen M, et al. De-escalation strategies in HER2-positive early breast cancer (EBC): final analysis of the WSG-ADAPT HER2+/HR- phase II trial: efficacy, safety, and predictive markers for 12 weeks of neoadjuvant dual blockade with trastuzumab and pertuzumab +/- weekly paclitaxel. *Ann Oncol.* 2017;28:2768−2772.

FURTHER READING

1. Sikov WM, Berry DA, Perou CM, et al. Impact of the addition of carboplatin and/or bevacizumab to neoadjuvant once-per-week paclitaxel followed by dose-dense doxorubicin and cyclophosphamide on pathologic complete response rates in stage II to III triple-negative breast cancer: CALGB 40603 (Alliance). *J Clin Oncol.* 2015;33:13−21.

2. von Minckwitz G, Procter M, de Azambuja E, et al. Adjuvant pertuzumab and trastuzumab in early HER2-positive breast cancer. *N Engl J Med.* 2017;377:122−131.

3. Stavenhagen JB, Gorlatov S, Tuaillon N, et al. Fc optimization of therapeutic antibodies enhances their ability to kill tumor cells in vitro and controls tumor expansion in vivo via low-affinity activating Fcgamma receptors. *Cancer Res.* 2007;67:8882−8890.

4. Shields RL, Namenuk AK, Hong K, et al. High resolution mapping of the binding site on human IgG1 for Fc gamma RI, Fc gamma RII, Fc gamma RIII, and FcRn and design of IgG1 variants with improved binding to the Fc gamma R. *J Biol Chem.* 2001;276:6591−6604.

5. Clynes RA, Towers TL, Presta LG, Ravetch JV. Inhibitory Fc receptors modulate in vivo cytotoxicity against tumor targets. *Nat Med.* 2000;6:443−446.

6. Hudis CA. Trastuzumab—mechanism of action and use in clinical practice. *N Engl J Med.* 2007;357:39−51.

7. Collins DM, Gately K, Hughes C, et al. Tyrosine kinase inhibitors as modulators of trastuzumab-mediated antibody-dependent cell-mediated cytotoxicity in breast cancer cell lines. *Cell Immunol.* 2017;319:35−42.

8. Deeks ED. Neratinib: first global approval. *Drugs.* 2017;77: 1695−1704.

9. Martin M, Holmes FA, Ejlertsen B, et al. Neratinib after trastuzumab-based adjuvant therapy in HER2-positive breast cancer (ExteNET): 5-year analysis of a randomised, double-blind, placebo-controlled, phase 3 trial. *Lancet Oncol.* 2017;18:1688−1700.

10. Harbeck N, Huang CS, Hurvitz S, et al. Afatinib plus vinorelbine versus trastuzumab plus vinorelbine in patients with HER2-overexpressing metastatic breast cancer who had progressed on one previous trastuzumab treatment (LUX-Breast 1): an open-label, randomised, phase 3 trial. *Lancet Oncol.* 2016;17:357−366.

11. Herbst RS, Baas P, Kim DW, et al. Pembrolizumab versus docetaxel for previously treated, PD-L1-positive, advanced non-small-cell lung cancer (KEYNOTE-010): a randomised controlled trial. *Lancet.* 2016;387:1540−1550.

12. Loi S, Giobbe-Hurder A, Gombos A, et al. Abstract GS2−06: phase Ib/II study evaluating safety and efficacy of pembrolizumab and trastuzumab in patients with trastuzumab-resistant HER2-positive metastatic breast cancer: results from the PANACEA (IBCSG 45-13/BIG 4-13/KEYNOTE-014) study. *Cancer Res.* 2018;78:GS2-06-GS02-06.

13. Mukai H, Saeki T, Aogi K, et al. Patritumab plus trastuzumab and paclitaxel in human epidermal growth factor receptor 2-overexpressing metastatic breast cancer. *Cancer Sci.* 2016;107:1465−1470.

14. Doi T, Shitara K, Naito Y, et al. Safety, pharmacokinetics, and antitumour activity of trastuzumab deruxtecan (DS-8201), a HER2-targeting antibody-drug conjugate, in patients with advanced breast and gastric or gastro-oesophageal tumours: a phase 1 dose-escalation study. *Lancet Oncol.* 2017;18:1512−1522.

15. Espelin CW, Leonard SC, Geretti E, et al. Dual HER2 targeting with trastuzumab and liposomal-encapsulated doxorubicin (MM-302) demonstrates synergistic antitumor activity in breast and gastric cancer. *Cancer Res.* 2016;76:1517−1527.

16. Miller K, Cortes J, Hurvitz SA, et al. HERMIONE: a randomized Phase 2 trial of MM-302 plus trastuzumab versus chemotherapy of physician's choice plus trastuzumab in patients with previously treated, anthracycline-naive, HER2-positive, locally advanced/metastatic breast cancer. *BMC Cancer.* 2016;16:352.

CHAPTER 7

Adjuvant Therapy

ANA CRISTINA SANDOVAL-LEON, MD • RESHMA MAHTANI, DO •
MOHAMMAD JAHANZEB, MD, FACP

INTRODUCTION

The human epidermal growth factor receptor 2 (HER2) is amplified in approximately 20% of breast cancers (BC).[1] The natural history of HER2-positive disease has changed with the development of HER2-targeted therapies. Once considered one of the most aggressive subtypes of BC, it now is associated with a better prognosis for those who receive guideline-compliant therapy. The approval of trastuzumab in the metastatic setting was based on significant improvements in progression-free and overall survival (OS) when added to cytotoxic chemotherapy.[2,3] This resulted in much enthusiasm and optimism for evaluation of this agent in the adjuvant setting. The objective of this chapter is to review the current data on the use of HER2-targeted therapy as treatment for early-stage BC with a focus on chemotherapy backbones, optimal length and timing of HER2-targeted regimens, and new agents recently approved and under investigation for the adjuvant treatment of BC. The data in the neoadjuvant setting and toxicity data are covered elsewhere in this text.

TRASTUZUMAB

Trastuzumab is a humanized monoclonal antibody that binds to the extracellular domain of HER2 and inhibits ligand-independent downstream signaling. Several pivotal studies were completed that demonstrated the addition of 1 year of adjuvant trastuzumab to standard chemotherapy improved invasive disease-free survival (IDFS) and OS as compared with chemotherapy alone, without compromising safety. An interim analysis of four of these large trials eventually led to FDA approval of trastuzumab in 2006 for the treatment of early-stage BC.[4–10] More recently, longer-term follow-up (8–11 years) confirms the previously demonstrated survival benefits afforded by the addition of trastuzumab to standard chemotherapy, with no new significant safety signals identified (Table 7.1).

Large Randomized Trials of Adjuvant Trastuzumab
Herceptin Adjuvant
The herceptin adjuvant (HERA) phase III, randomized trial evaluated the efficacy of trastuzumab in the adjuvant setting and also investigated the optimal duration of therapy (1 vs. 2 years). The study enrolled a total of 5102 patients with HER2-positive BC between 2001 and 2005 in 39 countries. After completion of all primary therapy (including surgery, chemotherapy, and radiotherapy as indicated), patients were randomly assigned (1:1:1) to receive trastuzumab for 1 year (once at 8 mg/kg of bodyweight intravenously and then 6 mg/kg once every 3 weeks) or for 2 years (with the same dose and schedule), or to the observation group. The primary endpoint was disease-free survival (DFS).[6]

Half of the patients had tumors with hormone receptor (HR) co-expression. This trial included patients with node-negative disease if tumors were larger than 1 cm. Most patients received an anthracycline (94%) and only 26% received a combination of an anthracycline and a taxane. Median time from the completion of chemotherapy to the initiation of trastuzumab was 89 days (46–112 days).[6]

A total of 5099 patients were in the intention-to-treat (ITT) population (1697 in observation, 1702 in 1-year trastuzumab, and 1700 in the 2-year trastuzumab groups). The most recently updated results, after a median follow-up of 11 years, continue to show that 1 year of trastuzumab significantly improved DFS (HR 0·76, 95% CI: 0·68–0·86) and OS (HR 0·74, 0·64–0·86) compared with observation. There was no DFS benefit with an additional year (total 2 years) of trastuzumab compared with the standard 1 year of therapy (HR 1·02, 95% CI: 0·89–1·17). Estimates of 10-year DFS were 69% for both 1 and 2 years of trastuzumab compared with 63% for observation. OS was 80%, 79%, and 73% in these groups, respectively. Fifty-two percent (n = 884) of the patients who were

TABLE 7.1
Efficacy Summary Randomized Adjuvant Trastuzumab Trials

Trial	Pts (N)	Treatment	DFS (%)	HR	P	OS (%)	HR	P
NSABP B-31/NCCTG	2028	AC → TH	73.7[a]	0.60	<.001	84[a]	0.63	<.001
N9831	2018	AC → T	62.2			75		
BCIRG 006	1074	AC → TH	74.6[b]	0.64	<.0001	85.9[b]	0.73	.0001
	1075	TCH	73.0	0.75	<.001	83.3	0.76	.0075
	1073	AC → T	67.9			78.7		
HERA	1697	Chemo → Obs	63	0.76	<.0001	81[c]	0.74	.0005
	1702	Chemo → T (1 year)	69[c]	1.02		76		
	1700	Chemo → T (2 years)	69					
FinHER	116	V/T + H → FEC	83.3	0.42	.01	96	0.41	.07
	116	V/T → FEC	73			90		
PACS04	260	FEC/ED → T	81	0.86	.42	92[a]	1.27	NR
	268	FEC/ED → Obs	78			93		

[a] At 8 years.
[b] At 10 years.
[c] At 11 years.
AC → T, doxorubicin plus cyclophosphamide followed by docetaxel; AC → TH, doxorubicin plus cyclophosphamide followed by docetaxel plus trastuzumab; Chemo → Obs, chemotherapy followed by observation; Chemo → T, chemotherapy followed by trastuzumab; DFS, disease-free survival; FEC/ET → FEC/ET, fluorouracil, epirubicin, and cyclophosphamide followed by epirubicin and trastuzumab; HR, hazard ratio; OS, overall survival; pts, patients; TCH, docetaxel, carboplatin, and trastuzumab; NR, not rated; V/T → FEC, vinorelbine or docetaxel/trastuzumab followed by fluorouracil, epirubicin, and cyclophosphamide; V/T + H → FEC, vinorelbine or docetaxel with trastuzumab followed by fluorouracil, epirubicin, and cyclophosphamide.
Figure reproduced from: Mahtani R, Sandoval A, Jahanzeb M. Update on HER2-positive adjuvant therapy. *AJHO*. 2017;13(8):16.

assigned to the observation group initially crossed over to receive trastuzumab, which likely narrowed the survival gap between the observation and the treatment groups in this updated 11-year analysis (Fig. 7.1). Cardiac toxicity remained low in all groups and occurred mainly during the treatment phase. The incidence of secondary cardiac endpoints was 7.3% in the 2-year trastuzumab group, 4.4% in the 1-year trastuzumab group, and 0.9% in the observation group. This trial clearly demonstrated that the sequential use of trastuzumab for 1 year after completion of chemotherapy improves both DFS and OS and also showed that there is no advantage to extending the duration of adjuvant trastuzumab beyond 1 year.[6]

North Central Cancer Treatment Group N9831 and National Surgical Adjuvant Breast and Bowel Project B-31 (Combined Analyses)

The North Central Cancer Treatment Group (NCCTG) N9831 and the National Surgical Adjuvant Breast and Bowel Project (NSABP) B-31 had a similar design and could therefore be analyzed together. These two studies tested the safety and efficacy of adjuvant trastuzumab with paclitaxel followed by trastuzumab alone for

1 year versus placebo after completion of chemotherapy with doxorubicin and cyclophosphamide.[4]

NCCTG N9831 compared three arms: a control arm of doxorubicin combined with cyclophosphamide every 3 weeks for four cycles (AC), followed by weekly paclitaxel (arm A) versus a sequential arm of AC followed by weekly paclitaxel followed by 1 year of trastuzumab (arm B), and a concurrent arm of AC followed by weekly paclitaxel for 12 weeks with concurrent trastuzumab (starting with the first dose of paclitaxel) and completing 1 year of trastuzumab administration. NSABP B-31 compared two arms: AC followed by paclitaxel for 12 weeks (given either weekly or every 3 weeks, group 1) versus the same regimen with trastuzumab initiated concurrently with paclitaxel (group 2).[4]

Both trials included patients with node-positive disease and N9831 also included patients with high-risk node-negative BC (tumors >2 cm or tumors >1 cm, which were estrogen receptor and progesterone receptor negative). These studies enrolled patients from 2000 to 2005. In the joint analysis, the control arm of 1679 patients included arm A of NCCTG N9831 and group 1 of NSABP B-31, and the experimental arm of 1672 patients included arm C and group 2 of the two studies,

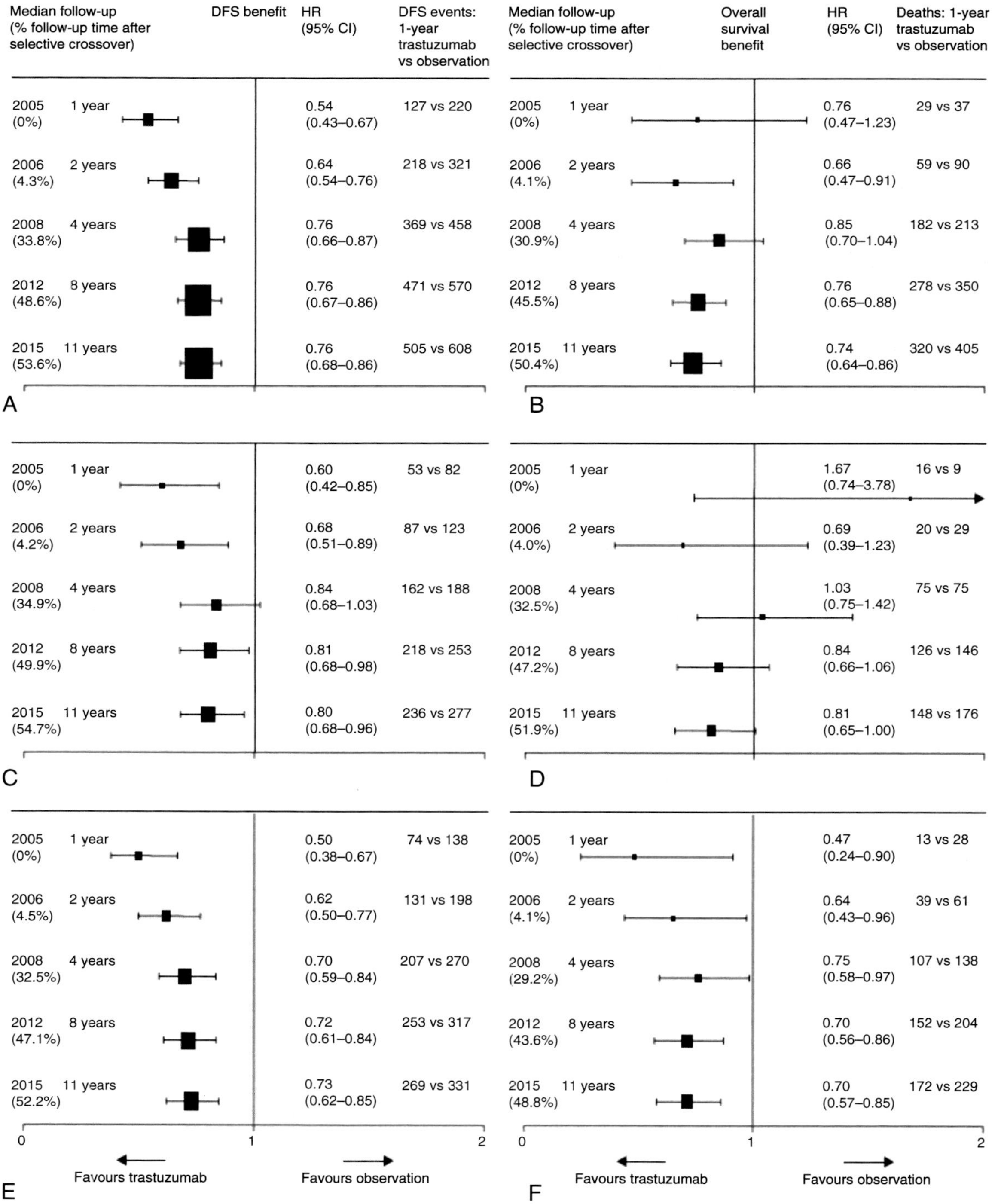

A

Median follow-up (% follow-up time after selective crossover)	DFS benefit	HR (95% CI)	DFS events: 1-year trastuzumab vs observation
2005 (0%) 1 year		0.54 (0.43–0.67)	127 vs 220
2006 (4.3%) 2 years		0.64 (0.54–0.76)	218 vs 321
2008 (33.8%) 4 years		0.76 (0.66–0.87)	369 vs 458
2012 (48.6%) 8 years		0.76 (0.67–0.86)	471 vs 570
2015 (53.6%) 11 years		0.76 (0.68–0.86)	505 vs 608

B

Median follow-up (% follow-up time after selective crossover)	Overall survival benefit	HR (95% CI)	Deaths: 1-year trastuzumab vs observation
2005 (0%) 1 year		0.76 (0.47–1.23)	29 vs 37
2006 (4.1%) 2 years		0.66 (0.47–0.91)	59 vs 90
2008 (30.9%) 4 years		0.85 (0.70–1.04)	182 vs 213
2012 (45.5%) 8 years		0.76 (0.65–0.88)	278 vs 350
2015 (50.4%) 11 years		0.74 (0.64–0.86)	320 vs 405

C

2005 (0%) 1 year		0.60 (0.42–0.85)	53 vs 82
2006 (4.2%) 2 years		0.68 (0.51–0.89)	87 vs 123
2008 (34.9%) 4 years		0.84 (0.68–1.03)	162 vs 188
2012 (49.9%) 8 years		0.81 (0.68–0.98)	218 vs 253
2015 (54.7%) 11 years		0.80 (0.68–0.96)	236 vs 277

D

2005 (0%) 1 year		1.67 (0.74–3.78)	16 vs 9
2006 (4.0%) 2 years		0.69 (0.39–1.23)	20 vs 29
2008 (32.5%) 4 years		1.03 (0.75–1.42)	75 vs 75
2012 (47.2%) 8 years		0.84 (0.66–1.06)	126 vs 146
2015 (51.9%) 11 years		0.81 (0.65–1.00)	148 vs 176

E

2005 (0%) 1 year		0.50 (0.38–0.67)	74 vs 138
2006 (4.5%) 2 years		0.62 (0.50–0.77)	131 vs 198
2008 (32.5%) 4 years		0.70 (0.59–0.84)	207 vs 270
2012 (47.1%) 8 years		0.72 (0.61–0.84)	253 vs 317
2015 (52.2%) 11 years		0.73 (0.62–0.85)	269 vs 331

F

2005 (0%) 1 year		0.47 (0.24–0.90)	13 vs 28
2006 (4.1%) 2 years		0.64 (0.43–0.96)	39 vs 61
2008 (29.2%) 4 years		0.75 (0.58–0.97)	107 vs 138
2012 (43.6%) 8 years		0.70 (0.56–0.86)	152 vs 204
2015 (48.8%) 11 years		0.70 (0.57–0.85)	172 vs 229

0 ← Favours trastuzumab   1   Favours observation → 2

0 ← Favours trastuzumab   1   Favours observation → 2

FIG. 7.1 **Herceptin adjuvant.** Disease-free survival (DFS) for the entire intention-to-treat (ITT) population **(A)**, for patients with hormone receptor–positive disease **(C)**, and for those with hormone receptor–negative disease **(E)**. Overall survival for the entire ITT population **(B)**, for the hormone receptor–positive cohort **(D)**, and

respectively. The sequential arm (B) of N9831 was excluded from this analysis. The trastuzumab containing experimental arm was associated with a reduced risk of a DFS event (HR 0.48, 95% CI: 0.39–0.59; $P < .0001$) and an OS event (HR 0.67, 95% CI: 0.48–0.95; $P = .015$) versus the chemotherapy alone control arm. Updated analyses after a median follow-up of 8.4 years indicated that the survival benefit associated with receipt of trastuzumab was maintained. The 10-year OS rate increased from 75.2% to 84%, and there was a 37% relative improvement in OS versus the control arm (HR 0.63, 95% CI: 0.54–0.73, $P < .001$). Treatment with trastuzumab + chemotherapy was also associated with a 40% improvement in DFS (HR0.60, 95% CI: 0.53–0.68; $P < .001$) versus chemotherapy alone. Despite a crossover of 20% after the first interim analysis and that 5% of the patients assigned to trastuzumab did not receive the drug because of safety concerns, there was a statistical improvement in both OS and DFS and benefitted all subgroups as defined by tumor size, age, and HR status.[4]

Breast Cancer International Research Group 006

Given the substantial cardiotoxicity demonstrated with the concurrent use of anthracyclines and trastuzumab in the pivotal trial, there was a strong rationale to try to develop effective non–anthracycline-containing regimens to combine with trastuzumab.[2] Thus, the safety and efficacy of trastuzumab was tested in combination with docetaxel and carboplatin in Breast Cancer International Research Group 006, after promising phase II data established it efficacy in metastatic disease.[11] This study enrolled a total of 3222 patients with HER2-positive BC between 2001 and 2004 in 41 countries. Patients were randomized to receive AC followed by docetaxel every 3 weeks (AC-T) or the same regimen plus concurrent trastuzumab starting with docetaxel (AC-TH) or with docetaxel and carboplatin every 3 weeks for six cycles given concurrently with trastuzumab (TCH). In both of the trastuzumab-containing

arms, trastuzumab alone was given to complete 1 year. The primary endpoint was DFS.[5]

Patients with node-positive and high-risk node-negative disease were included. High-risk node-negative disease was defined as age less than 35, tumor greater than 2 cm in size, or HR negative or histologic/nuclear grade 2–3.[12] Only 2.1% of the patients in the control arm crossed over to receive trastuzumab. The final analysis reported 10-year follow-up of this landmark trial. As expected, 10-year DFS was better in both trastuzumab-containing groups: 74.6% and 73% in the anthracycline and non–anthracycline-containing regimens, respectively, compared with 67.9% in the control group. There was no statistical advantage with regard to DFS or OS for AC-TH over TCH, although the study was not powered to detect equivalence between the two groups. There were only 10 DFS events separating the two arms, in favor of the anthracycline-containing regimen. However, this numerical advantage came at the cost of significantly more toxicity including a fivefold increase in congestive heart failure, higher rates of sustained left ventricular ejection fraction decline >10% from baseline, and higher leukemia rates. In terms of OS there were demonstrated improvements documented with the receipt of trastuzumab, with OS at 10 years 85.9%, 83.3%, and 78.7%, representing risk reductions of 27% ($P < .0001$) and 24% ($P = .0075$), respectively. Notably, in a subset analysis of node-positive patients, outcomes were similar to the entire study population, which suggests that the benefit of anthracyclines, even in a high-risk population, may be minimal.[5]

Small Randomized trials
Finland Herceptin Trial

This was an open-label, prospective phase III, multicenter study aimed to investigate a shorter duration of trastuzumab in the adjuvant setting, as well as the effect of receiving trastuzumab prior to anthracycline therapy. The trial enrolled a total of 1010 women with node-positive BC or who had node-negative tumors that were larger than 2 cm in diameter *and* had negative

for the hormone receptor–negative cohort (F). These ITT analyses are affected by selective crossover in 884 (52%) patients from the observation group who received trastuzumab after the first trial results 1 were published in 2005. *HR*, hazard ratio. *The percentages are of follow-up time in the ITT analysis, which was accrued after selective crossover for patients assigned to the observation group. (Figure reproduced and modified from Cameron D, Piccart-Gebhart MJ, Gelber RD, et al. 11 years' follow-up of trastuzumab after adjuvant chemotherapy in HER2-positive early breast cancer: final analysis of the HERceptin Adjuvant (HERA) trial. *Lancet (Lond Engl)*. 2017;389(10075):1195–1205; Goldhirsch A, Gelber RD, Piccart-Gebhart MJ, et al. 2 years versus 1 year of adjuvant trastuzumab for HER2-positive breast cancer (HERA): an open-label, randomised controlled trial. *Lancet (Lond, Engl)*. 2013;382(9897):1021–1028 by permission of Elsevier.)

staining for progesterone receptors. Patients were randomized to receive three cycles of either docetaxel or vinorelbine followed by three cycles of fluorouracil, epirubicin, and cyclophosphamide (FEC). Out of the entire study population, 232 patients were HER2 positive and they were further randomized to receive a short course trastuzumab for 9 weeks concurrently with either docetaxel or vinorelbine or no trastuzumab therapy during this time. Due to high rates of neutropenic fever, the dose of docetaxel was decreased from 100 mg/m^2 to 80 mg/m^2 in 59% of the patients assigned to this drug.[13]

Results for the HER2-positive subset at 5 years follow-up indicated those patients treated with trastuzumab tended to have better distant DFS than those treated with chemotherapy alone, although not statistically significant: 83.3% versus 73%, respectively (HR 0.65, 95% CI: 0.38–1.12; $P = .12$). The authors concluded that docetaxel improved distant DFS compared with vinorelbine in the entire population, and for those with HER2-positive disease, the combination of trastuzumab with docetaxel might be better than the combination with vinorelbine. The study had a small number of patients who were HER2 positive, thus had a limited power. As such, the authors concluded that chemotherapy regimens combined with shorter courses of trastuzumab should be explored in future studies.[13] These data have not led to widespread use of shorter courses of trastuzumab in the adjuvant setting but spawned additional trials aiming to study a shorter duration of therapy than a year (see Optimal Length of Therapy With Trastuzumab).

Federation Nationale des Centres de Lutte Contre le Cancer-Programe Adjuvant Cancer Sein (FNCLCC-PACS04) Trial
Between 2001 and 2004 a total of 3010 patients with operable BC from France and Belgium were enrolled in this trial that evaluated the efficacy of adjuvant trastuzumab in an exclusively node-positive group of patients. Patients were randomized to receive adjuvant anthracycline-based chemo with or without docetaxel. In the 528 patients who had HER2-positive BC, there was a further randomization to trastuzumab for 1 year (n = 260) or observation after completion of chemotherapy and radiotherapy.[14]

There was no statistically significant difference in DFS with a 3-year DFS of 80.9% versus 77.8% favoring the trastuzumab arm (HR of 0.86; 95% CI: 0.61–1.22). There was no significant difference in the risk of death between the trastuzumab arm and the observation arm (HR 1.27, 95% CI: 0.68–2.38; $P = .41$), with

3-year OS rates of 95% and 96%, respectively. The failure to find a difference could be due to the small sample size, sequential use of trastuzumab, or both and lack of strict adherence to protocol-specified therapy (10% of patients assigned to the trastuzumab arm did not receive the drug and 25% discontinued trastuzumab before the 16th dose).[14]

Concurrent Versus Sequential Trastuzumab
As detailed above, three trials have evaluated the sequential use of trastuzumab: HERA, NCCTG N9831, and PACS04.[6,14,15] HERA showed a statistical significant improvement in both DFS and OS when sequential trastuzumab was used compared with observation.[6] PACS04 failed to find statistical significant DFS with sequential use of trastuzumab versus observation.[14] N9831 was the only study to directly compare sequential trastuzumab concurrent use during the taxane portion of chemotherapy.[15] After a median of 3.9 years of follow-up, a strong trend toward increased 5-year DFS was noted with concurrent trastuzumab and paclitaxel relative to sequential administration (HR 0.77, 99.9% CI: 0.53–1.11; $P = .0216$), but the P value did not cross the prespecified O'Brien-Fleming boundary for the interim analysis.[15] Despite the lack of statistical difference, concurrent use of trastuzumab with a taxane is generally favored.

Optimal Length of Therapy With Trastuzumab
The current data support 1 year of trastuzumab. As previously described, the HERA study did not show a benefit of 2 years of trastuzumab over the standard 1 year of therapy.[6,16]

Protocol of Herceptin Adjuvant with Reduced Exposure
Another study evaluating the optimal duration of adjuvant trastuzumab was the Protocol of Herceptin Adjuvant with Reduced Exposure trial. This was a phase III French open-label, noninferiority trial that randomized 3384 patients to receive either 6 or 12 months of trastuzumab, following receipt of at least four cycles of chemotherapy.[16]

Patients with node-negative and node-positive disease were included and most received an anthracycline- and taxane-containing regimen. Approximately 55% received trastuzumab concurrently with chemotherapy. In the ITT analysis 3380 patients were included. The 2-year DFS was 91.1% and 93.8% in the 6- and 12-month groups, respectively (HR: 1.28; 95% CI: 1.05–1.56 $P = .29$). Therefore, the study failed to demonstrate noninferiority for the (shorter) investigational arm at the prespecified hazard ratio (1.15).[16]

The Hellenic Cooperative Oncology Research Group Study

This study also compared 6 versus 12 months of adjuvant trastuzumab in patients with axillary node-positive or high-risk node-negative disease. Patients received FEC followed by docetaxel in combination with trastuzumab. The primary endpoint was DFS. Between 2004 and 2012 a total of 240 patients were randomized to 6 months of trastuzumab and 241 to 1 year of trastuzumab. The 3-year DFS was 95.7% versus 93.3% favoring the 12-month trastuzumab group. OS and cardiac toxicity were not different between the groups.[17]

The Persephone Trial

This is a randomized, phase III trial that enrolled 2500 patients in the United Kingdom from 2007 to 2012. They were randomized to either 12 months or 6 months of trastuzumab given sequentially or concurrently with chemotherapy. Their primary endpoint was DFS. They demonstrated that 6 months of trastuzumab was no-inferior to 12 months with a 3% non-inferiority margin. They also showed that there were significant less cardiac events in the shorter duration group. They have only reported cardiac toxicity, which was one of their secondary endpoints, and it showed that there were significant less cardiac events in the shorter duration group.[18–19]

ShortHER

This phase III, multicenter study aimed to assess the efficacy of a shorter course of adjuvant trastuzumab (9 weeks) and establish noninferiority to standard 1 year of therapy. Investigators enrolled 1254 patients from December 2007 to October 2013. After receiving standard anthracycline and taxane-based treatment, patients were randomized to a long arm (1 year) or a short arm (9 weeks) of trastuzumab. Hormonal therapy started at the completion of chemotherapy for patients with HR-positive tumors. The primary endpoint was DFS and OS. Secondary endpoints included incidence of cardiac events. The primary endpoints were analyzed after 198 events or at a median follow-up of 5 years. There were 89 DFS events in the long arm (627 patients) and 100 in the short arm (626 patients). The study could not establish noninferiority for a shorter course of trastuzumab treatment, as the 5-year DFS did not reach noninferiority. However, a subgroup analysis of DFS comparing stage III with stage I and II patients and nodal status (0–1 nodes vs. 2–3) did reach

significance. In addition, there was an ongoing decline in left ventricular ejection fraction for the long arm but a much slower decline in the short arm over an 18-month period.[19] Taking these findings into consideration, a shorter course of trastuzumab may be considered safe and efficacious for a lower risk population (<3 positive nodes) when cardiac toxicity is of concern or where access to trastuzumab may be limited.

The Synergism or Long Duration

This was yet another trial that sought to establish whether a shorter course (9 weeks) of trastuzumab in the adjuvant setting was comparable with the standard 1 year of therapy. This was a randomized phase III study that compared 9 weeks of trastuzumab plus docetaxel followed by FEC with the same regimen followed by trastuzumab to complete 1 year. The primary outcome was DFS and secondary endpoints were distant DFS and OS. They enrolled 2168 patients between 2008 and 2014. Results were recently reported in the 2017 San Antonio Breast Cancer Symposium.[20,21] DFS after the shorter course of adjuvant trastuzumab was not comparable with DFS 12 months of adjuvant trastuzumab, supporting the current practice of 1 year of therapy. However, 5-year distant DFS was 88% versus 90.5% in the 9-week arm versus the 12-month arm. The 5-year OS was also similar between arms (94.7% vs. 95.9%, respectively). The shorter course of therapy was associated with less cardiac failure (3% and 2% of patients in the 1-year and 9-week arms, respectively).[21]

Anthracycline Versus Nonanthracycline Regimens

Although BICRG 006 and BETH trial (discussed below) were not powered to find a difference between an anthracycline and a nonanthracycline regimen, both studies showed a similar efficacy with non–anthracycline-based therapy.[5,22] Longer 10-year follow-up continues to demonstrate good disease control rates without the use of anthracycline-based therapy. The risk of cardiotoxicity and leukemia is higher with an anthracycline-containing regimen, and due to toxicity concerns many have started to incorporate nonanthracycline regimens into the adjuvant treatment of early-stage BC. For these reasons, the use on a nonanthracycline regimen is now considered an option.

DUAL HER2 BLOCKADE

Given the consistent rates of distant relapse postcompletion of standard adjuvant chemotherapy with trastuzumab and evidence of superiority of dual HER2 blockade by adding pertuzumab or a tyrosine kinase inhibitor in the metastatic setting, investigations have focused on studying similar approaches in the adjuvant setting.

PERTUZUMAB

Pertuzumab is a humanized monoclonal antibody that binds to the extracellular domain of HER2. Its binding prevents ligand-dependent dimerization of HER2 with other HER receptors. It acts complementary to trastuzumab as they bind to different epitopes. It is approved in combination with trastuzumab for the treatment of HER2-positive metastatic BC as first-line treatment in combination with a taxane and trastuzumab, based on impressive improvements in both PFS and OS (an unprecedented 56 months!) noted in the CLEOPATRA trial.[23] It is also approved for treatment in the neoadjuvant setting for tumors ≥2 cm or those with node-positive disease based on multiple studies that have demonstrated substantial improvements in pathologic complete response rates (pCR) with the incorporation of pertuzumab to chemotherapy and trastuzumab.[24]

Given these data, there was enthusiasm to investigate the incorporation of adjuvant pertuzumab in early-stage HER2-positive BC.

Adjuvant Pertuzuamb and Herceptin in Initial Therapy of Breast Cancer

This phase III, randomized trial evaluated whether adding pertuzumab to standard trastuzumab for 1 year after surgery improved outcomes. This trial enrolled 4805 women with HER2-positive BC who were randomized to receive standard adjuvant chemotherapy for 18 weeks plus 1 year of either trastuzumab and placebo or trastuzumab and pertuzumab. Chemotherapy consisted of a number of standard anthracycline-taxane sequences or a nonanthracycline (TCH) regimen (Fig. 7.2). Overall, 63% of patients had cancer that had node-positive disease and 36% had HR-negative disease; pT1-3 primary tumors were included. For patients with node-negative disease to be eligible, they required tumors larger than 1 cm, and midway through the study, the number of patients with node-negative disease was capped to allow a higher-risk population

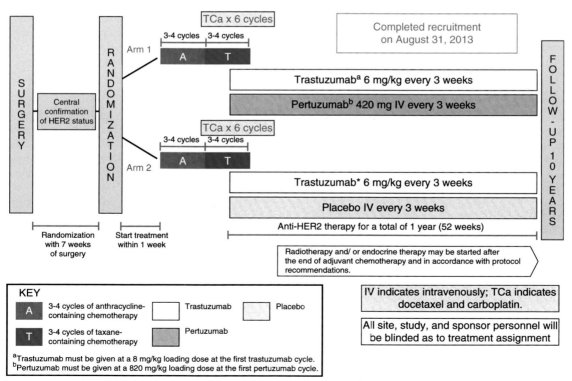

FIG. 7.2 **APHINITY trial.** (Mahtani R, Sandoval A, Jahanzeb M. Update on HER2-positive adjuvant therapy. *AJHO*. 2017;13(8):16.)

to be included to the study. The primary endpoint was DFS.[25]

The 3-year DFS was 94.1% versus 93.2% (HR: 0.81; 95% CI: 0.68–1.00, $P = .045$) favoring the pertuzumab arm by about 1%. At a median follow-up of almost 4 years, 171 (7.1%) patients in the pertuzumab group had developed invasive BC compared with 210 (8.7%) patients in the placebo group. The magnitude of benefit was greater for patients with node-positive disease with a 3-year DFS of 92.0% versus 90.2% (HR 0.77; 95% CI: 0.62–0.96, $P = .019$). In contrast, in the node-negative group no difference in DFS was noted at this early analysis point. Additionally, there was about a 2% difference in DFS in the HR-negative subgroup and no such difference could be discerned in the HR-positive subgroup. The cardiac toxicity was minimal, with no significant differences noted with the addition of pertuzumab. Increased rates of diarrhea were noted to a greater degree in the pertuzumab arm.[25]

Although there was a statistical significant improvement in DFS, the magnitude of benefit was marginal and must be weighed against the substantial cost. As such, incorporation of pertuzumab in the adjuvant setting may be considered for higher-risk patients (node-positive, ER-negative) The FDA recently approved the adjuvant use of pertuzumab in combination with chemotherapy and trastuzumab for patients with HER2-positive BC at high risk of recurrence.

Adjuvant Lapatinib
Lapatinib (Tykerb) is an oral, dual tyrosine kinase inhibitor that targets HER1 and HER2. It was approved in 2007 for second-line treatment of metastatic BC in combination with capecitabine. This was based on a phase III, randomized trial comparing lapatinib in combination with capecitabine with capecitabine alone, in which the combination demonstrated improvement in time to progression and overall response rates.[26]

Tykerb Evaluation After Chemotherapy Trial
Lapatinib has been evaluated in a patient population that was not treated with adjuvant trastuzumab because of lack of availability or the fact they were diagnosed with BC prior to the approval of trastuzumab as adjuvant therapy. This trial was a phase III, randomized, placebo-control trial done between 2006 and 2008 in 33 countries. It randomized 3161 patients with HER2-positive BC to receive either lapatinib for 1 year or placebo. Patients had stage I–IIIC BC, had received prior chemotherapy, and had no trastuzumab.[27]

A total of 3147 patients were in the ITT population (14 withdrew before treatment). The 4-year DFS was 87% in the lapatinib group and 83% in the placebo

group, but this difference was not statistically significant (HR: 0.83; 95% CI: 0.70–1.00; $P = .053$). The 4-year OS was 94% in both the groups. A caveat of this trial is that 29% of patients started lapatinib for more than 4 years after their initial diagnosis. Given these findings, adjuvant lapatinib alone is not an appropriate therapy in the adjuvant setting.[27]

The Adjuvant Lapatinib and/or Trastuzumab Treatment Optimization Trial
Combination therapy with lapatinib and trastuzumab has also been investigated. The Adjuvant Lapatinib and/or Trastuzumab Treatment Optimization trial was a phase III trial that randomized 8381 patients to receive concurrent lapatinib with trastuzumab, sequential trastuzumab followed by lapatinib, lapatinib alone, or trastuzumab alone. Forty-four countries participated in this trial. The single-agent lapatinib arm was closed early because of futility. The primary endpoint was DFS.[28]

HER2-directed therapy started sequentially or concurrently with chemotherapy. Patients with node-positive and node-negative disease were included. Cardiac toxicity was uncommon. The 4-year DFS with the concurrent lapatinib regimen was 88%, with the sequential lapatinib regimen 87%, and with trastuzumab alone 86%. These differences were not statistically significant and as such, lapatinib is not a recommended or approved therapy in the adjuvant setting.[28]

NERATINIB
Neratinib is an oral tyrosine kinase inhibitor. It is a pan-HER inhibitor that binds irreversible to the epidermal growth factor receptor (HER1), HER2, and HER4. This binding leads to decrease phosphorylation and activation of downstream signaling pathways.[29] It differs from monoclonal antibodies such as trastuzumab, as it blocks the ATP-binding site on the intracellular domain of the HER2 molecule, thereby inhibiting downstream signal transduction through the AKT-PI3 kinase pathway. It also differs from other tyrosine kinase inhibitors such as lapatinib because it binds not only to HER1 and HER2 but also to HER4 and does so irreversibly.[29] This agent has shown promising activity for patients with HER2-positive metastatic breast cancer (MBC).[30,31]

ExteNET Trial
Although as previously described, there is no benefit in the adjuvant setting to 2 years of trastuzumab over 1 year, a switch to a different HER2-targeted therapy after the first year or so called "extended adjuvant

therapy" may be of benefit and thus the premise for the ExteNET trial. This was a double-blind, placebo-controlled, multicenter, phase III trial that enrolled a total of 2840 women in 495 centers around the world between 2009 and 2011. Patients were randomized to receive neratinib for 1 year or placebo after completing 1 year of standard adjuvant treatment with trastuzumab. Patients were permitted to enroll on study and had to be randomized no more than 2 years postcompletion of adjuvant trastuzumab, although 81% of patients were randomized within 1 year, and none had received prior pertuzumab in the neoadjuvant or adjuvant setting. Patients with stage I—III node-positive and node-negative patients with tumors greater than 1 cm in size were included. The primary endpoint was IDFS.[32]

The 5-year IDFS was 90.2% versus 87.7% favoring the neratinib arm (HR 0.73; 95% CI: 0.57—0.92; $P = .008$). A subgroup analysis that was prespecified suggested that patients with HR-positive disease had greater benefit (HR 0.60; CI: 0.43—0.83; $P = .002$). Cardiac events were very low. The main side effect was diarrhea, and antidiarrheal prophylaxis was not uniformly given.[33] The CONTROL trial is assessing the use of loperamide alone or in combination with antiinflammatory treatment (budesonide, colestipol) to decrease the incidence of grade 3 or higher diarrhea, and this prophylactic regimen was successful. The incidence of grade ≥ 3 diarrhea in the ExteNET study was 39.9%. In the CONTROL trial, the incidence of grade ≥ 3 diarrhea was 30% in the loperamide group, 26.6% in the loperamide + budesonide group, and 10.8% in the loperamide + colestipol group.[34—36] In July 2017, the FDA approved neratinib for the extended adjuvant treatment of HER2 BC.

BEVACIZUMAB

Bevacizumab is an inhibitor of angiogenesis. It binds to the vascular endothelial growth factor A (VEGF-A). In 2008, it was approved for the treatment of metastatic BC. In 2011 the FDA withdrew its approval because of lack of evidence of consistent efficacy and safety.[37] Preclinical studies have shown that the overexpression of HER2 is associated with upregulation of VEGF. These observations led to the development of clinical trials in patients with HER2-positive BC.[38]

BETH Trial

This was an open-label, phase III trial that randomized 3509 women with HER2-positive BC around the world to receive chemotherapy plus trastuzumab with or without bevacizumab. It had two cohorts. In cohort one (nonanthracycline regimen), 3231 patients were randomized to docetaxel, carboplatin, and trastuzumab with or without bevacizumab. In cohort two, 278 women were randomized to FEC followed by docetaxel and trastuzumab with or without bevacizumab.

This trial included node-positive and high-risk node-negative patients. The primary endpoint was IDFS. After a median follow-up of 38 months, the rate of IDFS in cohort one was 92% for both groups. In cohort two it was 91% versus 87% favoring the bevacizumab arm, but this difference was not statistically significant. As previously stated, although this trial was not designed to find a difference between an anthracycline and non—anthracycline-containing regimen, both regimens had similar IDFS.[22]

ONGOING STUDIES

Ado-Trastuzumab Emtansine

Ado-trastuzumab emtansine (T-DM1) is an antibody drug conjugate of trastuzumab with emtansine. It was approved in 2013 for the second-line treatment of metastatic BC based on improved progression-free and OS when compared with lapatinib with capecitabine.[39] Due to the favorable toxicity profile, considerable efforts are ongoing to investigate its use in the adjuvant setting.

Katherine Trial

This is a phase III, open-label study that is randomizing women with HER2-positive BC who do not achieve a pCR after neoadjuvant chemotherapy to receive either adjuvant trastuzumab or T-DM1 for 14 cycles. The primary endpoint is IDFS. Accrual started in 2013 and the estimated time to complete the study is 2023.[40]

ATEMPT Trial

T-DM1 is being tested in the adjuvant setting in the ATEMPT trial. This is a phase II study that is randomizing patients with stage I HER2-positive BC to either paclitaxel in combination trastuzumab or T-DM1.[41]

Trial of Adjuvant T-DM1 for Older Patients With HER2-Positive BC

This is a phase II, single-arm trial that is enrolling patients who are 60 years or older and have stage I—III HER2-positive BC who decline chemotherapy or are not candidates for standard chemotherapy. They will receive a total of 17 courses of T-DM1 every 3 weeks. The primary endpoint is IDFS. The study started in 2015 and is expected to finish in 2022.[42]

NSABP-B47

In the pivotal adjuvant trastuzumab trials, some patients were found to be HER2-negative after central testing. Efficacy of adjuvant trastuzumab was still seen in these patients, despite the fact they were not confirmed to be HER2 positive by immunihistochemistry (IHC) or fluorescent in situ hybridization (FISH) in a central lab. As such, NSABP-B47 aimed to explore whether weak expressions of HER2 (1+ or 2+ by immunohistochemistry but are FISH negative) may benefit from the addition of trastuzumab. This was an open-label, phase III trial that randomized women with node-positive or high-risk node-negative HER2-low BC to chemotherapy alone or chemotherapy with trastuzumab. The primary outcome was IDFS. One must recognize that these patients were not identical to the pivotal trial participants who were HER2 positive by local testing but only found to be negative at the central testing. Accrual started in 2011 and was completed in 2015. A total of 3270 patients were enrolled, worldwide. After a median follow-up of 46.1 months, the 5-year invasive DFS was 89.2% for the patients who did not receive trastuzumab and 89.6% for the ones who received it. With this finding, we can conclude that patients with weak HER2 expression do not benefit from the addition of trastuzumab to their chemotherapeutic regimen.[43]

CONCLUSIONS

HER2-targeted therapy has changed the landscape of treating HER2-positive BC. The discovery of this target led to the development of many other molecules that block this pathway and improve not only DFS but, in case of trastuzumab, also OS when used in combination with adjuvant chemotherapy. Currently, many oncologists prefer to use a non—anthracycline-containing regimen in combination with trastuzumab because of similar efficacy and less cardiotoxicity. Although adjuvant pertuzumab significantly improved IDFS, the effect was minimal and it has not become standard practice to uniformly use it in this setting. On the other hand, neratinib was recently FDA approved for extended adjuvant treatment of HER2-positive BC after completing 1 year of trastuzumab, where the benefit was limited to patients with HR-positive disease. The main side effect is diarrhea, which is manageable with the use of prophylactic loperamide. Currently studies are testing the use of adjuvant T-DM1 in early-stage BC and elderly patients to avoid the use of chemotherapy. Its incremental efficacy is also being tested when added to trastuzumab to improve outcomes. Finally, NSABP-B47

showed that patients with low expression of HER2 do not benefit from HER2-directed therapy.

Although all of this progress is exciting and rewarding, 15%—30% of patients who present with potentially curable disease relapse and are no longer curable.[4,6] Studying mechanisms of resistance and associated biomarkers to identify these patients at diagnosis will be essential in the quest to incrementally improve outcomes for this subset of BC patients.

REFERENCES

1. Moasser MM, Krop IE. The evolving landscape of HER2 targeting in breast cancer. *JAMA Oncol.* 2015;1(8): 1154—1161.
2. Slamon DJ, Leyland-Jones B, Shak S, et al. Use of chemotherapy plus a monoclonal antibody against HER2 for metastatic breast cancer that overexpresses HER2. *N Engl J Med.* 2001;344(11):783—792.
3. Marty M, Cognetti F, Maraninchi D, et al. Randomized phase II trial of the efficacy and safety of trastuzumab combined with docetaxel in patients with human epidermal growth factor receptor 2-positive metastatic breast cancer administered as first-line treatment: the M77001 study group. *J Clin Oncol.* 2005;23(19):4265—4274.
4. Perez EA, Romond EH, Suman VJ, et al. Trastuzumab plus adjuvant chemotherapy for human epidermal growth factor receptor 2-positive breast cancer: planned joint analysis of overall survival from NSABP B-31 and NCCTG N9831. *J Clin Oncol.* 2014;32(33):3744—3752.
5. Slamon DJ, Eiermann W, Robert NJ, et al. Ten year follow-up of BCIRG-006 comparing doxorubicin plus cyclophosphamide followed by docetaxel with doxorubicin plus cyclophosphamide followed by docetaxel and trastuzumab with docetaxel, carboplatin, and trastuzumab in HER2-positive early breast cancer. In: *Presented at: San Antonio breast cancer symposium.* December 11, 2015.
6. Cameron D, Piccart-Gebhart MJ, Gelber RD, et al. 11 years' follow-up of trastuzumab after adjuvant chemotherapy in HER2-positive early breast cancer: final analysis of the HERceptin Adjuvant (HERA) trial. *Lancet (Lond Engl).* 2017;389(10075):1195—1205.
7. Slamon D, Eiermann W, Robert N, et al. Phase III trial comparing AC-T with AC-TH and with TCH in the adjuvant treatment of HER2 positive early breast cancer patients: first interim analysis. In: *Presented at the 28th San Antonio breast cancer symposium; San Antonio, TX, USA.* December 7—10, 2005.
8. O'Sullivan CC, Bradbury I, Campbell C, et al. Efficacy of adjuvant trastuzumab for patients with human epidermal growth factor receptor 2-positive early breast cancer and tumors </= 2 cm: a meta-analysis of the randomized trastuzumab trials. *J Clin Oncol.* 2015;33(24):2600—2608.
9. Piccart-Gebhart MJ, Procter M, Leyland-Jones B, et al. Trastuzumab after adjuvant chemotherapy in HER2-positive breast cancer. *N Engl J Med.* 2005;353(16):1659—1672.

10. Slamon D, Eiermann W, Robert N, et al. Adjuvant trastuzumab in HER2-positive breast cancer. *N Engl J Med.* 2011; 365(14):1273–1283.
11. Valero V, Forbes J, Pegram MD, et al. Multicenter phase III randomized trial comparing docetaxel and trastuzumab with docetaxel, carboplatin, and trastuzumab as first-line chemotherapy for patients with HER2-gene-amplified metastatic breast cancer (BCIRG 007 study): two highly active therapeutic regimens. *J Clin Oncol.* 2011;29(2): 149–156.
12. Au HJ, Eiermann W, Robert NJ, et al. Health-related quality of life with adjuvant docetaxel- and trastuzumab-based regimens in patients with node-positive and high-risk node-negative, HER2-positive early breast cancer: results from the BCIRG 006 Study. *Oncologist.* 2013;18(7): 812–818.
13. Joensuu H, Bono P, Kataja V, et al. Fluorouracil, epirubicin, and cyclophosphamide with either docetaxel or vinorelbine, with or without trastuzumab, as adjuvant treatments of breast cancer: final results of the FinHer Trial. *J Clin Oncol.* 2009;27(34):5685–5692.
14. Spielmann M, Roche H, Delozier T, et al. Trastuzumab for patients with axillary-node-positive breast cancer: results of the FNCLCC-PACS 04 trial. *J Clin Oncol.* 2009;27(36): 6129–6134.
15. Perez EA, Suman VJ, Davidson NE, et al. Sequential versus concurrent trastuzumab in adjuvant chemotherapy for breast cancer. *J Clin Oncol.* 2011;29(34):4491–4497.
16. Pivot X, Romieu G, Debled M, et al. 6 months versus 12 months of adjuvant trastuzumab for patients with HER2-positive early breast cancer (PHARE): a randomised phase 3 trial. *Lancet Oncol.* 2013;14(8):741–748.
17. Mavroudis D, Saloustros E, Malamos N, et al. Six versus 12 months of adjuvant trastuzumab in combination with dose-dense chemotherapy for women with HER2-positive breast cancer: a multicenter randomized study by the Hellenic Oncology Research Group (HORG). *Ann Oncol.* 2015;26(7):1333–1340.
18. Earl HM, Vallier AL, Dunn J, et al. Trastuzumab-associated cardiac events in the Persephone trial. *Br J Cancer.* 2016; 115(12):1462–1470.
19. Earl HM, Hiller L, Vallier AL, et al. PERSEPHONE: 6 versus 12 months (m) of adjuvant trastuzumab in patients (pts) with HER2 positive (+) early breast cancer (EBC): Randomised phase 3 non-inferiority trial with definitive 4-year (yr) disease-free survival (DFS) results. *J Clin Oncol.* 2018;36 (suppl; abstr 506).
20. Conte PF, Bisagni G, Frassoldati A, et al. 9 weeks vs 1 year adjuvant trastuzumab in combination with chemotherapy: results of the phase III multicentric Italian study Short-HER. *J Clin Oncol.* 2017;35(suppl 15):501.
21. *The synergism or long duration (SOLD) study - full text view;* 2017. ClinicalTrials.gov. https://clinicaltrials.gov/ct2/show/ NCT00593697.
22. Joensuu H, Fraser J, Wildiers H, et al. A randomized phase III study of adjuvant trastuzumab for a duration of 9 weeks versus 1 year, combined with adjuvant taxane-anthracycline chemotherapy, for early HER2-positive breast cancer (the SOLD study). In: *Presented at: San Antonio breast cancer symposium; San Antonio, TX, USA.* Dec 7. 2017.
23. Slamon D, Swain S, Buyse M, et al. Primary results from BETH, a phase 3 controlled study of adjuvant chemotherapy and trastuzumab ± bevacizumab in patients with HER2-positive, node-positive or high risk node-negative breast cancer. In: *Presented at: San Antonio Breast Cancer Symposium; Presented.* December 11, 2013.
24. Baselga J, Cortés J, Kim S-B, et al. Pertuzumab plus trastuzumab plus docetaxel for metastatic breast cancer. *N Engl J Med.* 2012;366(2):109–119.
25. Gianni L, Pienkowski T, Im Y-H, et al. 5-year analysis of neoadjuvant pertuzumab and trastuzumab in patients with locally advanced, inflammatory, or early-stage HER2-positive breast cancer (NeoSphere): a multicentre, open-label, phase 2 randomised trial. *Lancet Oncol.* 2016; 17(6):791–800.
26. Von Minckwitz G, Procter M, de Azambuja E, et al. Adjuvant pertuzumab and trastuzumab in early HER2-positive breast cancer. *N Engl J Med.* 2017;377(2):122–131.
27. Geyer CE, Forster J, Lindquist D, et al. Lapatinib plus capecitabine for HER2-positive advanced breast cancer. *N Engl J Med.* 2006;355(26):2733–2743.
28. Goss PE, Smith IE, O'Shaughnessy J, et al. Adjuvant lapatinib for women with early-stage HER2-positive breast cancer: a randomised, controlled, phase 3 trial. *Lancet Oncol.* 2013;14(1):88–96.
29. Piccart-Gebhart MJ, Holmes AP, Baselga J, et al. First results from the phase III ALTTO trial (BIG 2-06; NCCTG [Alliance] N063D) comparing one year of anti-HER2 therapy with lapatinib alone (L), trastuzumab alone (T), their sequence (T→L), or their combination (T+L) in the adjuvant treatment of HER2-positive early breast cancer (EBC). *J Clin Oncol.* 2014;32(suppl 18):LBA4–LBA4.
30. Feldinger K, Kong A. Profile of neratinib and its potential in the treatment of breast cancer. *Breast Cancer (Dove Med Press).* 2015;7:147–162.
31. Tiwari SR, Mishra P, Abraham J. Neratinib, a novel HER2-targeted tyrosine kinase inhibitor. *Clin Breast Cancer.* 2016; 16(5):344–348.
32. Saura C, Garcia-Saenz JA, Xu B, et al. Safety and efficacy of neratinib in combination with capecitabine in patients with metastatic human epidermal growth factor receptor 2–positive breast cancer. *J Clin Oncol.* 2014;32(32): 3626–3633.
33. Chan A, Delaloge S, Holmes FA, et al. Neratinib after trastuzumab-based adjuvant therapy in patients with HER2-positive breast cancer (ExteNET): a multicentre, randomised, double-blind, placebo-controlled, phase 3 trial. *Lancet Oncol.* 2016;17(3):367–377.

34. Jimenez MM, Holmes FA, Ejlersten B, et al. Neratinib after trastuzumab (T)-based adjuvant therapy in early-stage HER2+ breast cancer (BC): 5-year analysius of the phase III ExteNET trial. *Ann Oncol.* 2017;28(suppl 5):v43–v67. https://doi.org/10.1093/annonc/mdx362.

35. *A study looking the incidence and severity of diarrhea in patients with early-stage HER2+ breast cancer treated with Neratinib and Loperamide - full text view;* 2017. ClinicalTrials.gov. https://clinicaltrials.gov/ct2/show/NCT02400476.

36. Ibrahim E, Tripathy D, Wilkinson M, et al. Abstract CT128: effects of adding budesonide or colestipol to loperamide prophylaxis on neratinib-associated diarrhea in patients (pts) with HER2+ early-stage breast cancer (eBC): the CONTROL trial. *Cancer Res.* 2017;77(suppl 13):CT128.

37. Hurvitz S, Chan A, Iannotti N, et al. Effects of adding budesonide or colestipol to loperamide prophylaxis on neratinib-associated diarrhea in patients with HER2+ early-stage breast cancer: the CONTROL trial. In: *Presented at: San Antonio breast cancer symposium.* TX, USA: San Antonio; Dec 7, 2017.

38. Research CfDEa. *Drug safety and availability - Avastin (Bevacizumab) information;* 2017 [WebContent] https://www.fda.gov/Drugs/DrugSafety/ucm193900.htm.

39. Konecny GE, Meng YG, Untch M, et al. Association between HER-2/neu and vascular endothelial growth factor expression predicts clinical outcome in primary breast cancer patients. *Clin Cancer Res.* 2004;10(5):1706–1716.

40. Verma S, Miles D, Gianni L, et al. Trastuzumab emtansine for HER2-positive advanced breast cancer. *N Engl J Med.* 2012;367(19):1783–1791.

41. *A study of trastuzumab emtansine versus trastuzumab as adjuvant therapy in patients with HER2-positive breast cancer who have residual tumor in the breast or axillary lymph nodes following preoperative therapy (KATHERINE) -full text view;* 2017. ClinicalTrials.gov. https://clinicaltrials.gov/ct2/show/NCT01772472.

42. *T-DM1 Vs paclitaxel/trastuzumab for breast (ATEMPT Trial) - full text view;* 2017. ClinicalTrials.gov. https://clinicaltrials.gov/ct2/show/NCT01853748.

43. *Trastuzumab emtansine in treating older patients with human epidermal growth factor receptor 2-positive stage I-III breast cancer - full text view;* 2017. ClinicalTrials.gov. https://clinicaltrials.gov/ct2/show/NCT02414646.

44. Fehrenbacher L, Cecchini R, Geyer C, et al. NSABP B-47 (NRG oncology): phase III randomized trial comparing adjuvant chemotherapy with adriamycin (A) and cyclophosphamide (C) → weekly paclitaxel (WP), or docetaxel (T) and C with or without a year of trastuzumab (H) in women with node-positive or high-risk node-negative invasive breast cancer (IBC) expressing HER2 staining intensity of IHC 1+ or 2+ with negative FISH (HER2-Low IBC). In: *Presented at: San Antonio breast cancer symposium.* TX, USA: San Antonio; December 6, 2017.

CHAPTER 8

Hormone Receptor and Human Epidermal Growth Factor Receptor 2 Co-expressing Tumors: Overview of Clinical Practical Implications and Treatment Strategies

DEBORA DE MELO GAGLIATO, MD • JESUS SOBERINO, MD •
JOSE MANUEL PEREZ-GARCIA, MD, PHD • JAVIER CORTES, MD, PHD

INTRODUCTION

Hormone receptor (HR) and human epidermal growth factor receptor 2 (HER2) are important drivers of breast cancer (BC) biology. Amplification or overexpression of HER2 is found in approximately 15%−20% of human BCs. Of note, approximately half of tumors that harbor HER2 amplification also display HR positivity.[1,2] On the basis of genomic profiling, HER2+ tumors are highly heterogeneous. Different intrinsic molecular subtypes, including luminal A and B, can be found among HR+ and HER2+ BC patients, enabling delineation of distinct treatment strategies for each specific subtype.

Both estrogen receptor (ER) and HER2 signaling pathways might interact through a bidirectional cross talk. In this interaction, ER can be activated regardless of direct estrogen interaction with ER α and β, over a variety of kinases, including mitogen-activated protein kinases and protein kinase B (Akt), resulting in phosphorylation of specific sites of the ER.[3] In this process, ligand-independent ER activation is achieved, leading to the transcription of genes that may promote proliferation, cell survival, and resistance to treatment.[3−5]

Observation of in vitro cell line experiments and analysis of published trial data suggest that HER2 expression might confer resistance and poor response to antiestrogen therapies.[5,6] As an example, a small retrospective analysis of a neoadjuvant (NAT) trial suggested that women with HER2+ tumors (by fluorescence in situ hybridization [FISH]), who received NAT letrozole, experienced significantly less Ki-67 suppression compared with the FISH-negative cohort.[7]

The paradigm of "intrinsic" endocrine resistance, combined with the doctrine of treating all HER2+ BC patients equally, has lead to a plethora of clinical trials in which the combination of HER2 therapy with chemotherapy was the mainstay of treatment in different disease scenarios, regardless of ER status and biologic characterization. Indeed, many large phase III randomized clinical trials demonstrated that patients with HR-positive disease derived as much benefit as those with HR-negative disease from the addition of trastuzumab to chemotherapy.[8,9] Therefore, there is no evidence that the efficacy of trastuzumab is different according to the HR status of the primary tumor, and the benefit of trastuzumab is also noted in overall survival in both subgroups of ER status.[9−11]

Although the majority of clinical trials in HER2+ explored HER2-targeting strategies in combination with cytotoxic agents, strategies focused on the combination of ER and other targeted therapies in combination with anti-HER2 therapies are being increasingly explored. This strategy might have the potential to spare patients from short- and long-term toxicities from cytotoxic agents.[12−15]

In term of prognosis, compared with patients with HR-negative tumors, patients with co-expressing HR and HER2 tumors seem to have better disease-free survival (DFS) and overall survival. This finding appeared to be independent of therapy received and of classical anatomic pathologic characteristics.[16,17] Despite overexpression of the HER2 oncogene, HR status is still a determinant of disease outcome, with many trials demonstrating more recurrences and deaths in women with HER2+ HR-negative disease and also differences in time patterns of disease recurrence.[9,18]

Taking into account our current knowledge of tumor biology, the approach of considering all HER2+ BCs as a uniform disease group, with no distinction based on ER status, should change. This chapter will discuss different treatment strategies and provide a detailed characterization of the group of HR+/HER2+ tumors.

PROGNOSTIC IMPLICATIONS OF PATHOLOGIC COMPLETE RESPONSE AMONG PATIENTS WITH HR+/HER2+ BREAST CANCER

Different new drugs, such as HER2-targeted agents, platinum agents,[19] Poly (ADP-ribose) Polymerase Inhibitor (PARP) inhibitors,[20] anti–PD1-targeted therapies,[21] and others, are being tested in combination with standard NAT (presurgical) systemic regimens in the curative setting, some of which result in increased rates of pathologic complete response (pCR). The achievement of a pCR, defined as the absence of any residual invasive carcinoma on hematoxylin and eosin of the resected breast specimen and lymph nodes after NAT or preoperative systemic treatment, might be informative of prognosis, classifying patients into distinct risk of recurrence groups. While pCR rates do not appear to correlate with survival outcomes in HR+ HER2-negative tumors, it may predict long-term outcome in HER2+ BC.[22]

Several trials found that pCR rates are far less common in HR/HER2 co-expressing tumors compared with those tumors without HR co-expression, regardless of whether single-agent trastuzumab or dual HER2 blockade was given.[23–26] New strategies and treatments other than chemotherapy are currently being explored in this BC subtype and will be discussed later in this chapter.

A previous pooled analysis investigated the potential of pCR as a surrogate end point for long-term outcomes in primary BC patients treated with preoperative chemotherapy followed by surgery.[27] The main finding from this study was the observation that pCR, as defined by the description previously presented, had the strongest correlation with survival outcomes in aggressive BC subtypes, such as triple receptor negative and HR-negative, HER2+ groups.

Another pooled analysis conducted by the German group also found that there was a weaker association between pCR and long-term outcomes in HR and HER2 co-expressing tumors. Authors classified patients into different groups, namely luminal A, luminal B (divided into HER2+ and negative), HER2+ nonluminal, and triple negative. The classification utilized by authors was in alignment with clinicopathologic criteria recommended by the St. Gallen[28] consensus. Factors such as ER, progesterone receptor, and HER2 status, as well as histologic grade, were evaluated. Ultimately, final analysis revealed that pCR was not prognostic in the luminal B/HER2+ subgroup, irrespective of trastuzumab treatment.[22]

In contrast, a recent patient-level metaanalysis focused only on stage I–III HER2+ BC patients who received NAT demonstrated a clear association between pCR and long-term outcomes in all subgroup of patients, regardless of ER status. In this report, a major interest was the evaluation of the relationship between HR status and anti-HER2 therapy to the impact of pCR rates on event-free survival (EFS). A cohort of 5768 patients was included, revealing that the advantage of experiencing a pCR was greater in the HR-negative subgroup (median Hazard Ratio, 0.29 [95% PI, 0.24–0.36]) compared with the HR+ subgroup (median Hazard Ratio, 0.52 [95% PI, 0.40–0.66]). Nevertheless, pCR was associated with substantially longer times to recurrence and death in both cohorts.[29]

Evidence accumulated through several pooled- and metaanalyses suggested that tumor response to NAT and pCR is an adequate surrogate end point for survival outcomes. Overall, the achievement of pCR is strongly correlated with favorable long-term survival rates. Nevertheless, when inspecting data more carefully, this relationship is less robust for co-expressing HR and HER2 tumors. Altogether, surrogate markers alternative to pCR are desperately warranted for this group of patients, and novel surrogate markers are needed for long-term outcome prediction. After chemotherapy-based NAT therapy, these less-proliferative tumors can derive a greater benefit to hormone therapy, given in the adjuvant setting. In addition, chemotherapy-free regimens are also being developed for this group of patients with interesting results (this topic will be further discussed later).

CORRELATION BETWEEN IMMUNOHISTOCHEMISTRY AND BC MOLECULAR SUBTYPES AMONG HR+/HER2+ TUMORS

Studies have demonstrated that BC can be grouped into different molecular subtypes on the basis of distinct gene expression profiles. Gene expression arrays, with measurements of important gene clusters, allowed the foundation of a molecular portrait of the tumor, with the characterization of the different molecular subtypes in BC. Five subtypes of BCs (basal-like, HER2-enriched, luminal A, luminal B, and normal breast-like) have been proposed based on an intrinsic gene set.[30–32]

Distinct prognosis, treatment sensitivity, and epidemiology are associated with each BC subtype.[33–36] Among HER2+ tumors, all intrinsic molecular subtypes can be found. Therefore, not all clinically defined HER2+ tumors are HER2 enriched by mRNA analysis, and not all HER2 enriched by mRNA analysis are clinically HER2+ by immunohistochemistry or FISH.

Overall, the HER2-enriched subtype comprises most tumors with amplification or overexpression of HER2+ tumors. Nevertheless, the proportion of HER2-enriched subtype drastically varies according to HR status. The HER2-enriched subtype is characterized by overexpression of genes in the ERBB2 amplicon, such as GRB7.[30] Also, TP53 mutations are typically found in HER2-enriched or ER-negative HER2+ tumors, whereas GATA3 mutations were predominantly observed in luminal subtypes or HR+ samples.[30]

In a previous NAT trial, in patients who have HR+ and HER2+ tumors, 40%–50% are classified as HER2 enriched, with luminal A and B tumors found in approximately half of the remaining cases. Contrasting, in the HR-negative cohort, 80%–90% are HER2-E and 10%–20% are basal-like.[37] Combining data generated in several NAT trials, approximately half of HER2+ tumor samples are molecularly characterized as HER2 enriched, approximately 40%–45% are luminal A and B, and 10% are basal-like.[38] This information could be important, as molecular subtype might predict response to anti-HER2 and other therapies.

CALGB 40601, a trial designed to evaluate pCR to NAT weekly paclitaxel with trastuzumab plus lapatinib compared to weekly paclitaxel with trastuzumab alone, demonstrated a markedly higher pCR among the HER2-enriched tumors compared with any other subtype of HER2+ tumors, regardless of treatment arm. Patients with the HER2-enriched subtype who received paclitaxel combined with trastuzumab experienced a pCR in the breast of 70% compared with 34% and 36% for luminal A and B, respectively.[39] Intrinsic subtype was more important than HR status in predicting pCR. Also, CALGB 40601 demonstrated that among the tumors with residual disease after NAT, molecular subtype distribution considerable differed from the pretreatment overall cohort. The major striking difference was the lower rate of HER2-enriched subtype group

and proportionally more luminal tumors. In samples with matched pre- and posttreatment tumor samples, excluding normal-like posttreatment samples, the most frequent posttreatment subtype alteration was to the luminal A subtype.

In alignment with these findings, the expression of ERBB2/HER2 using RNA sequencing was the most significant predictor of pCR in an analysis of the NeoALTTO trial. The second most important predictor of pCR was the HER2-enriched subtype.[40] Other studies also associated the HER2-enriched subtype with a greater likelihood of achieving a pCR following anti-HER2-based treatment, compared with the other subtypes.[41,42]

The precise molecular subtype may thus have important implications for clinical practice and patient management, though prospective clinical trials are needed. Selection of patients that might be adequately treated with dual HER2 blockade only, in the absence of chemotherapy, is one of greatest applications for this knowledge. The PAMELA trial illustrates this hypothesis. In this study, patients with stage I–IIIA HER2+ BC were recruited regardless of HR status. Patients were given lapatinib combined with trastuzumab for 18 weeks in a chemotherapy-free regimen.[37] Intrinsic molecular subtypes of biopsy samples were taken at baseline and day 14 with the PAM50 molecular signature. The pCR in the breast of the HER2-enriched subtype was 40.2% versus 10.0% in non-HER2-enriched tumors, suggesting that this particular group of patients might be exclusively managed with anti-HER2 therapy, sparing patients from the toxic side effects from chemotherapy.

Other NAT trials also tested chemotherapy-free regimens in HER2+ BC patients. TBCRC006 evaluated the combination of trastuzumab and lapatinib. Treatment included letrozole in women with co-expressing HER2 and HR tumors. Overall breast pCR was 27%, with ER-positive and ER-negative patients experienced a pCR rate of 21% and 36%, respectively.[14] Another NAT trial, NeoSphere, tested the impact of adding pertuzumab to trastuzumab in a cohort of patients with predominantly locally advanced HER2+ BC, including inflammatory tumors. One arm consisted of the pertuzumab and trastuzumab combination, with no chemotherapy or hormonal therapy. Among the intention to treat patient population, pCR was obtained in 16.8%, contrasting with 5.9% for the group with HR and HER2 co-expression and 27.3% for the group without HR expression.[23]

In summary, profiling of HER2+ BC with molecular expression arrays illustrates the heterogeneity found in this BC subtype. The diversity is reflected clinically, as response to different therapies is observed in the context of several NAT trials, and survival outcomes may vary between different subgroups. Diverse genetic alterations with distinct genomic drivers might generate therapeutic advances and interventions tailored to each specific group.

EFFICACY OF ANTI–HER2-BASED NEOADJUVANT THERAPY IN HR+/HER2+ PATIENTS

NAT therapy in the early disease setting has focused on the use of a variety of anti–HER2-targeted agents, such as trastuzumab, lapatinib, pertuzumab, and trastuzumab emtansine (T-DM1). Several potential advantages can be achieved with this approach. Tumor downsizing, with conversion of a mastectomy candidate to lumpectomy, is traditionally an indication for NAT. Also, as previously discussed above, pCR is a surrogate marker for EFS. Another potential advantage of NAT in the context of clinical trials is the opportunity to collect tissue biopsy, assessing for potential predictors of treatment response and resistance, enabling the development of new treatment strategies.

Tables 8.1–8.5 illustrate pCR rates according to a variety of NAT trials that evaluated different anti–HER2-treatment strategies in patients with HER2+ BC.

The NOAH trial was a pioneer study, incorporating trastuzumab in the treatment of HER2+ BC patients.[25] Patients were randomly allocated to receive anthracycline, taxane, and CMF chemotherapy with or without trastuzumab. Patients who received trastuzumab had a pCR in the breast of 43% compared with 22% for the chemotherapy only group. Other trials explored the addition of trastuzumab to NAT chemotherapy backbones and demonstrated similar findings. The addition of trastuzumab consistently resulted in higher pCR rates.[43,44]

Lapatinib, a dual reversible tyrosine kinase inhibitor, targeted against Epidermal Growth Factor receptor (EGFR) and HER2, was also tested in the NAT setting. Combined with trastuzumab, an increase in pCR rate was obtained with the addition of lapatinib. Of note, in several trials this small augmentation in pCR was not statistically significant.[24,26,39,42] The most significant findings of these trials are summarized in Table 8.2. Contrasting with the NOAH trial, in which the use of trastuzumab with chemotherapy was associated with a significant improvement in EFS, the incorporation of lapatinib did not result in better survival outcomes. The NeoALTTO trial evaluated a 18-week treatment duration consisting of paclitaxel plus lapatinib or paclitaxel plus trastuzumab, or paclitaxel plus

trastuzumab and lapatinib. Among patients with HR and HER2+ co-expressing tumors, pCR was obtained in 16.1%, 22.7%, and 41.6% in patients who received lapatinib, trastuzumab, and trastuzumab combined with lapatinib, respectively. Endocrine therapy (ET) was not added to the NAT treatment.

Although pCR rates were considerably higher in lapatinib plus trastuzumab combination, EFS neither differed between the lapatinib and the trastuzumab groups (Hazard Ratio 1·06, 95% CI 0·66–1·69, $P = 0·81$) nor between the combination and trastuzumab groups (Hazard Ratio 0·78, 0·47–1·28, $P = 0·33$).[45] However, it should be noted that the trial was not powered enough for long-term outcomes.

Pertuzumab, a monoclonal antibody that binds to the HER2 receptor in a different domain than trastuzumab, is another anti-HER2 drug that was evaluated in the NAT setting. The pivotal trial that led to pertuzumab approval in this setting was the NeoSphere trial.[23] Patients were randomized to receive docetaxel combined with one of the three different treatment arms: trastuzumab, trastuzumab and pertuzumab, or pertuzumab alone. This study also had a chemotherapy-free arm, consisting of trastuzumab and pertuzumab combination. There was a clear increase in pCR with chemotherapy, trastuzumab plus pertuzumab compared with trastuzumab alone, from 29% to 46%. Of note, compared with the HR-negative cohort of patients, the HR+ group experienced lower pCR rates. Among patients with HR+ BC, pCR rates were 20%, 26%, 5.9%, and 17.4% in patients who received trastuzumab plus docetaxel, trastuzumab plus pertuzumab plus docetaxel, pertuzumab plus trastuzumab, and pertuzumab plus docetaxel, respectively. Contrasting to these numbers, in patients with HR-negative BC, pCR rates were obtained in 36.8%, 63.2%, 27.3%, and 30% in patients who received trastuzumab plus docetaxel, trastuzumab plus pertuzumab plus docetaxel, pertuzumab plus trastuzumab, and pertuzumab plus docetaxel, respectively. Similarly to previously discussed trials, ET was not added to the NAT treatment in this study. Other trials that incorporated pertuzumab in the trastuzumab–chemotherapy treatment schema also demonstrated a higher pCR in the group of patients treated with pertuzumab.[46] These data are summarized in Table 8.4.

As commented before, a homogeneous finding among all trials that evaluated NAT drug combinations in patients with HER2+ is the observation that the HR-negative cohort of patients experienced higher rates of pCR compared with HR-positive patients. Therefore, new treatment strategies based on tumor characteristics, namely HR and HER2 status, are being developed. The trials described below are strategies focused on sparing patients from the toxic effects from chemotherapy.

TABLE 8.1
Trials that Evaluated the Addition of Trastuzumab to Neoadjuvant Therapy in HER2+ BC Patients

Clinical Study	Study Treatment	pCR Definition	pCR (Breast-Axilla; Overall)	pCR (Breast-Axilla; ER-)	pCR (Breast-Axilla; ER+)	pCR (Breast; Overall)	pCR (Breast, ER-)	pCR (Breast, ER+)	Reference
NOAH	AP × 3 c + H → P × 4 c + H → CMF × 3 c + H	ypT0/is	38%			43%			25
GEPARQUATTRO	EC × 4 c + H → D ± X × 4 c + H	ypT0N0	31.7%	43.5%	23.4%				43
GEPARQUINTO	EC × 4 c + H → D × 4 c + H	ypT0N0	30.3%	38.7%	25.8%				68
ACOSOG Z1041	FEC × 4 c → P × 12 w + H	ypT0/isN0	56.5%	70.4%	47.6%				69
HannaH	D × 4 c + H → FEC × 4 c + H	ypT0/is	34.2%			40.7%			70
NeoALTTO	H × 2 c → P × 12 w + H	ypT0/is	27.6%			29.5%	36.5%	22.7%	24
CHERLOB	P × 12 w + H → FEC × 4 c + H	ypT0/isN0	25%	26.6%	25%				71
NSABP B41	AC × 4 c + H → P × 12 w + H	ypT0/is	49.4%	58.2%	45.5%	52.5%	65.5%	46.7%	26
CALGB 40601	P × 16 w + H	ypT0/is				46%	54%	41%	39
TRIO B07	H × 1 c → Cb + D × 6 c + H	ypT0/isN0	47%	57%	40%				72

A, adriamycin; C, cyclophosphamide; c, cycle; Cb, carboplatin; CMF, cyclophosphamide, methotrexate, 5-fluorouracil; D, docetaxel; E, epirubicin; FEC, 5-fluorouracil, epirubicin, cyclophosphamide; H, trastuzumab; P, paclitaxel; pCR, pathologic complete response; X, capecitabine.

TABLE 8.2
Trials that Evaluated the Addition of Lapatinib to Neoadjuvant Therapy in HER2+ BC Patients

Clinical Study	Study Treatment	pCR Definition	pCR (Breast-Axilla; Overall)	pCR (Breast-Axilla; ER-)	pCR (Breast; Axilla; ER+)	pCR (Breast; Overall)	pCR (Breast, ER-)	pCR (Breast, ER+)	Reference
GEPARQUINTO	EC × 4 c + L → D ± X × 4 c + L	ypT0N0	22.7%	28.3%	16.2%				68
NeoALTTO	L × 2 c → P × 12 w + L	ypT0/is	20%			24.7%	33.7%	16.1%	24
CHERLOB	P × 12 w + L → FEC × 4 c + L	ypT0/isN0	26.3%	35.7%	22.7%				71
NSABP B41	AC × 4 c + L → P × 12 w + L	ypT0/is	47.4%	54.9%	42%	53.2%	60.6%	48%	26
CALGB 40601	P × 16 w + L	ypT0/is				32%	37%	29%	39
TRIO B07	L × 1 c → Cb + D × 6 + L	ypT0/isN0	25%	41%	11%				72

A, adriamycin; *C*, cyclophosphamide; *c*, cycle; *Cb*, carboplatin; *D*, docetaxel; *E*, epirubicin; *FEC*, 5-fluorouracil, epirubicin, cyclophosphamide; *L*, lapatinib; *P*, paclitaxel; *pCR*, pathologic complete response; *X*, capecitabine.

TABLE 8.3
Trials that Evaluated the Addition of Trastuzumab and Lapatinib to the Neoadjuvant Treatment in HER2+ BC Patients

Clinical Study	Study Treatment	pCR Definition	pCR (Breast-Axilla; Overall)	pCR (Breast-Axilla; ER-)	pCR (Breast-Axilla; ER+)	pCR (Breast; Overall)	pCR (Breast, ER-)	pCR (Breast, ER+)	Reference
NeoALTTO	L + H × 2 c → P × 12 w + L + H	ypT0/is	46.8%			51.3%	61.3%	41.6%	24
CHERLOB	P × 12 w + L + H → FEC × 4 c + L + H	ypT0/isN0	46.7%	56.2%	35.7%				71
NSABP B41	AC × 4 c + L + H → P × 12 w + L + H	ypT0/is	60.2%	69.8%	54.6%	62%	73%	55.6%	26
CALGB 40601	P × 16 w + L + H	ypT0/is				56%	79%	41%	39
TRIO B07	L + H × 1 c → Cb + D × 6 c + L + H	ypT0/isN0	52%	67%	40%				72

A, adriamycin; *C*, cyclophosphamide; *c*, cycle; *Cb*, carboplatin; *FEC*, 5-fluorouracil, epirubicin, cyclophosphamide; *H*, herceptin; *L*, lapatinib; *P*, paclitaxel; *pCR*, pathologic complete response; *w*, weeks.

TABLE 8.4
Trials that Evaluated the Addition of Trastuzumab and Pertuzumab to the Neoadjuvant Treatment in HER2+ BC Patients

Clinical Study	Study Treatment	pCR Definition	pCR (Breast-Axilla; Overall)	pCR (Breast-Axilla; ER-)	pCR (Breast-Axilla; ER+)	pCR (Breast; Overall)	pCR (Breast, ER-)	pCR (Breast, ER+)	Reference
NeoSphere	D + H + P × 4 c	ypT0/is	45.8%			39.3%	63.2%	26%	23
TRYPHAENA	↓FEC × 3 c D × 3 c + H + P	ypT0/is	45.3%			57.3%	65%	48.6%	46
	FEC × 3 c + H + P → D × 3 c + H + P		50.7%			61.6%	79.4%	46.2%	
	Cb + D × 6 c + H + P		51.9%			66.2%	83.8%	50%	
BERENICE	AC × 4 c → T × 12 w + H + P	ypT0/isN0	61.8%						73
	FEC × 4 c → D × 4 c + H + P		60.7%						
KRISTINE	Cb + D × 6 c + H + P	ypT0/isN0	55.7%	72.4%	44.8%				74
TRAIN2	Cb + T × 9 c + H + P	ypT0/isN0	68%	84%	55%				74
	FEC × 3 c + H + P → Cb + T × 6 c + H + P		67%	89%	51%				

A, adriamycin; C, cyclophosphamide; c, cycle; Cb, carboplatin; D, docetaxel; FEC, 5-fluorouracil, epirubicin, cyclophosphamide; H, herceptin; P, pertuzumab; pCR, pathologic complete response; T, paclitaxel; w, weeks.

TABLE 8.5
Trials that Evaluated a Chemotherapy-Free Regimen, Based on Dual Anti-HER2 Blockage, to the Neoadjuvant Treatment in HER2+ BC Patients

Clinical Study	Study Treatment	pCR Definition	pCR (Breast-Axilla; Overall)	pCR (Breast-Axilla; ER-)	pCR (Breast-Axilla; ER+)	pCR (Breast; Overall)	pCR (Breast, ER-)	pCR (Breast, ER+)	Reference
TBCRC 006	L+H × 12 w ± ExT if ER+	ypT0/is	22%	28%	18%	27%	36%	21%	14
TBCRC023	L+H × 12 w ± ExT if ER+	ypT0/is				12%	20%	9%	53
	L+H × 24 w ± ExT if ER+					28%	18%	33%	
NeoSphere	H+P × 4 c	ypT0/is	11.2%			16.8%	27.3%	5.9%	23
ADAPT	H+P × 4 c	ypT0/isN0		36.3%					48
PAMELA	L+H × 18 w ± ExT if ER+	ypT0/isN0				30%	43%	18%	37

c, cycle; ER, estrogen receptor; E × T, endocrine therapy; H, herceptin; L, lapatinib; P, pertuzumab; pCR, pathologic complete response; w, weeks.

The West German Study Group Adjuvant Dynamic Marker-Adjusted Personalized Therapy Trial Optimizing Risk Assessment and Therapy Response Prediction in Early Breast Cancer (ADAPT) trial is an ongoing "umbrella" trial in which the different BC subtypes are being divided into distinct therapy groups.[47] Early surrogate markers of therapy success in each established subgroup is being evaluated, as the trial progresses. In the HR+/HER2+ group of patients, T-DM1, an antibody drug conjugate of trastuzumab with the cytotoxic antimicrotubule compound DM1 with or without ET was evaluated.[48] This drug was strategic chosen because of less toxicity compared with chemotherapy, particularly alopecia, polyneuropathy, myelotoxicity, and febrile neutropenia[49] and also because of important drug activity in the metastatic setting. Patients were randomized to T-DM1, T-DM1 plus ET, or trastuzumab plus ET. Patients who received T-DM1 (arm A), T-DM1 plus ET (arm B), or trastuzumab plus ET (arm C) experienced a pCR of 40.1%, 41.5%, and 15.1%, respectively. Both T-DM1 containing arms achieved a statistically significantly higher pCR compared with the trastuzumab arm.

An exploratory analysis demonstrated that patients who were postmenopausal versus premenopausal achieved pCR rates of 44.1% versus 37.9%, respectively (T-DM1); 45.0% versus 38.1%, respectively, (T-DM1 plus ET); and 16.7% versus 13.6%, respectively, (trastuzumab plus ET). Of note, pCR rates were numerically higher in postmenopausal women, but differences were not statistically significant. Overall, the addition of ET to T-DM1 was not shown to improve pCR in this 4 cycle, 12-week treatment. On the other hand, there was no indication of a detrimental effect of the addition of ET to the antibody drug conjugate T-DM1.

T-DM1 was also evaluated in the randomized phase III KRISTINE trial.[50] In this trial, patients with HER2-overexpressing tumors larger than 2 cm in diameter were randomly assigned to receive T-DM1 plus pertuzumab (T-DM1 + P arm) or docetaxel plus carboplatin plus trastuzumab and pertuzumab (TCH + P arm), each given every 3 weeks for 6 cycles, followed by definitive breast surgery, followed by 12 more cycles of the same HER2-directed regimen as adjuvant treatment. The pCR rate in the breast and axillary lymph nodes was 56% in the TCH + P arm and 44% in the T-DM1 + P arm (P 0.0155). Among patients with both HR and HER2+ tumors, pCR responses were 44% and 35% for TCH + P and T-DM1 + P arms, respectively. In the cohort of patients with HR-negative tumors, pCR rate was 73% for TCH + P and 54% for those receiving T-DM1 + P.

The addition of ET to the TCH + P regimen was evaluated in the phase III NRG Oncology/NSABP B-52 trial.[51] In this study, patients with locally advanced nonmetastatic ER+ HER2+ tumors were randomized to TCH + P with or without estrogen deprivation therapy with an aromatase inhibitor. Premenopausal women were allowed in this trial, with an Luteinizing hormone releasing hormone (LHRH) agonist added to the aromatase inhibitor therapy. pCR rates in breast and nodes were 40.9% for TCH + P alone, compared with 46.1% TCH + P plus estrogen deprivation therapy ($P = .36$). Although there was not an antagonistic effect from adding ET to chemotherapy and anti-HER2 therapy, the numerical improvement in pCR was not statistically significant. Tissue sample analysis of patients who may benefit from the addition of ET is important.

Generally, NAT endocrine-based trials have demonstrated that longer treatment duration is associated with a better tumor response. A phase II trial aimed to determine the optimal treatment duration with NAT letrozole demonstrated that more than one third of responders reached maximal tumor reduction after 6 months of therapy.[52] TBCRC023 was a randomized phase II study, investigating lapatinib combined with trastuzumab, with or without ET for 12 versus 24 weeks.[53] Patients who received the 24-week treatment regimen experienced a near double pCR rate compared with the 12-week treatment group (overall pCR rate of 12.2% vs. 24.2%).

Overall, NAT trials that contained chemotherapy-free regimens arms, as previously discussed, demonstrated that a proportion of patients are able to achieve pCR.[14,23,37,48] Once again, the HR-negative cohort of patients is able to achieve higher rates of pCR compared with HR-positive tumors, even when ET is added to anti-HER2 therapy.

NOVEL THERAPIES ON THE HORIZON FOR HR/HER2 CO-EXPRESSING TUMORS

PIK3CA mutations are the most common somatic mutations found in HR+BC[54] and might interfere with the capability of NAT to result in pCR. Previous research demonstrated that activating mutations in the PIK3CA gene of HER2+ BCs are associated with reduced sensitivity to anti-HER2 therapy.[55] Activation of the AKT kinase, mediated by PIK3CA mutation, with transmission of a network of intracellular signals mediates tumor cell proliferation. A previous patient-level analysis from five NAT trials demonstrated that tumors that harbored PIK3CA mutation had a significantly lower rate of pCR, compared with those with PIK3CA wild type, namely 16.2% versus 29.6%, respectively $(P < .001)$.[56] An important observation from this analysis was that among patients with tumors co-expressing HR and HER2, the association between PIK3CA mutations and lower rates of pCR was even stronger, with pCR rates of 24.2% versus 7.6% for wild type and mutated PIK3CA, respectively $(P < .001)$. Contrasting with these findings, in the HR-negative cohort, pCR rates in the PIK3CA wild-type group was 36.4% versus 27.2% for PIKCA mutant (P 0.125). The development of novel-targeted therapies specific to treat HER2+ tumors harboring PIK3CA mutations is ongoing. β sparing or α-specific PIK3CA inhibitors are of great interest.

Another important aspect is the potential for late recurrences among luminal tumors, with implications for treatment duration. Risk of recurrence may persist from the first few years after treatment to at least 20 years later.[57–59] In a recent update of a large randomized trial that evaluated the benefit of adding trastuzumab to conventional cytotoxic adjuvant chemotherapy in localized HER2+ BC, time to recurrence was different in the HR-positive and -negative cohorts, with an initial higher frequency of DFS events in patients in the HR-negative group, compared with HR+.[9] Nevertheless, events still occurred up to 10 years after randomization in both cohorts. Thus the evaluation of extending anti-HER2 therapy beyond the recommended 1 year is of great interest in this group.

Neratinib, an irreversible small-molecule tyrosine kinase inhibitor of HER1, HER2, and HER4,[60] was evaluated in this setting. The ExteNET trial investigated the addition of neratinib after completion of 1 year of adjuvant trastuzumab in patients with early-stage HER2+ BC, regardless of HR status.[61] The study demonstrated that patients in the neratinib group achieved better invasive disease-free survival (IDFS) compared with the placebo group, with a 5-year IDFS of 90·2% versus 87·7% in the neratinib and placebo groups, respectively. The benefit was particularly observed in the subgroup of patients with HR+ disease, with a Hazard Ratio for IDFS in the neratinib group compared with the placebo group of 0.60 (95% CI 0.43−0.83), contrasting with patients in the HR-negative disease, in which the Hazard Ratio for IDFS was 0.95 (0.66−1.35). Bidirectional cross talk between estrogen and HER2 pathways might have resulted with the benefit achieved with extended anti-HER2 therapy observed in the HR+ cohort of patients from ExteNET. ER function depends not only on the receptor activation itself but also on the levels of growth factor receptors and their ligands. Malignant cells that have amplification or overexpression of tyrosine kinase receptors

such as HER2 might depend on this interaction to activate receptor and to proliferate.[3]

Another promising therapeutic intervention in the subgroup of HER2 and HR co-expressing tumors is the CDK4/6 inhibitors. There are three CDK4/6 inhibitors approved for HR+ and HER2-negative metastatic BC: ribociclib, palbociclib, and abemaciclib. As previously discussed, a substantial proportion of co-expressing HR and HER2 tumors is luminal A or B. Preclinical data indicate that this molecular subtype is particularly sensitive to CDK4/6 inhibitors, while nonluminal/basal subtypes are mostly resistant.[62] Of note, a preclinical study identified that CDK4/6 inhibitors were capable of inhibiting growth in luminal HR+ and HER2-amplified BC cell lines.[62] Many trials evaluating the combination of ET with anti-HER2 drugs and CDK4/6 inhibitors are currently ongoing (NCT03054363, NCT02947685, NCT02448420, NCT02657343).

Androgen receptor (AR), a steroid ligand-activated receptor, is another target of interest in HER2+ BC, especially in the cohort of patients with HR co-expression. AR signaling is required for androgen- and estrogen-induced tumor cell growth in vitro and in vivo.[63] A previous cell line experiment evaluated the combination of trastuzumab with enzalutamide, an antiandrogen. Researchers were able to demonstrate that AR might interplay with HER2+ by cross talking with the HER2 signaling.[64] A phase II study evaluating enzalutamide combined with trastuzumab in patients with metastatic or locally advanced HER2+ and AR+ BC is ongoing (NCT02091960).

A field that has been the focus of great scientific progress and new discoveries is the area of immunology. Several studies have shown that tumor-infiltrating lymphocytes (TILs) are associated with better survival outcomes in some subtypes of primary BC tumors, such as triple negative and HER2+.[65] Also, evidence is accumulating in the sense that TILs can act as predictive indicators for improved rates of pCR to NAT.[66] A recent study evaluated immune signatures in BC tissue collected after a short course of trastuzumab or nanoparticle albumin-bound (nab)-paclitaxel from patients who achieved pCR.[67] PAM50 subtypes were assigned and immune cell activation was measured based on gene expression profile. The HER2-enriched subtype had a significantly higher pCR rate compared with other subtypes. Importantly, there was a marked increase in immune cell activation in HER2-enriched tumors. As many co-expressing HR and HER2 are characterized as HER2 enriched, a strategy to develop potential clinically useful biomarkers in this particular molecular subtype might be of interest.

CONCLUSION

Knowledge about the complex interaction between hormone and HER2 pathways are constantly evolving, enabling a better understanding of the molecular characterization of this unique BC group, distinct from the so-called "HER2 pure" ER-negative subtype. Consequently, clinical behavior and outcomes can be more accurately predicted response to treatment tailored to specific drugs that target molecular aberrations and protein upregulation found among the triple positive cohort of patients.

REFERENCES

1. Press MF, Pike MC, Chazin VR, et al. Her-2/neu expression in node-negative breast cancer: direct tissue quantitation by computerized image analysis and association of overexpression with increased risk of recurrent disease. *Cancer Res.* 1993;53:4960–4970.
2. Konecny G, Pauletti G, Pegram M, et al. Quantitative association between HER-2/neu and steroid hormone receptors in hormone receptor-positive primary breast cancer. *J Natl Cancer Inst.* 2003;95:142–153.
3. Shou J, Massarweh S, Osborne CK, et al. Mechanisms of tamoxifen resistance: increased estrogen receptor-HER2/neu cross-talk in ER/HER2-positive breast cancer. *J Natl Cancer Inst.* 2004;96:926–935.
4. Osborne CK, Zhao H, Fuqua SA. Selective estrogen receptor modulators: structure, function, and clinical use. *J Clin Oncol.* 2000;18:3172–3186.
5. Benz CC, Scott GK, Sarup JC, et al. Estrogen-dependent, tamoxifen-resistant tumorigenic growth of MCF-7 cells transfected with HER2/neu. *Breast Cancer Res Treat.* 1992;24:85–95.
6. Lipton A, Ali SM, Leitzel K, et al. Elevated serum Her-2/neu level predicts decreased response to hormone therapy in metastatic breast cancer. *J Clin Oncol.* 2002;20:1467–1472.
7. Ellis MJ, Tao Y, Young O, et al. Estrogen-independent proliferation is present in estrogen-receptor HER2-positive primary breast cancer after neoadjuvant letrozole. *J Clin Oncol.* 2006;24:3019–3025.
8. Untch M, Gelber RD, Jackisch C, et al. Estimating the magnitude of trastuzumab effects within patient subgroups in the HERA trial. *Ann Oncol.* 2008;19:1090–1096.
9. Cameron D, Piccart-Gebhart MJ, Gelber RD, et al. 11 years' follow-up of trastuzumab after adjuvant chemotherapy in HER2-positive early breast cancer: final analysis of the HERceptin adjuvant (HERA) trial. *Lancet.* 2017;389:1195–1205.
10. Hayes DF, Thor AD, Dressler LG, et al. HER2 and response to paclitaxel in node-positive breast cancer. *N Engl J Med.* 2007;357:1496–1506.
11. Perez EA, Romond EH, Suman VJ, et al. Trastuzumab plus adjuvant chemotherapy for human epidermal growth factor receptor 2-positive breast cancer: planned joint analysis of overall survival from NSABP B-31 and NCCTG N9831. *J Clin Oncol.* 2014;32:3744–3752.
12. Johnston S, Pippen Jr J, Pivot X, et al. Lapatinib combined with letrozole versus letrozole and placebo as first-line therapy for postmenopausal hormone receptor-positive metastatic breast cancer. *J Clin Oncol.* 2009;27:5538–5546.
13. Kaufman B, Mackey JR, Clemens MR, et al. Trastuzumab plus anastrozole versus anastrozole alone for the treatment of postmenopausal women with human epidermal growth factor receptor 2-positive, hormone receptor-positive metastatic breast cancer: results from the randomized phase III TAnDEM study. *J Clin Oncol.* 2009;27:5529–5537.
14. Rimawi MF, Mayer IA, Forero A, et al. Multicenter phase II study of neoadjuvant lapatinib and trastuzumab with hormonal therapy and without chemotherapy in patients with human epidermal growth factor receptor 2-overexpressing breast cancer: TBCRC 006. *J Clin Oncol.* 2013;31:1726–1731.
15. Marcom PK, Isaacs C, Harris L, et al. The combination of letrozole and trastuzumab as first or second-line biological therapy produces durable responses in a subset of HER2 positive and ER positive advanced breast cancers. *Breast Cancer Res Treat.* 2007;102:43–49.
16. Perez EA, Romond EH, Suman VJ, et al. Four-year follow-up of trastuzumab plus adjuvant chemotherapy for operable human epidermal growth factor receptor 2-positive breast cancer: joint analysis of data from NCCTG N9831 and NSABP B-31. *J Clin Oncol.* 2011;29:3366–3373.
17. Vaz-Luis I, Ottesen RA, Hughes ME, et al. Impact of hormone receptor status on patterns of recurrence and clinical outcomes among patients with human epidermal growth factor-2-positive breast cancer in the National Comprehensive Cancer Network: a prospective cohort study. *Breast Cancer Res.* 2012;14:R129.
18. Gomez HL, Castaneda CA, Vigil CE, et al. Prognostic effect of hormone receptor status in early HER2 positive breast cancer patients. *Hematol Oncol Stem Cell Ther.* 2010;3:109–115.
19. von Minckwitz G, Schneeweiss A, Loibl S, et al. Neoadjuvant carboplatin in patients with triple-negative and HER2-positive early breast cancer (GeparSixto; GBG 66): a randomised phase 2 trial. *Lancet Oncol.* 2014;15:747–756.
20. Rugo HS, Olopade OI, DeMichele A, et al. Adaptive randomization of veliparib-carboplatin treatment in breast cancer. *N Engl J Med.* 2016;375:23–34.
21. Nanda R, Liu MC, Yau C, et al. *Pembrolizumab Plus Standard Neoadjuvant Therapy for High-Risk Breast Cancer (BC): Results from I-SPY 2.* Chicago, IL: ASCO Annual Meeting; 2017.
22. von Minckwitz G, Untch M, Blohmer JU, et al. Definition and impact of pathologic complete response on prognosis after neoadjuvant chemotherapy in various intrinsic breast cancer subtypes. *J Clin Oncol.* 2012;30:1796–1804.
23. Gianni L, Pienkowski T, Im YH, et al. Efficacy and safety of neoadjuvant pertuzumab and trastuzumab in women

with locally advanced, inflammatory, or early HER2-positive breast cancer (NeoSphere): a randomised multicentre, open-label, phase 2 trial. *Lancet Oncol.* 2012;13: 25−32.

24. Baselga J, Bradbury I, Eidtmann H, et al. Lapatinib with trastuzumab for HER2-positive early breast cancer (Neo-ALTTO): a randomised, open-label, multicentre, phase 3 trial. *Lancet.* 2012;379:633−640.

25. Gianni L, Eiermann W, Semiglazov V, et al. Neoadjuvant chemotherapy with trastuzumab followed by adjuvant trastuzumab versus neoadjuvant chemotherapy alone, in patients with HER2-positive locally advanced breast cancer (the NOAH trial): a randomised controlled superiority trial with a parallel HER2-negative cohort. *Lancet.* 2010; 375:377−384.

26. Robidoux A, Tang G, Rastogi P, et al. Lapatinib as a component of neoadjuvant therapy for HER2-positive operable breast cancer (NSABP protocol B-41): an open-label, randomised phase 3 trial. *Lancet Oncol.* 2013;14: 1183−1192.

27. Cortazar P, Zhang L, Untch M, et al. Pathological complete response and long-term clinical benefit in breast cancer: the CTNeoBC pooled analysis. *Lancet.* 2014;384:164−172.

28. Goldhirsch A, Wood WC, Coates AS, et al. Strategies for subtypes−dealing with the diversity of breast cancer: highlights of the St. Gallen International Expert Consensus on the Primary Therapy of Early Breast Cancer 2011. *Ann Oncol.* 2011;22:1736−1747.

29. Broglio KR, Quintana M, Foster M, et al. Association of pathologic complete response to neoadjuvant therapy in HER2-positive breast cancer with long-term outcomes: a meta-analysis. *JAMA Oncol.* 2016;2:751−760.

30. Perou CM, Sorlie T, Eisen MB, et al. Molecular portraits of human breast tumours. *Nature.* 2000;406:747−752.

31. Sorlie T, Perou CM, Tibshirani R, et al. Gene expression patterns of breast carcinomas distinguish tumor subclasses with clinical implications. *Proc Natl Acad Sci USA.* 2001;98: 10869−10874.

32. Sorlie T, Tibshirani R, Parker J, et al. Repeated observation of breast tumor subtypes in independent gene expression data sets. *Proc Natl Acad Sci USA.* 2003;100:8418−8423.

33. O'Brien KM, Cole SR, Tse CK, et al. Intrinsic breast tumor subtypes, race, and long-term survival in the Carolina Breast Cancer Study. *Clin Cancer Res.* 2010;16:6100−6110.

34. Voduc KD, Cheang MC, Tyldesley S, Gelmon K, Nielsen TO, Kennecke H. Breast cancer subtypes and the risk of local and regional relapse. *J Clin Oncol.* 2010;28: 1684−1691.

35. van 't Veer LJ, Dai H, van de Vijver MJ, et al. Gene expression profiling predicts clinical outcome of breast cancer. *Nature.* 2002;415:530−536.

36. Rouzier R, Perou CM, Symmans WF, et al. Breast cancer molecular subtypes respond differently to preoperative chemotherapy. *Clin Cancer Res.* 2005;11:5678−5685.

37. Llombart-Cussac A, Cortes J, Pare L, et al. HER2-enriched subtype as a predictor of pathological complete response following trastuzumab and lapatinib without chemotherapy in early-stage HER2-positive breast cancer

(PAMELA): an open-label, single-group, multicentre, phase 2 trial. *Lancet Oncol.* 2017;18:545−554.

38. Prat A, Pascual T, Adamo B. Intrinsic molecular subtypes of HER2+ breast cancer. *Oncotarget.* 2017;8:73362−73363.

39. Carey LA, Berry DA, Cirrincione CT, et al. Molecular heterogeneity and response to neoadjuvant human epidermal growth factor receptor 2 targeting in CALGB 40601, a randomized phase III trial of paclitaxel plus trastuzumab with or without lapatinib. *J Clin Oncol.* 2016;34: 542−549.

40. Fumagalli D, Venet D, Ignatiadis M, et al. RNA sequencing to predict response to neoadjuvant anti-HER2 therapy: a secondary analysis of the NeoALTTO randomized clinical trial. *JAMA Oncol.* 2016:227−234.

41. Prat A, Bianchini G, Thomas M, et al. Research-based PAM50 subtype predictor identifies higher responses and improved survival outcomes in HER2-positive breast cancer in the NOAH study. *Clin Cancer Res.* 2014;20: 511−521.

42. Dieci MV, Prat A, Tagliafico E, et al. Integrated evaluation of PAM50 subtypes and immune modulation of pCR in HER2-positive breast cancer patients treated with chemotherapy and HER2-targeted agents in the CherLOB trial. *Ann Oncol.* 2016;27:1867−1873.

43. Untch M, Rezai M, Loibl S, et al. Neoadjuvant treatment with trastuzumab in HER2-positive breast cancer: results from the GeparQuattro study. *J Clin Oncol.* 2010;28: 2024−2031.

44. Buzdar AU, Ibrahim NK, Francis D, et al. Significantly higher pathologic complete remission rate after neoadjuvant therapy with trastuzumab, paclitaxel, and epirubicin chemotherapy: results of a randomized trial in human epidermal growth factor receptor 2-positive operable breast cancer. *J Clin Oncol.* 2005;23:3676−3685.

45. de Azambuja E, Holmes AP, Piccart-Gebhart M, et al. Lapatinib with trastuzumab for HER2-positive early breast cancer (NeoALTTO): survival outcomes of a randomised, open-label, multicentre, phase 3 trial and their association with pathological complete response. *Lancet Oncol.* 2014; 15:1137−1146.

46. Schneeweiss A, Chia S, Hickish T, et al. Pertuzumab plus trastuzumab in combination with standard neoadjuvant anthracycline-containing and anthracycline-free chemotherapy regimens in patients with HER2-positive early breast cancer: a randomized phase II cardiac safety study (TRYPHAENA). *Ann Oncol.* 2013;24:2278−2284.

47. Hofmann D, Nitz U, Gluz O, et al. WSG ADAPT - adjuvant dynamic marker-adjusted personalized therapy trial optimizing risk assessment and therapy response prediction in early breast cancer: study protocol for a prospective, multi-center, controlled, non-blinded, randomized, investigator initiated phase II/III trial. *Trials.* 2013;14:261.

48. Harbeck N, Gluz O, Christgen M, et al. De-escalation strategies in human epidermal growth factor receptor 2 (HER2)-positive early breast cancer (BC): final analysis of the west German study group adjuvant dynamic marker-adjusted personalized therapy trial optimizing risk assessment and therapy response prediction in early

BC HER2- and hormone receptor-positive phase II randomized trial-efficacy, safety, and predictive markers for 12 weeks of neoadjuvant trastuzumab emtansine with or without endocrine therapy (ET) versus trastuzumab plus ET. *J Clin Oncol.* 2017;35:3046−3054.

49. Barok M, Joensuu H, Isola J. Trastuzumab emtansine: mechanisms of action and drug resistance. *Breast Cancer Res.* 2014;16:209.

50. Hurvitz SA, Martin M, Symmans WF, et al. *Pathologic Complete Response Rates after Neoadjuvant Trastuzumab Emtansine (T-DM1) + Pertuzumab vs. Docetaxel + Carboplatin + Trastuzumab + Pertuzumab (TCH+P)Treatment in Patients with HER2-Positive (HER2+) Early Breast Cancer(KRISTINE/TRIO-021)*. Chicago, IL: ASCO Annual Meeting; 2016.

51. Rimawi MF, Cecchini RS, Rastogi P, et al. *A Phase III Trial Evaluating PCR in Patients with HR+, HER2-Positive Breast Cancer Treated with Neoadjuvant Docetaxel, Carboplatin, Trastuzumab, and Pertuzumab (TCHP) +/- Estrogen Deprivation: NRG Oncology/NSABP B-52*. San Antonio, TX: SABCS; 2016.

52. Llombart-Cussac A, Guerrero A, Galan A, et al. Phase II trial with letrozole to maximum response as primary systemic therapy in postmenopausal patients with ER/PgR [+] operable breast cancer. *Clin Transl Oncol.* 2012;14:125−131.

53. Rimawi MF, Niravath PA, Wang T, et al. *TBCRC023: A Randomized Multicenter Phase II Neoadjuvant Trial of Lapatinib Plus Trastuzumab, with Endocrine Therapy and without Chemotherapy, for 12 vs. 24 Weeks in Patients with HER2 Overexpressing Breast Cancer*. San ANtonio, TX, US: San Antonio Breast Cancer Symposium; 2015.

54. Roy-Chowdhuri S, de Melo Gagliato D, Routbort MJ, et al. Multigene clinical mutational profiling of breast carcinoma using next-generation sequencing. *Am J Clin Pathol.* 2015;144:713−721.

55. Goel S, Krop IE. Deciphering the role of phosphatidylinositol 3-kinase mutations in human epidermal growth factor receptor 2-positive breast cancer. *J Clin Oncol.* 2015;33:1407−1409.

56. Loibl S, Majewski I, Guarneri V, et al. PIK3CA mutations are associated with reduced pathological complete response rates in primary HER2-positive breast cancer: pooled analysis of 967 patients from five prospective trials investigating lapatinib and trastuzumab. *Ann Oncol.* 2016;27:1519−1525.

57. Saphner T, Tormey DC, Gray R. Annual hazard rates of recurrence for breast cancer after primary therapy. *J Clin Oncol.* 1996;14:2738−2746.

58. Anderson WF, Chen BE, Jatoi I, Rosenberg PS. Effects of estrogen receptor expression and histopathology on annual hazard rates of death from breast cancer. *Breast Cancer Res Treat.* 2006;100:121−126.

59. Pan H, Gray R, Braybrooke J, et al. 20-year risks of breast-cancer recurrence after stopping endocrine therapy at 5 years. *N Engl J Med.* 2017;377:1836−1846.

60. Rabindran SK, Discafani CM, Rosfjord EC, et al. Antitumor activity of HKI-272, an orally active, irreversible inhibitor of the HER-2 tyrosine kinase. *Cancer Res.* 2004;64:3958−3965.

61. Martin M, Holmes FA, Ejlertsen B, et al. Neratinib after trastuzumab-based adjuvant therapy in HER2-positive breast cancer (ExteNET): 5-year analysis of a randomised, double-blind, placebo-controlled, phase 3 trial. *Lancet Oncol.* 2017:1688−1700.

62. Finn RS, Dering J, Conklin D, et al. PD 0332991, a selective cyclin D kinase 4/6 inhibitor, preferentially inhibits proliferation of luminal estrogen receptor-positive human breast cancer cell lines in vitro. *Breast Cancer Res.* 2009; 11:R77.

63. Cochrane DR, Bernales S, Jacobsen BM, et al. Role of the androgen receptor in breast cancer and preclinical analysis of enzalutamide. *Breast Cancer Res.* 2014;16:R7.

64. He L, Du Z, Xiong X, et al. Targeting androgen receptor in treating HER2 positive breast cancer. *Sci Rep.* 2017;7: 14584.

65. Loi S, Sirtaine N, Piette F, et al. Prognostic and predictive value of tumor-infiltrating lymphocytes in a phase III randomized adjuvant breast cancer trial in node-positive breast cancer comparing the addition of docetaxel to doxorubicin with doxorubicin-based chemotherapy: BIG 02-98. *J Clin Oncol.* 2013;31:860−867.

66. Denkert C, Loibl S, Noske A, et al. Tumor-associated lymphocytes as an independent predictor of response to neoadjuvant chemotherapy in breast cancer. *J Clin Oncol.* 2010;28:105−113.

67. Varadan V, Gilmore H, Miskimen KL, et al. Immune signatures following single dose trastuzumab predict pathologic response to preoperative trastuzumab and chemotherapy in HER2-positive early breast cancer. *Clin Cancer Res.* 2016;22:3249−3259.

68. Untch M, Loibl S, Bischoff J, et al. Lapatinib versus trastuzumab in combination with neoadjuvant anthracycline-taxane-based chemotherapy (GeparQuinto, GBG 44): a randomised phase 3 trial. *Lancet Oncol.* 2012;13:135−144.

69. Buzdar AU, Suman VJ, Meric-Bernstam F, et al. Fluorouracil, epirubicin, and cyclophosphamide (FEC-75) followed by paclitaxel plus trastuzumab versus paclitaxel plus trastuzumab followed by FEC-75 plus trastuzumab as neoadjuvant treatment for patients with HER2-positive breast cancer (Z1041): a randomised, controlled, phase 3 trial. *Lancet Oncol.* 2013;14:1317−1325.

70. Ismael G, Hegg R, Muehlbauer S, et al. Subcutaneous versus intravenous administration of (neo)adjuvant trastuzumab in patients with HER2-positive, clinical stage I-III breast cancer (HannaH study): a phase 3, open-label, multicentre, randomised trial. *Lancet Oncol.* 2012;13: 869−878.

71. Guarneri V, Frassoldati A, Bottini A, et al. Preoperative chemotherapy plus trastuzumab, lapatinib, or both in human epidermal growth factor receptor 2-positive operable breast cancer: results of the randomized phase II CHER-LOB study. *J Clin Oncol.* 2012;30:1989−1995.

72. Hurvitz S, Miller JM, Dichmann R, et al. Final analysis of a phase II 3-arm, randomized trial of neoadjuvant trastuzumab or lapatinib or the combination of trastuzumab and lapatinib, followed by six cycles of docetaxel and carboplatin with trastuzumab and/or lapatinib in patients with

HER2+ breast cancer (TRIO-US B07). *Cancer Res.* 2013; 73(suppl 24).

73. Swain SM, Ewer MS, Viale G, et al. Pertuzumab, trastuzumab, and standard anthracycline- and taxane-based chemotherapy for the neoadjuvant treatment of patients with HER2-positive localized breast cancer (BERENICE): a phase II, open-label, multicenter, multinational cardiac safety study. *Ann Oncol.* 2017:646−653.

74. Van Ramshorst MS, van Werkhoven E, Mandjes IA, et al. A phase III trial of neoadjuvant chemotherapy with or without anthracyclines in the presence of dual HER2-blockade for HER2+ breast cancer: the TRAIN-2 study (BOOG 2012-03). *J Clin Oncol.* 2017;35(suppl 15), 507−507.

CHAPTER 9

Deescalating Treatment in the Adjuvant Setting in Low-Risk HER2-Positive Breast Cancer

ROMUALDO BARROSO-SOUSA, MD, PHD • SARA M. TOLANEY, MD, MPH

INTRODUCTION

In 2006, based on the results of the joint analysis of the NSABP B-31 and the N9831 studies,[1] the Food and Drug Administration approved the use of the anti-human epidermal growth factor receptor 2 (HER2) monoclonal antibody (mAb) trastuzumab for the treatment of patients with early-stage breast cancer, classified as HER2-positive tumors. Together with data from the HERA[2] and the BCIRG-006[3] studies, data from four phase III randomized studies, evaluating more than 10,000 patients, showed that when trastuzumab was administered in combination with or after chemotherapy for 1 year, the risk of recurrence decreased by approximately 40% and overall survival (OS) was improved.[1-3] These pivotal trials established 1 year of trastuzumab plus comprehensive chemotherapy regimens (ACTH or TCH) as the standard of care for most women with early-stage HER2-positive breast cancer. Notably, such regimens can be associated with both short- and long-term adverse events, including alopecia, fatigue, neuropathy, febrile neutropenia, cardiac failure, and leukemia.

However, the patients included in those above mentioned clinical trials were mainly high-risk patients with stage II or stage III HER2-positive breast cancer (Table 9.1), and consequently, the population who will derive the largest absolute benefit from the combined trastuzumab and chemotherapy regimen. Of note, only the BCIRG-006 included patients with pT1abN0 tumors, and this subset of patients represented less than 5% of the study population.[3] The benefit of adjuvant therapy for patients with stage I HER2-positive tumors is less clear. Thus, different groups launched clinical trials evaluating the possibility of deescalating systemic therapy in patients with low-risk early-stage HER2-positive breast cancer and treating these patients with a less intense chemotherapy regimen.

In this chapter, we will discuss the data regarding different approaches to deescalating adjuvant systemic in patients with low-risk HER2-positive breast cancer. We will also discuss additional biomarkers, other than TNM stage, that could predict which patients could be candidates for deescalating approaches and spared from more toxic cytotoxic chemotherapy regimens.

DEESCALATING THERAPY FOR SMALL TUMORS

Before the approval of trastuzumab, even patients with stage I HER2-positive tumors used to have a poor prognosis compared with other subtypes of breast cancer (Table 9.2).[4-10] A study using data from 117 patients with node-negative, HER2-positive breast cancer measuring up to 2 cm in the greatest dimension included in the tumor registry of British Columbia, Canada, showed a 10-year rate of relapse-free survival of 68.3% among patients with hormone receptor (HR)—negative tumors and 77.5% among patients with HR—positive tumors.[5] Another study from the MD Anderson Cancer Center including 98 patients with T1a—bN0 HER2-positive tumors showed a 5-year rate of recurrence-free survival (RFS) of 77.1%.[6] The largest study evaluating small (up to 1 cm in the greatest dimension) HER2-positive tumors evaluated the outcomes of 520 patients utilizing the NCCN database.[10] The 5-year rate of survival free from distant recurrence was 94% for patients with T1bN0 HR—negative tumors, 93% for T1aN0 HR—negative tumors, and 94%—96% for patients with T1a—bN0 HR—positive disease. The biases associated with retrospective designs should be taken into consideration when examining the risk of

TABLE 9.1

Pivotal Trials Evaluating the Efficacy of Adding One Year of Trastuzumab to Adjuvant Chemotherapy for Patients With Early-Stage HER2-Positive Breast Cancer

Study (reference), Sample Size in Primary Analysis	Treatment Regimens Compared	Inclusion of pT1N0 Patients?	Number of pT1 Patients in Primary Analysis	Number of N0 Patients in Primary Analysis
HERA,[9] N = 3387	Multiple trial-approved chemotherapy regimens +/− H	Only pT1c	1347	1100
NSABP B31,[10] N = 1736	AC-T vs. AC-TH	No	677	0
NCCTG N9831,[10] N = 1615	AC-T vs. AC-TH	Only pT1c if ER/PR-negative No pT1 if ER/PR-positive	630	191
BCIRG 006,[11] N = 3322	AC-T vs. AC-TH vs. TCH	148 pT1ab patients, pT1N0 subset not specified	1283	922

AC-T, doxorubicin/cyclophosphamide-paclitaxel; AC-TH, doxorubicin/cyclophosphamide-paclitaxel/trastuzumab; ER, estrogen receptor; H, trastuzumab; PR, progesterone receptor; TCH, docetaxel/carboplatin/trastuzumab.
Data reported are from original trial publications, as referenced.

breast cancer recurrence in patients with small HER2-positive disease in the absence of trastuzumab adjuvant therapy, but these studies showed that patients with T1N0 (≤2 cm) have more than just a minimal risk of disease recurrence. Thus, efforts have been made to investigate the outcomes of patients with small HER2-positive tumors treated with less toxic adjuvant systemic regimens.

Jones et al.[11] evaluated the efficacy of four cycles of docetaxel and cyclophosphamide administered every 3 weeks, given concomitantly with weekly trastuzumab, followed by trastuzumab administered every 3 weeks for the remainder of 1 year. Among the 493 patients enrolled in the multicenter, single arm, phase II study, approximately 58% of patients had stage I tumors, and approximately 79% had node-negative tumors. After a median follow-up of 36.1 months, the 3-year disease-free survival (DFS) and OS rate were 96.9% (95% confidence interval [CI], 94.8–98.1) and 98.7% (95% CI, 97.1–99.4), respectively. The most common grade 3–4 toxic effects were neutropenia (47.1%), febrile neutropenia (6.2%), fatigue (4.3%), and diarrhea (3.3%); only two patients developed symptomatic congestive heart failure (0.5%) on study.

Tolaney et al.[12] conducted a multicenter, single arm study evaluating 12 weeks of adjuvant paclitaxel and trastuzumab (TH) followed by 9 months of trastuzumab monotherapy in 406 patients with HER2-positive,

node-negative tumors measuring up to 3 cm. The primary endpoint of the so called APT trial was DFS. Recurrence-free interval (RFI), breast cancer–specific survival (BCSS), and OS were also analyzed. Remarkably, approximately 50% of patients in this trial had tumors that were ≤1 cm; 9% of patients had tumors between 2 and 3 cm. Six patients had a nodal micrometastasis. The regimen was very well tolerated overall. A total of 13 patients (3.2%; 95% CI, 1.7 to 5.4) reported at least one episode of grade 3 neuropathy, and two patients had symptomatic congestive heart failure (0.5%; 95% CI, 0.1 to 1.8), both of whom had normalization of the left ventricular ejection fraction after discontinuation of trastuzumab. A total of 13 patients had significant asymptomatic declines in ejection fraction (3.2%; 95% CI, 1.7 to 5.4), as defined by the study, but 11 of these patients could resume trastuzumab therapy after a brief interruption. After a median follow-up period of 4 years, the 3-year rate of survival free from invasive disease was 98.7% (95% CI, 97.6 to 99.8). Recently, an updated analysis with a median follow-up of 6.5 years was presented at the American Society for Clinical Oncology 2017 Annual Meeting.[13] At the time, there were 23 DFS events observed, including 4 (1.0%) distant recurrences, 5 local/regional recurrences (1.2%), 6 new contralateral breast cancer cases (1.5%), and 8 deaths without documented recurrence (2.0%). Additionally, the 7-year DFS was 93.3% (95% CI, 90.4–96.2); the

TABLE 9.2
Outcomes of Patients With Small (T1N0) HER2-Positive Breast Cancer

Study (reference)/ Sample Size	Study Population			Follow-Up	Outcomes (%)			
	Stage	HR+ (%)	CT-treated(%)/ H-treated(%)	Time Period (Years)	DFS/ RFS	DDFS/ DRFS	BCSS	OS
RETROSPECTIVE DESIGN								
Joensuu et al.[4] N = 65	pT1abc	NR	NR/0	9	NR	72	NR	NR
Chia et al.[5] N = 117	pT1abc	34	NR/0	10	71.6	77.5	81.3	70.9
Gonzalez-Angulo et al.[6] N = 98	pT1ab	61	0/0	5	77.1	86.4	NR	NR
Curigliano et al.[7] N = 71	pT1ab	100	25.4/0	5	92	NR	NR	NR
Curigliano et al.[7] N = 79	pT1ab	0	43.7/0	5	91	NR	NR	NR
Fehrenbacher et al.[8] N = 234	pT1ab	59	25.6/8.1	5	94.1[a]	96.5[b]	NR	NR
Rouanet et al.[9] N = 44	pT1ab	59	10/0	10	73	80[b]	NR	84
Vaz-Luis et al.[10] N = 89	pT1b	100	0/0	5	NR	94	98	95
Vaz-Luis et al.[10] N = 17	pT1b	0	0/0	5	NR	94	100	100
Vaz-Luis et al.[10] N = 102	pT1a	100	0/0	5	NR	96	99	95
Vaz-Luis et al.[10] N = 49	pT1a	0	0/0	5	NR	94	100	100
PROSPECTIVE DESIGN								
Jones et al.[11,c] N = 493	79.3% N0 67.1% pT1bc	64.9%	100/100	3	96.9	NR	NR	98.7
Tolaney et al.[13,c] N = 406	100% N0 91% pT1bc	67	100/100	7	93.3	NR	98.6	95
ATEMPT (NCT02246621) N = 500	pT1abc	NR	100	Ongoing	Ongoing	Ongoing	Ongoing	Ongoing

BCSS, breast cancer–specific survival; *CI*, confidence interval; *CT*, chemotherapy; *DDFS*, distant disease–free survival; *DFS*, disease-free survival; *DRFS*, distant recurrence–free survival; *H*, trastuzumab; *NR*, not recorded; *OS*, overall survival; *RFI*, recurrence-free interval; *RFS*, recurrence-free survival.

[a] Data reported are RFI (invasive disease only).
[b] Data reported is metastasis-free survival.
[c] These trials also included tumors more than 2 cm and/or node-positive.
Data reported are from original publications, as referenced. Point estimates for outcomes are included in table; original publications include CI. Point estimates must be interpreted in context of confidence intervals.

7-year RFI was 97.5% (95% CI, 95.9–99.1); the 7-year BCSS was 98.6% (95% CI, 97.0–100); and the 7-year OS was 95.0% (95% CI, 92.4–97.7).

There are several caveats when interpreting data from the APT trial. First, it is a single arm trial, and there is no randomized data available from a trial that focuses on the stage I HER2+ population. Given the perceived benefits of trastuzumab-based therapy, a control arm without trastuzumab would have been difficult to accrue to. Moreover, a standard chemotherapy approach, such as ACTH or TCH, seemed excessively toxic as a possible control for this relatively lower risk population. Furthermore, this study enrolled very few patients with tumors larger than 2 cm, so results cannot be generalized to this population. Additionally, approximately two-thirds of patients had hormone receptor–positive tumors, which are generally associated with later recurrences, but the follow-up data now out to 7 years are reassuring. Given the favorable TH regimen safety profile, and the remarkable survival outcomes with 7-year RFI of 97.5%, we do believe this should be considered a reasonable treatment approach for the majority of patients with stage I HER2-positive breast cancer for whom adjuvant systemic therapy is indicated. Moreover, given the low event rate with TH, it seems unlikely that adding other biologic agents, such as pertuzumab or neratinib, will add substantial benefit in this patient population. Conversely, we also recognize that there are some patients with T1aN0 disease for whom adjuvant treatment is not required, especially those with estrogen receptor–positive disease.

Researchers have also been investigating methods of further reducing the toxicity of adjuvant therapy in patients with stage I HER2-positive breast cancer. The ATEMPT trial (NCT02246621), a multicenter, randomized, phase II trial, has just recently completed accrual (n = 500). This study randomized stage I HER2-positive breast cancer patients in a 3:1 fashion to 1 year of the antibody-drug conjugate transtuzumab emtansine (T-DM1) administered every 3 weeks versus TH administered for 12 weeks followed by trastuzumab given every 3 weeks for 9 additional months. The two primary endpoints of ATEMPT are to compare clinically relevant toxicities between the two arms and to evaluate the 3-year DFS among those enrolled to the T-DM1 treatment arm. Results from this study are anticipated to be available in 2019.

USING BIOMARKERS TO DEESCALATE THERAPY

A large effort has been made to develop reliable biomarkers, other than TNM stage, that could not only identify low- versus high-risk HER2-positive tumors but also predict benefit from anti-HER2 therapy, allowing the deescalation of therapy.

Intrinsic Breast Cancer Molecular Subtypes

Oncogenic HER2 addiction, a term used to express the dependency on HER2 signaling itself for the maintenance of their malignant phenotype (sustained cell survival and proliferation), has been recognized as one of the most important determinants of responsiveness to anti-HER2 therapies.[14] In the case of HER2 dependency, this factor is associated with high levels of HER2 gene amplification, RNA expression, and downstream signaling.

Although thought to be a unique disease, Prat et al.[15] used the dataset from The Cancer Genome Atlas (n = 495) and from the Molecular Taxonomy of Breast Cancer International Consortium dataset (n = 1730) and confirmed that clinical HER2-positivity (cHER2), assessed by Immunohistochemistry (IHC) or Fluorescence In Situ Hybridization (FISH), comprises a heterogeneous disease. While cHER2 largely overlaps with the molecular intrinsic subtype genomic-enriched HER2 subtype (HER2E), all the intrinsic subtypes (luminal A, luminal B, HER2E, and basal-like) can be found within this subtype of breast cancer. Conversely, there are some cHER2-negative tumors that are molecularly classified as HER2E tumors.[15]

Of note, different studies have shown that these intrinsic molecular subtypes of breast cancer predict different responses to therapy. In the neoadjuvant setting, studies have shown that the rates of pathologic complete response (pCR) to different anti-HER2 therapies were markedly higher among HER2E tumors compared with any other intrinsic subtype, both when anti-HER2 therapy was combined with (NeoALTTO[16] and CALGB 40601[17]) and without (PAMELA[18]) chemotherapy. In the adjuvant setting, data from the N9831 study showed that patients with HER2E had similar long-term outcomes to those with luminal subtypes. Conversely, basal-like tumors did not derive a better RFS when treated with trastuzumab plus chemotherapy compared with chemotherapy alone.[19] Although these data do not allow intrinsic subtype to replace cHER2 status to predict the benefit of trastuzumab therapy, they inform us that intrinsic subtypes can improve the selection of patients who may benefit from dual anti-HER2 therapy without chemotherapy.

PI3K-AKT Pathway Alterations

PI3K-AKT pathway is a major downstream component of HER2 signaling.[20] Following the HER2 receptor tyrosine kinase activation, the lipid kinase phosphoinositide 3-kinase (PI3K) is stimulated to phosphorylate phosphatidylinositol (4,5)-bisphosphate (PIP2) to phosphatidylinositol (3,4,5)-trisphosphate (PIP3) at the plasma membrane. Ultimately, this will lead to the activation of the AKT kinase that will trigger intracellular signals mediating tumor cell proliferation, survival, metabolism, and growth.[21] Therefore, deregulation of elements in this pathway—including activating mutations in *PIK3CA*, the gene encoding the p110a catalytic subunit of PI3K, or partial/complete loss of the tumor suppressor PTEN, that negatively regulates the PI3K pathway—have been suggested to be associated with resistance to anti-HER2 treatments.[22–24]

Using individual patient data from five neoadjuvant trials including a total of 967 patients with HER2-positive breast cancer, Loibl et al.[25] showed that PIKCA mutations were present in 21.7% of this population. Moreover, *PIK3CA* mutation was associated with a significantly lower rate of pCR (wild-type pCR 29.6% vs. mutant pCR 16.2%, P < .001), although it was not accompanied by an inferior DFS. Regarding PTEN protein loss, which is found in approximately 20%–25% HER2-positive tumors, and in response to anti-HER2 therapy in the neoadjuvant setting, there are conflicting results. While in the German GeparQuattro study PTEN levels predicted pCR after anti-HER2 treatment combined with chemotherapy,[26] a subanalysis of NeoALTTO trial failed to demonstrate such correlation.[27]

In the adjuvant setting, while retrospective analysis of FINHER[28] and NSABP B-31[29] showed no correlation between PIK3CA mutation and lack of benefit associated with the addition of trastuzumab, data from the adjuvant N9831[30] trial also did not demonstrate a correlation between PTEN status and trastuzumab benefit. Notably, all these data are confounded by the fact that anti-HER2 therapies were given concomitantly with chemotherapy.

Immune Biomarkers
Recently, both preclinical and clinical data suggest that the interaction between the immune system and breast cancer cells is critical for disease outcome.[31] As such, there is increased interest in identifying immune biomarkers that could help to select patients with early-stage HER2-positive breast cancer who may be candidates for deescalating therapy.

In this context, tumor-infiltrating lymphocytes (TILs) have been shown to be predictive for response to neoadjuvant therapy in HER2-positive breast cancer.[32] A recent metaanalysis of six prospective neoadjuvant

clinical trials, including 1379 patients with HER2-positive breast cancer, showed that increased stromal TILs were observed in 19% of HER2-positive tumors.[33] Increased TILs were significantly associated with increased pCR rates (P < .0005) and with improved DFS (P = .02). Both the NeoALTTO[34] and NeoSphere[35] trials found that only tumors with less than 5% of TILs had lower pCR rates. Conversely, survival data from the adjuvant N9831 study suggested that the presence of high stromal TILs was associated with an improvement in RFS of patients treated with chemotherapy alone but not among patients treated with chemotherapy plus trastuzumab in the adjuvant setting.[36]

Another biomarker of interest is the immune-related gene expression profile, or simply the immune signature of the tumor. In another subanalysis of the N9831 study, Perez et al.[37] showed that the benefit in terms of RFS from the addition of trastuzumab to chemotherapy was restricted to those patients whose tumors presented an increased expression of a subset of immune function genes (P < .001). Conversely, the same immune signature was not associated with increased RFS in the arm treated with chemotherapy only (P = .64).

Given the contrasting data between the predictive role of TILs and immune signatures regarding survival benefits with trastuzumab, it is difficult to make definitive conclusions on the utility of these biomarkers, and further work is needed.

NEW CLINICAL TRIAL DESIGNS: USING RESPONSE TO PREOPERATIVE THERAPY TO DEESCALATE THERAPY
Despite the fact that response rates are higher when chemotherapy is added to anti-HER2 therapies, data from the NeoSphere,[38] PAMELA,[18] and WSG-ADAPT[39] studies show that there is a subgroup of patients very sensitive to anti-HER2 treatment even in the absence of chemotherapy. Therefore, it is important to launch clinical trials assessing whether patients who achieve pCR to different combinations of less toxic regimens could receive less therapy after surgery. A large metaanalysis of 12 international trials,[40] including 11,955 patients, confirmed the prognostic value of pCR for use in clinical practice; however, the study did not find an association of the magnitude of difference in pCR rates between treatment arms (study level) and differences in long-term outcome. The study failed to validate pCR as an established surrogate endpoint for improved event-free survival and OS,[40] and trials with

long-term follow-up are still needed to address survival outcomes for specific therapies.

More recently, attention has been directed toward whether plasma tumor DNA (ptDNA) can be used to determine the presence of micrometastatic disease following neoadjuvant therapy and if this information could predict if further therapy is needed. To validate this rationale, the Translational Breast Cancer Research Consortium launched the 040 study (NCT02743910), which is evaluating whether ptDNA can be used to predict pCR in newly diagnosed patients with invasive HER2-positive or triple-negative breast cancer receiving preoperative therapy. Blood collection will be performed at baseline (before starting preoperative therapy), during preoperative treatment, immediately before surgery, and after completion of any adjuvant therapy. The study will also investigate the prognostic value of ptDNA for 5-year invasive DFS and distant DFS in patients following completion of locoregional and systemic therapy. Depending on its results, this ptDNA could be used to deescalate therapy, selecting patients suitable for avoiding additional chemotherapy following a pCR.

CONCLUSION
The investigation of the feasibility of deescalating adjuvant systemic therapy in patients with low-risk HER2-positive breast cancer without impairing their survival outcomes is important to spare patients from unnecessary toxicities related to regimens using polychemotherapy in combination with anti-HER-2 therapy. In patients with stage I tumors, TH can be considered a standard treatment approach for the majority of patients. That being said, there may be some patients with particularly high-risk features for whom more standard approaches, such as ACTH or TCH, can be considered. The clinical development of biomarkers other than anatomic stage is critical, and possible candidates include intrinsic biomarkers, components of PIK3-AKT pathway, and immune biomarkers. Additional work is needed to determine if the achievement of a pCR to preoperative therapy can help us identify patients who may not need further adjuvant treatment, and whether ptDNA can identify patients with low risk of disease recurrence.

DISCLOSURE STATEMENT
S.M.T. receives research funding (institutional) from Genentech, Exelixis, Novartis, Pfizer, Eli Lilly, Nektar, AstraZeneca, Eisai, and Merck. S.M.T has also served as an advisor to Novartis, Pfizer, Nektar, AstraZeneca, Merck, Puma, and Nanostring. R.BS has no conflicts of interest.

REFERENCES
1. Romond EH, Perez EA, Bryant J, et al. Trastuzumab plus adjuvant chemotherapy for operable HER2-positive breast cancer. *N Engl J Med.* 2005;353:1673−1684.
2. Piccart-Gebhart MJ, Procter M, Leyland-Jones B, et al. Trastuzumab after adjuvant chemotherapy in HER2-positive breast cancer. *N Engl J Med.* 2005;353:1659−1672.
3. Slamon D, Eiermann W, Robert N, et al. Adjuvant trastuzumab in HER2-positive breast cancer. *N Engl J Med.* 2011; 365:1273−1283.
4. Joensuu H, Isola J, Lundin M, et al. Amplification of erbB2 and erbB2 expression are superior to estrogen receptor status as risk factors for distant recurrence in pT1N0M0 breast cancer: a nationwide population-based study. *Clin Cancer Res.* 2003;9:923−930.
5. Chia S, Norris B, Speers C, et al. Human epidermal growth factor receptor 2 overexpression as a prognostic factor in a large tissue microarray series of node-negative breast cancers. *J Clin Oncol.* 2008;26:5697−5704.
6. Gonzalez-Angulo AM, Litton JK, Broglio KR, et al. High risk of recurrence for patients with breast cancer who have human epidermal growth factor receptor 2-positive, node-negative tumors 1 cm or smaller. *J Clin Oncol.* 2009;27:5700−5706.
7. Curigliano G, Viale G, Bagnardi V, et al. Clinical relevance of HER2 overexpression/amplification in patients with small tumor size and node-negative breast cancer. *J Clin Oncol.* 2009;27:5693−5699.
8. Fehrenbacher L, Capra AM, Quesenberry Jr CP, Fulton R, Shiraz P, Habel LA. Distant invasive breast cancer recurrence risk in human epidermal growth factor receptor 2-positive T1a and T1b node-negative localized breast cancer diagnosed from 2000 to 2006: a cohort from an integrated health care delivery system. *J Clin Oncol.* 2014;32: 2151−2158.
9. Rouanet P, Roger P, Rousseau E, et al. HER2 overexpression a major risk factor for recurrence in pT1a-bN0M0 breast cancer: results from a French regional cohort. *Cancer Med.* 2014;3:134−142.
10. Vaz-Luis I, Ottesen RA, Hughes ME, et al. Outcomes by tumor subtype and treatment pattern in women with small, node-negative breast cancer: a multi-institutional study. *J Clin Oncol.* 2014;32:2142−2150.
11. Jones SE, Collea R, Paul D, et al. Adjuvant docetaxel and cyclophosphamide plus trastuzumab in patients with HER2-amplified early stage breast cancer: a single-group, open-label, phase 2 study. *Lancet Oncol.* 2013;14: 1121−1128.
12. Tolaney SM, Barry WT, Dang CT, et al. Adjuvant paclitaxel and trastuzumab for node-negative, HER2-positive breast cancer. *N Engl J Med.* 2015;372:134−141.

13. Tolaney SM, Barry WT, Guo H, et al. Seven-year (yr) follow-up of adjuvant paclitaxel (T) and trastuzumab (H) (APT trial) for node-negative, HER2-positive breast cancer (BC). *J Clin Oncol.* 2017;35(suppl 15):511.
14. Veeraraghavan J, De Angelis C, Reis-Filho JS, et al. De-escalation of treatment in HER2-positive breast cancer: determinants of response and mechanisms of resistance. *Breast.* 2017;34(suppl 1):S19–S26.
15. Prat A, Carey LA, Adamo B, et al. Molecular features and survival outcomes of the intrinsic subtypes within HER2-positive breast cancer. *J Natl Cancer Inst.* 2014; 106:dju152.
16. Fumagalli D, Venet D, Ignatiadis M, et al. RNA Sequencing to predict response to neoadjuvant anti-HER2 therapy: a secondary analysis of the NeoALTTO randomized clinical trial. *JAMA Oncol.* 2016. [Epub ahead of print].
17. Carey LA, Berry DA, Cirrincione CT, et al. Molecular heterogeneity and response to neoadjuvant human epidermal growth factor receptor 2 targeting in CALGB 40601, a randomized phase III trial of paclitaxel plus trastuzumab with or without lapatinib. *J Clin Oncol.* 2016;34:542–549.
18. Llombart-Cussac A, Cortes J, Pare L, et al. HER2-enriched subtype as a predictor of pathological complete response following trastuzumab and lapatinib without chemotherapy in early-stage HER2-positive breast cancer (PAMELA): an open-label, single-group, multicentre, phase 2 trial. *Lancet Oncol.* 2017;18:545–554.
19. Perez EA, Ballman KV, Mashadi-Hossein A, et al. Intrinsic subtype and therapeutic response among HER2-positive breast tumors from the NCCTG (Alliance) N9831 trial. *J Natl Cancer Inst.* 2017;109:djw207.
20. Mayer IA, Arteaga CL. The PI3K/AKT pathway as a target for cancer treatment. *Ann Rev Med.* 2016;67:11–28.
21. Manning BD, Cantley LC. AKT/PKB signaling: navigating downstream. *Cell.* 2007;129:1261–1274.
22. Berns K, Horlings HM, Hennessy BT, et al. A functional genetic approach identifies the PI3K pathway as a major determinant of trastuzumab resistance in breast cancer. *Cancer Cell.* 2007;12:395–402.
23. Fujita T, Doihara H, Kawasaki K, et al. PTEN activity could be a predictive marker of trastuzumab efficacy in the treatment of ErbB2-overexpressing breast cancer. *Br J Cancer.* 2006;94:247–252.
24. Moasser MM, Krop IE. The evolving landscape of HER2 targeting in breast cancer. *JAMA Oncol.* 2015;1: 1154–1161.
25. Loibl S, Majewski I, Guarneri V, et al. PIK3CA mutations are associated with reduced pathological complete response rates in primary HER2-positive breast cancer: pooled analysis of 967 patients from five prospective trials investigating lapatinib and trastuzumab. *Ann Oncol.* 2016; 27:1519–1525.
26. Loibl S, Darb-Esfahani S, Huober J, et al. Integrated analysis of PTEN and p4EBP1 protein expression as predictors for pCR in HER2-positive breast cancer. *Clin Cancer Res.* 2016;22:2675–2683.
27. Nuciforo PG, Aura C, Holmes E, et al. Benefit to neoadjuvant anti-human epidermal growth factor receptor 2 (HER2)-targeted therapies in HER2-positive primary breast cancer is independent of phosphatase and tensin homolog deleted from chromosome 10 (PTEN) status. *Ann Oncol.* 2015;26:1494–1500.
28. Loi S, Michiels S, Lambrechts D, et al. Somatic mutation profiling and associations with prognosis and trastuzumab benefit in early breast cancer. *J Natl Cancer Inst.* 2013;105: 960–967.
29. Pogue-Geile KL, Song N, Jeong JH, et al. Intrinsic subtypes, PIK3CA mutation, and the degree of benefit from adjuvant trastuzumab in the NSABP B-31 trial. *J Clin Oncol.* 2015; 33:1340–1347.
30. Perez EA, Dueck AC, McCullough AE, et al. Impact of PTEN protein expression on benefit from adjuvant trastuzumab in early-stage human epidermal growth factor receptor 2-positive breast cancer in the North Central Cancer Treatment Group N9831 trial. *J Clin Oncol.* 2013;31:2115–2122.
31. Kroemer G, Senovilla L, Galluzzi L, Andre F, Zitvogel L. Natural and therapy-induced immunosurveillance in breast cancer. *Nat Med.* 2015;21:1128–1138.
32. Ingold Heppner B, Untch M, Denkert C, et al. Tumor-infiltrating lymphocytes: a predictive and prognostic biomarker in neoadjuvant-treated HER2-positive breast cancer. *Clin Cancer Res.* 2016;22:5747–5754.
33. Denkert C, von Minckwitz G, Darb-Esfahani S, et al. Abstract S1-09: evaluation of tumor-infiltrating lymphocytes (TILs) as predictive and prognostic biomarker in different subtypes of breast cancer treated with neoadjuvant therapy - a metaanalysis of 3771 patients. *Cancer Res.* 2017;77(suppl 4):S01–S09.
34. Salgado R, Denkert C, Campbell C, et al. Tumor-infiltrating lymphocytes and associations with pathological complete response and event-free survival in HER2-positive early-stage breast cancer treated with lapatinib and trastuzumab: a secondary analysis of the NeoALTTO trial. *JAMA Oncol.* 2015;1:448–454.
35. Bianchini G, Pusztai L, Pienkowski T, et al. Immune modulation of pathologic complete response after neoadjuvant HER2-directed therapies in the NeoSphere trial. *Ann Oncol.* 2015;26:2429–2436.
36. Perez EA, Ballman KV, Tenner KS, et al. Association of stromal tumor-infiltrating lymphocytes with recurrence-free survival in the N9831 adjuvant trial in patients with early-stage HER2-positive breast cancer. *JAMA Oncol.* 2016;2:56–64.
37. Perez EA, Thompson EA, Ballman KV, Anderson SK, Asmann YW. Genomic analysis reveals that immune function genes are strongly linked to clinical outcome in the North Central Cancer Treatment Group N9831 Adjuvant Trastuzumab Trial. *J Clin Oncol.* 2015;33:701–708.
38. Gianni L, Pienkowski T, Im YH, et al. Efficacy and safety of neoadjuvant pertuzumab and trastuzumab in women with locally advanced, inflammatory, or early HER2-positive breast cancer (NeoSphere): a randomised multicentre, open-label, phase 2 trial. *Lancet Oncol.* 2012;13:25–32.

39. Harbeck N, Gluz O, Christgen M, et al. De-escalation strategies in human epidermal growth factor receptor 2 (HER2)-positive early breast cancer (BC): final analysis of the West German Study Group Adjuvant Dynamic Marker-Adjusted Personalized Therapy Trial Optimizing Risk Assessment and Therapy Response Prediction in Early BC HER2- and hormone receptor-positive phase II randomized trial-efficacy, safety, and predictive markers for 12 weeks of neoadjuvant trastuzumab emtansine with or without endocrine therapy (ET) versus trastuzumab plus ET. *J Clin Oncol.* 2017;35:3046–3054.

40. Cortazar P, Zhang L, Untch M, et al. Pathological complete response and long-term clinical benefit in breast cancer: the CTNeoBC pooled analysis. *Lancet.* 2014;384:164–172.

CHAPTER 10

Cardiac Toxicity of HER-2 Targeted Regimens

MIRELA TUZOVIC, MD • MEGHA AGARWAL, MD • NIDHI THAREJA, MD • ERIC H. YANG, MD

INTRODUCTION

The advent of anti-HER2 cancer therapies has heralded significantly improved survival rates along with decreased recurrence in breast cancer and is being increasingly used in other malignancies, including gastrointestinal tumors. However, a known effect that has been well documented is the onset of cardiomyopathy during treatment, which may potentially alter or delay critical treatment to these patients. This chapter reviews the proposed mechanisms of HER2-related cardiotoxicity, its incidence in major cancer trials and in the postapproval era—much of it related to trastuzumab—and proposed cardioprotective and surveillance strategies to potentially reduce the risk of developing cardiotoxicity.

PROPOSED MECHANISM OF HER2 CARDIOTOXICITY

In recent American and European cardiology society Expert Consensus statements, Cancer therapeutics—related cardiac dysfunction (CTRCD) is defined as a decline in left ventricular ejection fraction (LVEF) of >10% to a value of <53% and confirmed on repeat study after 2—3 weeks.[1] A "multiple-hit hypothesis" has been proposed as a potential explanation for the development of cardiotoxicity. This hypothesis states that patients with breast cancer, who are already at a higher risk of cardiovascular disease due to overlapping risk factors, develop subclinical or clinical cardiotoxicity due to subsequent serial or concurrent injury from various chemotherapeutics as well as maladaptive lifestyle changes during chemotherapy (Fig. 10.1).[2] Cardiac injury is generally classified into two types: Type I, as seen with anthracycline-induced cardiotoxicity, and Type II, caused by trastuzumab and other similar agents. This classification is likely

an oversimplification and does not account for many complex mechanistic effects of both traditional and novel chemotherapeutic agents; however, it provides a useful framework by highlighting some of the key differences in the pathophysiology, histologic appearance,[3] and prognosis of cardiotoxicity due to different chemotherapeutic agents (Table 10.1).

Although cardiotoxicity was recognized as a complication from trastuzumab more than a decade ago, the mechanism of cardiac injury remains unclear. The epidermal growth factor receptors (HER, EGFR, or ErbB) constitute a family of cell-surface receptor tyrosine kinases, which are essential to normal cell function, growth, and survival. A number of different receptors exist in the human body, including HER1 (EGFR), HER2 (erbB2), HER3 (erbB3), and HER4 (erbB4). Trastuzumab binds the HER2/erbB2 and has antineoplastic effects in tumors that overexpress those receptors.

Studies in animal models provide insight into the importance of HER/erbB receptors for cardiac development, maintenance of cardiac function, and enactment of compensatory mechanisms in the setting of cardiac stress. Mice with absence of erbB2/HER2 die in utero during embryogenesis secondary to abnormal cardiac development and loss of ventricular trabeculae.[4] Similar findings have also been reported for the erbB4 receptor.[5] In contrast, mice that are deficient in cardiac HER2/erbB2 have normal cardiac structure at birth; however, over several subsequent months, they demonstrate progressive ventricular dilation, reduced contractility, impaired relaxation, and overexpression of molecular markers of hypertrophy, all consistent with cardiomyopathy.[6,7] These mice hearts also demonstrate impaired compensatory and survival mechanisms in the setting of stressors and are more vulnerable to anthracycline toxicity. Similarly, mice

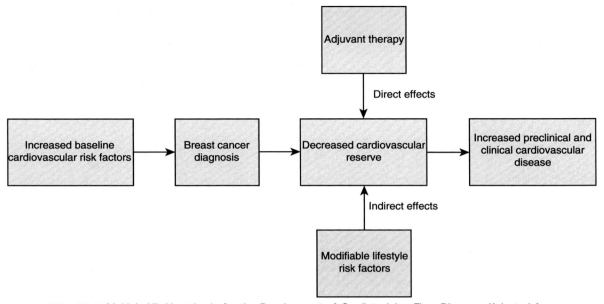

FIG. 10.1 Multiple-Hit Hypothesis for the Development of Cardiotoxicity. Flow Diagram. (Adapted from Jones LW, Haykowsky MJ, Swartz JJ, Douglas PS, Mackey JR. Early breast cancer therapy and cardiovascular injury. *J Am Coll Cardiol*. 2007;50:1435–1441.)

TABLE 10.1
Characteristics of Type I and Type II Cardiotoxicity

	Type I	Type II
Characteristic agent	Doxorubicin, daunorubicin, epirubicin	Trastuzumab, lapatinib
Dose effect	Dose dependent	Not dose dependent
Ultrastructural abnormalities	Vacuoles, myofibrillar disarray, myocyte necrosis	No apparent abnormalities
Reversibility	Permanent myocyte injury	Largely reversible
Prognosis	Variable, may stabilize after treatment	Good
Effect of rechallenge	High likelihood of recurrent cardiac dysfunction which may be progressive	Generally well tolerated

deficient in erbB4 are born with normal ventricular walls. They subsequently develop ventricular cavity dilation, reduced contractility, abnormal conduction systems and have reduced life expectancy.[8]

Human studies also indicate that HER2 signaling may be an important part of cardiac response and compensatory mechanisms in the setting of stress. One study looked at patients with HER2-negative tumors who were treated with anthracycline therapy. Radioactively labeled ^{111}In trastuzumab was infused after anthracycline treatment, and 50% (5/10) of patients showed cardiac uptake of trastuzumab. There was no uptake in the control group of patients with chronic heart failure.[9] In addition, chronic heart failure, a disease characterized by chronic activation of compensatory mechanisms and the sympathetic nervous system in response to cardiac stress eventually leading to myocardial destruction and disease progression, is associated with elevated HER2 levels. Higher HER2 levels also correlate with lower LVEF and higher New York Heart Association (NYHA) functional class.[10]

In conclusion, HER/erbB receptors appear to be essential for normal cardiac function and survival mechanisms in the setting of cardiac stressors. Patients treated with anthracyclines have increased trastuzumab binding, suggesting that upregulation of HER/erbB receptors may be an important compensatory mechanism to anthracycline toxicity. The fact that trastuzumab cardiotoxicity is largely seen in combination or following anthracycline administration supports the idea that trastuzumab acts as a modifier to anthracycline-induced cardiotoxicity[9] (Fig. 10.2). Nonetheless, it remains unclear whether trastuzumab simply acts as a modifier to anthracycline-induced cardiotoxicity or if it independently impairs normal cardiac function as well.

CLINICAL TRIALS AND INCIDENCE OF HER2 CARDIOTOXICITY
Clinical Incidence
Based on a metaanalysis of eight randomized-controlled trials (RCTs) of trastuzumab therapy, the overall incidence of congestive heart failure (CHF) is 2.5%, with a relative risk of 5.11[12] at a median follow up of 18—65 months. The definition of CHF varied among the trials and included the following: (1) determined to be symptomatic by a cardiologist with a decrease in LVEF ≥10% to <50%, (2) NYHA class III/IV either with or without a decrease in LVEF ≥10% from baseline to <50%, (3) heart failure grades 3 or 4, or (4) definition was not reported (Table 10.2).[12] These eight RCTs included 11,991 women with early breast cancer with a median age of 49 years (range 22—80 years). They concluded that if 1000 low-risk women are treated with conventional therapy (including anthracyclines), 900 would survive and 5 would experience CHF. With trastuzumab treatment, 933 would survive but 26 would experience CHF, although this cardiotoxicity is often reversible. Compared with development of CHF, the incidence of LVEF reduction was higher with 11.2% of patients showing left ventricular (LV) systolic dysfunction; however, there was substantial variation among studies in the definition of LVEF reduction.[12] The majority of patients included in the eight RCTs were also treated with anthracyclines. In the BCIRG 006 trial, there was one arm randomized to treatment with

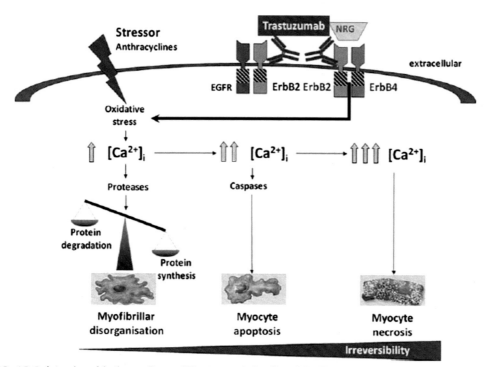

FIG. 10.2 Interplay of Anthracycline and Trastuzumab Cardiotoxicity. Trastuzumab Blocks the ErbB2-ErbB4 Repair Mechanism Enabling Anthracycline-Induced Oxidative Stress to Cause Cardiomyocyte Injury and Necrosis. (Reproduced from Tocchetti CG, Ragone G, Coppola C, et al. Detection, monitoring, and management of trastuzumab-induced left ventricular dysfunction: an actual challenge. *Eur J Heart Fail.* 2012;14:130—137 with permission.)

TABLE 10.2
Different Classification Schemes for Cardiac Toxicity and Heart Failure

Classification System	Severity			
	Low	**Intermediate**	**High**	
ONCOLOGY DERIVED				
LV systolic dysfunction (CTCAE, version 4.03)	—	Symptomatic as a result of a drop in EF; responsive to intervention	Refractory or poorly controlled HF owing to EF drop; intervention such as LVAD, vasopressor support, or heart transplantation indicated	Death
Heart failure (CTCAE, version 4.03)	Asymptomatic with abnormal biomarkers or imaging	Symptoms with mild to moderate activity or exertion	Severe with symptoms at rest or with minimal activity or exertion; intervention indicated	Life-threatening consequences; urgent intervention indicated (e.g., continuous IV therapy or mechanical hemodynamic support)	Death
Decreased ejection fraction (CTCAE, version 4.03)	—	Resting EF 40%–50%; 10%–19% drop from baseline	Resting EF 20%–39%; >20% drop from baseline	Resting EF <20%	—
Cardiac review and evaluation committee	Any of the four criteria confirms cardiac dysfunction: cardiomyopathy, reduced LVEF (global or more severe in the septum); symptoms of HF; signs associated with HF (S3 gallop and/or tachycardia); and decrease in LVEF from baseline ≥5% to <55% with accompanying signs or symptoms of HF or decline in LVEF ≥10% to <55% without accompanying signs of symptoms of HF			–
CARDIOLOGY DERIVED				
Heart failure stage (ACC/AHA)	Stage A, at risk (e.g., patients receiving cardiotoxic medications but without structural heart disease or symptoms)	Stage B, structural heart disease (hypertrophy, low EF, valve disease)	Stage C, structural heart disease with prior or current symptoms	Stage D, refractory HF requiring specialized interventions	—
NYHA symptom classification	Grade I, no limitations of activity	Grade II, mild limitation of activity; grade III, marked limitation of activity	Grade IV, confined to bed or chair	—

CTCAE, common terminology criteria for adverse events; *EF*, ejection fraction; *HF*, heart failure; *IV*, intravenous; *LV*, left ventricular; *LVAD*, left ventricular assist device; *LVEF*, left ventricular ejection fraction.
Adapted from Khouri MG, Douglas PS, Mackey JR, et al. Cancer therapy-induced cardiac toxicity in early breast cancer: addressing the unresolved issues. *Circulation.* 2012;126:2749–2763.

docetaxel, carboplatin, and trastuzumab without anthracyclines; this group of patients notably had the lowest incidence of cardiotoxicity (0.4%).[13]

Data from clinical trials may not reflect the incidence of cardiotoxicity in community practice, however. One population-based, retrospective cohort study of 12,500 women, which sought to show the real-world rates of cardiotoxicity, showed that the incidence may be higher than reported in the clinical trials. The risk of heart failure or cardiomyopathy in patients treated with trastuzumab with or without anthracyclines was 6.2% at 1 year following therapy and increased to 20.1% at 5 years.[14] The difference in incidence of cardiotoxicity is likely multifactorial, both due to different outcome definitions, concomitant usage of anthracyclines, as well as different age and comorbidity profiles of patients treated in the community.

Incidence of trastuzumab-induced cardiotoxicity (TIC) in breast cancer patients with metastatic disease may be higher than those with early disease; however, this has been less well defined. The pivotal trastuzumab studies H0649g, H0650g, and H0648g retrospectively noted an incidence of symptomatic heart failure of 8.5%, 2.6%, and 8.8%, respectively, in patients with HER2-positive metastatic breast cancer.[15] Another study looking at patients with HER2-positive metastatic breast cancer with progressive disease despite one to two cytotoxic chemotherapy regimens and who received recombinant humanized anti-HER2 antibody reported an incidence of cardiotoxicity of 4.7% (10/213 patients).[16]

Most of the cardiotoxicity appears to occur during or shortly after trastuzumab administration. In the B31 trial, for example, at 7 years, the incidence of cardiac events was 4.0% (37/947) in patients treated with trastuzumab versus 1.3% in the control group. Only 2 of the 37 events occurred after 2 years of follow-up.[17] A retrospective cohort study from the Ontario Cancer Registry that looked at 19,074 women with breast cancer showed that the risk of cardiotoxicity was much higher during the initial 1.5 years after treatment compared with patients receiving conventional chemotherapy (hazard ratio 5.77, CI 4.38−7.62, $P < .001$). However, the cardiotoxicity risks were not significantly different in the trastuzumab and control arms after 1.5 years (hazard ratio 0.87, CI 0.57−1.33, $P = .53$).[18]

Risk Factors

Risk factors which have thus far been associated with developing cardiotoxicity include anthracycline use,[15] previous administration of anthracyclines,[15]

age[17] ($\geq$50 years,[15] $\geq$60 years[19]), black race,[20] NYHA >II before enrollment,[15] higher cancer stage,[18] being on antihypertensive medications,[17,19] and low LVEF[21] (or less than 55% but above the lower limit of normal[19] and marginally normal LVEF 50%−54%[17]). Obesity and being overweight have also been shown to be associated with increased risk of cardiotoxicity (BMI >25[21]) in patients receiving anthracyclines or anthracyclines and trastuzumab,[21,22] although this risk factor is less accepted due to concerns regarding the methodology of the data interpretation.[23] Increased number of comorbidities[18,20] appear to increase risk of cardiotoxicity, and these include hyperlipidemia,[15] diabetes,[18,20] coronary artery disease,[20] stroke or transient ischemic attack,[20] hypertension,[20] renal failure,[20] atrial fibrillation/flutter.[20] Radiation therapy has not been found to be an independent risk factor for TIC.[17,24] Longer duration of trastuzumab (defined as >6 months) is associated with a significant increase in CHF; however, it is nonetheless associated with improved overall survival in patients with early breast cancer.[12]

Prior anthracycline administration appears to be the biggest risk factor for TIC by far.[15,24] One study looking at patients with HER2-positive metastatic breast cancer showed that trastuzumab alone has a risk of 3.6% versus 28% for anthracyclines in combination with trastuzumab. The risk for anthracyclines only was about 9.6%.[15] A population-based, retrospective cohort study of 12,500 women treated across 14 nonprofit research centers showed considerable variation in cardiotoxicity between patients who did and did not receive anthracyclines in addition to trastuzumab. The adjusted hazard ratio for patients with trastuzumab without anthracyclines was 4.12, 95% CI = 2.30 to 7.42, whereas the adjusted HR for patients with trastuzumab and anthracyclines was 7.19, 95% CI = 5.00 to 10.35.[14] Sequential and concurrent administration of anthracycline and trastuzumab are associated with a similar increase in risk of CHF.[12]

Age appears to be a big risk factor as well. A retrospective study looking at heart failure and cardiomyopathy incidence in breast cancer patients found that the event rate increased with age, such that patients who got anthracyclines and trastuzumab had an event rate as follows: <55 years old 7.5%, 55−64 years old 11.4%, 65−74 years old 35.6%, $\geq$75 years old 40.7%.[14]

A risk score was developed to predict which patients with nonmetastatic breast cancer are at high risk of developing cardiotoxicity including heart failure and cardiomyopathy using the surveillance, epidemiology, and end result medicare dataset (Fig. 10.3). Based on a cohort of 1664 women with mean age 73.6 ± 5.3,

Risk Factor	Hazard Ratio (95% Confidence Interval)	Regression Coefficient	P Value	Points Assigned
Adjuvant therapy				
Anthracycline chemotherapy	1.93 (1.11 to 3.36)	0.66	0.020	2
Non-anthracycline chemotherapy	1.64 (0.99 to 2.73)	0.50	0.055	2
No identified chemotherapy	Reference	Reference		
Age category, y				
67 to 74	Reference	Reference		
75 to 79	1.36 (0.92 to 2.01)	0.31	0.125	1
80 to 94	2.04 (1.29 to 3.24)	0.71	0.003	2
Cardiovascular conditions and risk factors				
Coronary artery disease	2.16 (1.21 to 3.86)	0.77	0.009	2
Atrial fibrillation/flutter	1.69 (0.98 to 2.91)	0.53	0.058	2
Diabetes mellitus	1.50 (1.03 to 2.18)	0.41	0.034	1
Hypertension	1.44 (0.99 to 2.08)	0.36	0.054	1
Renal failure	1.99 (0.96 to 4.14)	0.69	0.065	2

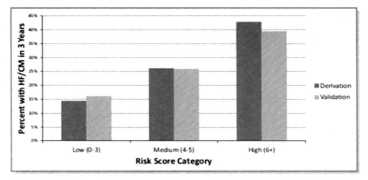

FIG. 10.3 Risk Prediction Model for Development of Heart Failure (HF) and Cardiomyopathy (CM) After Trastuzumab Therapy. (Reproduced from Ezaz G, Long JB, Gross CP, Chen J. Risk prediction model for heart failure and cardiomyopathy after adjuvant trastuzumab therapy for breast cancer. *J Am Heart Assoc.* 2014;3 with permission.)

predominantly Caucasian, they created a risk score of low (0–3 points), medium (4–5 points), and high (≥6 points). The risk factors included were anthracycline chemotherapy (2 points), nonanthracycline chemotherapy (2 points), age 75–79 (1 point), age 80–94 (2 points), coronary artery disease (2 points), atrial fibrillation/flutter (2 points), diabetes mellitus (1 point), hypertension (1 point), renal failure (2 points). The 3 year rates of heart failure and cardiomyopathy were 16.2%, 26.0%, and 39.5%, respectively.[25]

Cardiac Recovery
TIC has been shown to be a predominantly reversible disease in numerous studies. In the pivotal trials

evaluating the effects of trastuzumab for the treatment of HER2-positive metastatic breast cancer, the majority of patients with symptomatic cardiac dysfunction who were started on medical therapy (78%, or 32/41 patients) had significant improvement. The majority (68%, or 28/41 patients) also continued to receive trastuzumab, and of those, 75% (21/28 patient) showed improvement in cardiac symptoms nonetheless. For patients who stopped trastuzumab therapy, 85% (11/13 patients) showed improvement.[15] Patients with cardiac dysfunction were treated with diuretics (78%), angiotensin-converting enzyme inhibitors (ACEi, 58%), cardiac glycosides (58%), and other inotropic agents (10%). β-blockers use and nitrates were not quantified, although some patients did use those medications as well.[24]

A retrospective study at the University of Texas MD Anderson Cancer Center also suggests that there is typical reversibility seen with TIC.[26] They identified 38 patients with HER2-positive breast cancer treated at their institution who were suspected of having TIC based on either a drop in LVEF and/or development of CHF. Almost all, 92% (35/38), of the patients had a normal LVEF before initiation of trastuzumab (mean 61% ± 13). The mean LVEF decreased to 43% ± 16 at a median of 4.5 months. The majority of patients (97% or 37/38) discontinued therapy. Eighty-four percent of patients (31/37) were treated with medications for cardiac dysfunction including ACE-I and β-blockers. The mean LVEF improved to 55% ± 11 after about 1.5 months. More than half of these patients (66% or 25/38) were re-challenged with trastuzumab after stabilization of symptoms and LVEF while being on maximal medical therapy with ACE-I and β-blockers. LV reduction and/or heart failure symptoms were only seen in three patients (12%), while the majority (88% or 22/25 of patients) did not have any recurrence of heart failure.[26]

Two other RCTs (B31[17] and HERA[21]) showed similar findings. In the B31 study, over 50% of patients had LVEF recovery (58% or 21/36) and 92% (33/36) of patients were asymptomatic at ≥6 months.[17] In the HERA trial, of the patients with symptomatic CHF, 67% (24/36) recovered the LVEF within 151 days (median), and 69% (35/51) of patients who had an LVEF drop recovered in 191 days on average (median).[21]

A multitude of data shows that TIC is reversible in the majority of cases. However long-term data looking at patients who are >10 years out from trastuzumab are lacking.

CARDIOTOXICITY OF OTHER HER2 BLOCKING AGENTS

Other HER2 signaling pathway inhibitors are used in breast cancer either in place of or in combination with trastuzumab to strengthen the antineoplastic effect. In general, the incidence of cardiotoxicity associated with these agents is similar to or less than that seen with trastuzumab.

Monoclonal Antibodies: Trastuzumab Emtansine and Pertuzumab

Ado-trastuzumab emtansine (T-DM1) is an antibody drug conjugate consisting of trastuzumab, a thioether linker, and the antimitotic agent maytansine. When T-DM1 is administered following anthracycline-based chemotherapy in patients with early-stage HER2-positive breast cancer, cardiac event rate appears low. One study reported a 2.7% incidence of asymptomatic reduction in LVEF (≥10% from baseline to <50%).[27] Prior treatment with trastuzumab does not appear to significantly increase the rate of T-DM1-associated cardiotoxicity. Two studies that looked at patients with advanced HER2-positive breast cancer who had prior treatment with trastuzumab showed low rate of cardiac adverse events. In one study, there were no instances of LVEF decline to ≤45% or symptomatic congestive heart,[28] whereas in the second study, the rate of LVEF reduction to below 50% and ≥15% from baseline occurred in 8/481 patients (or 1.7%).[29]

A comparison of trastuzumab versus T-DM1 shows that the rate of cardiotoxicity is similar between the two drugs. In a phase II, multicenter study, patient with HER2-positive breast cancer, which was either locally advanced and unresectable or metastatic, 4.4% (or 3/67 patients) treated with T-DM1 experienced an asymptomatic decline in LVEF compared with 4.3% (or 3/70 patients) treated with trastuzumab and docetaxel.[30] No patients experienced symptomatic CHF in either arm.

Pertuzumab is a monoclonal antibody that targets the HER2 receptor but binds to a different epitope than trastuzumab; therefore, using a trastuzumab and pertuzumab combination can potentially cause a synergistic effect on tumor inhibition. This combination was initially tested in a multicenter phase II, single-arm study in patients with advanced HER2-positive breast cancer who experienced progression of disease during prior trastuzumab therapy. These patients received a combination of both trastuzumab and pertuzumab with 24.2% of patients showing an objective response to treatment regarding their cancer progression. Overall, the cardiac events were rare with only 4.5% (or 3/66 patients) developing an asymptomatic decline in LVEF to ≥10% and <50%.[31] Pertuzumab was subsequently tested in a randomized, double-blind, placebo-controlled trial which compared pertuzumab/trastuzumab/docetaxel to placebo/trastuzumab/docetaxel in patients as a first-line treatment. LV systolic dysfunction of ≥10% to below 50% was actually more common in the placebo group: 3.8% of patients in the pertuzumab arm (including all grades of dysfunction) versus 6.6% of patients in the placebo arm. Symptomatic LV systolic dysfunction was low, occurring in 1.0% of patients in the pertuzumab arm versus 1.8% of patients in the placebo group.[32]

Most recently, patients with node-positive or high-risk node-negative HER2-positive breast cancer were randomized to receive pertuzumab with standard chemotherapy and trastuzumab for 1 year in a multicenter, double-blind, placebo-controlled trial and showed even lower rates of cardiotoxicity. Pertuzumab did portend a slightly worse rate of cardiotoxicity with 17 patients (or 0.7%) experiencing a primary cardiac event (NYHA class III or IV heart failure or LVEF drop >10% and below 50%) with a median follow up of 45.4 months. The placebo group had an event rate of 0.3%.[33]

Tyrosine Kinase Inhibitors: Lapatinib, Afatinib, and Neratinib

Several tyrosine kinase inhibitors (TKIs) that block different parts of the HER2 signaling pathway also have therapeutic benefit in patients with breast cancer. The best studied is lapatinib, a small molecule and reversible inhibitor of HER2 and ErbB1 tyrosine kinase. Lapatinib has been evaluated as treatment for patients with HER2-positive breast cancer who have progression despite treatment with anthracyclines, taxane, and trastuzumab. Patients randomized to receive lapatinib and capecitabine had very few cardiac events (2.6% or 4/155 patients), all of which were asymptomatic.[34] A Mayo pooled analysis of patients who received lapatinib for a number of different cancers across 44 clinical studies including 10% healthy volunteers showed that the rate of cardiac events was also low (1.6% or 60/3689). The majority of patients with LVEF decline showed recovery in systolic function, and the recovery seemed similar between patients who discontinued lapatinib and those who did not.[35]

Combination HER2 blocking therapy does not appear to significantly increase cardiotoxicity with respect to monotherapy. Lapatinib and trastuzumab result in cardiotoxicity rates similar to those reported for trastuzumab alone (Table 10.3). One study showed that in patients with HER2-positive breast cancer with progression despite trastuzumab, patients treated with lapatinib and trastuzumab had a cardiac event rate of 3.4%. The group who received lapatinib alone in this study had an event rate of 1.4%.[38] A metaanalysis of six trials was done to look at the rates of cardiac events in dual HER2 therapy (pertuzumab and trastuzumab or trastuzumab and lapatinib) versus monotherapy (either lapatinib, trastuzumab, or pertuzumab). The overall odds ratio of developing CHF or decline in LVEF was not significantly different between dual and monotherapy.[39]

Two TKIs of HER2/ErbB2 with irreversible inhibition include afatinib and neratinib. Both TKIs have been studied as therapy in patients with HER2-positive breast cancer who had already been treated with trastuzumab, and both showed minimal to no significant cardiotoxicity. Afatinib was studied in a phase III, open-label study of 508 patients with two treatment arms: afatinib and vinorelbine versus trastuzumab and vinorelbine. Only one patient in the afatinib arm had a decline in ejection fraction (EF) (0.3% compared with 1.8% in the trastuzumab arm), and no patient developed CHF.[40] Neratinib was studied in a phase III multicenter trial of patients with early-stage HER2-positive breast cancer who completed trastuzumab therapy were randomized to receive neratinib versus placebo for a year. Neratinib improved invasive disease-free survival and showed minimal cardiotoxicity with only 1% of patients in both arms showing a decrease in LVEF at a 2 year follow-up.[41]

DETECTION OF CARDIOTOXICITY

Several diagnostic modalities have been investigated over the years to detect cardiac dysfunction from chemotherapeutic agents. Assessment of LV structure and function, which is central to the diagnosis of cardiotoxicity,[1] can be evaluated using multiple different imaging modalities including multigated cardiac blood pool acquisition (MUGA), cardiac magnetic resonance imaging (CMR), and transthoracic echocardiography (TTE). The advantages and disadvantages of the different modalities are described in the following section (Table 10.4).

Multigated Cardiac Blood Pool Acquisition

A MUGA study is performed by using a radiotracer to label a patient's red blood cell pool and detecting a change in counts of the tracer as the blood circulates through the heart. The LVEF is calculated based on the principle that the changes in count density are proportional to the changes in the LV volumes. MUGA scans are highly accurate, reproducible, and reliable, making them a very useful tool to assess LVEF; however, valvular and pericardial functions are not assessed. In addition, due to ongoing radiation exposure for baseline and follow-up assessments, risks and benefits of this technique should be weighed.

Cardiac Magnetic Resonance Imaging

CMR imaging is considered the gold standard of noninvasive assessment of ventricular volumes and systolic function. It can also be used to assess other cardiac

TABLE 10.3
Cardiotoxicity Induced by Trastuzumab in Five Randomized Controlled Trials

Trial	NCCTG N9831[19]	NSABP B31[17]	BCIRG 006[13]	HERA[36]	FinHer[37]
Number of patients	1944	2119	3222	3401	Total 1010, HER2+ 232
Age	49 years (median)	49 years (mean)	Majority of patients were <50 years	49 ± 10 years (median)	50.9 (25.5–65.8) years (median)
Breast cancer	HER2+, and node+ or high-risk node-invasive cancer	HER2+ and primary breast cancer	HER2+, and node+ or high-risk node-cancer	HER2+ early-stage cancer	HER2+ or HER2-, and node+ or high-risk node-cancer
Follow-up time	3.75 years	87 months (median)	65 months (median)	3.6 years	62 months
Treatment arms	1. AC >paclitaxel 2. AC ->paclitaxel >trastuzumab 3. AC >paclitaxel + trastuzumab >trastuzumab	1. AC + paclitaxel 2. AC + paclitaxel + trastuzumab	1. AC >docetaxel 2. AC >docetaxel >trastuzumab 3. Docetaxel + carboplatin >trastuzumab	1. Standard (neo)adjuvant chemotherapy[a] ± radiotherapy >observation 2. Standard (neo)adjuvant chemotherapy[a] ± radiotherapy >1 year of trastuzumab 3. Standard (neo)adjuvant chemotherapy[a] ± radiotherapy >2 years of trastuzumab	1. Docetaxel >FEC >no trastuzumab 2. Docetaxel >FEC >trastuzumab 3. Vinorelbine >FEC >no trastuzumab 4. Vinorelbine >FEC >trastuzumab
Definition of cardiac events	Symptomatic CHF Definite cardiac death Probable cardiac death	CHF (dyspnea + drop in LVEF) Definite cardiac death Probable cardiac death	CHF	Cardiac death Severe (Class III–VI) CHF Symptomatic CHF	LVEF decrease >20% Symptomatic heart failure Myocardial infarction
Total cardiac event rate based on treatment arm	1) 0.3% 2) 2.8% 3) 3.3%	1) 1.3% 2) 4.0%	1. 0.7% 2. 2.0% 3. 0.4%	LVEF reduction ≥10% and <50% 1. 0.7% 2. 4.3% Data not available	1&3. 7.8% 2&4. 12.2%
Cardiac imaging modality	MUGA	MUGA	MUGA	MUGA	Isotope cardiography
	Echocardiography	Echocardiography	Echocardiography	Echocardiography	Echocardiography
Cardiac improvement	"Majority" of patients improved	LVEF recovered to ≥50% in 57% of patients	Asymptomatic reduction in LVEF persisted in 33%	Acute recovery[b] occurred in 80.8% of patients within a median of 6.4 mos	—

AC, doxorubicin + cyclophosphamide; BCIRG, Breast Cancer International Research Group; CHF, congestive heart failure; FEC, flourourail + epirubicin + cyclophosphamide; FinHer, Finland Herceptin trial; HERA, Herceptin adjuvant trial; LVEF, left ventricular ejection fraction; MUGA, multigated cardiac blood pool acquisition; NCCTG, North Central Cancer Treatment Group; NSABP, National Surgical Adjuvant Breast and Bowel Project.

[a]94% of chemotherapy was anthracycline based.

[b]Acute recovery is defined as two or more sequential normal LVEFs.

TABLE 10.4
Imaging Modalities Currently Used to Evaluate Cardiotoxicity

Modality	Pros	Cons
MUGA	Reproducibility	Involves radiation
	Accuracy	Not able to evaluate other cardiac structures
CMR	Accuracy	Not easily available at all centers
	Can evaluate other cardiac structures	Higher costs
	Can evaluate myocardial perfusion, viability, and fibrosis	
TTE (2D/3D)	Easy accessibility	Not as accurate in evaluating LVEF when compared with MUGA and CMR and can miss small changes in LV contractility (use of contrast is recommended in 2D images if two contiguous segments are not well visualized in apical views)
	Portability	
	No radiation	
	Can evaluate other cardiac structures and pulmonary hypertension	
	Can use speckle tracking to evaluate for subclinical markers such as myocardial deformation	

2D, two-dimensional imaging; *3D,* three-dimensional imaging; *CMR,* cardiac magnetic resonance imaging; *LV,* left ventricular; *LVEF,* left ventricular ejection fraction; *MUGA:* multigated cardiac blood pool acquisition; *TTE,* transthoracic echocardiogram.

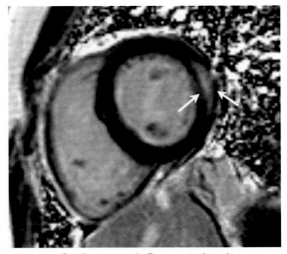

FIG. 10.4 Cardiac magnetic Resonance Imaging Demonstrates a Short Axis View of the Left and Right Ventricles, With a Short Axis Phase-Sensitive Reconstructed Inversion Recovery-True Fast Imaging With Steady-State Procession Image Through the Midventricle at the Level of the Papillary Muscle, Demonstrating mid-myocardial Delayed Enhancement (*arrows*) in the Lateral Wall of a Patient Who Developed Trastuzumab-Induced Cardiotoxicity. (Reproduced from Fallah-Rad N1, Walker JR, Wassef A, et al. The utility of cardiac biomarkers, tissue velocity and strain imaging, and cardiac magnetic resonance imaging in predicting early left ventricular dysfunction in patients with human epidermal growth factor receptor II-positive breast cancer treated with adjuvant trastuzumab therapy. *J Am Coll Cardiol.* 2011;57:2263–2270 with permission.)

chambers, valves, myocardium, and the pericardium. It is useful in evaluating myocardial perfusion, viability, and fibrosis in certain circumstances as well. Its utility is restricted by a lack of widespread availability and higher costs than other noninvasive imaging. In addition to an LVEF decrease as a sign of cardiotoxicity, presence of delayed enhancement of the midlateral wall after treatment with trastuzumab has also been noted in smaller studies[42] (Fig. 10.4).

Transthoracic Echocardiography

Echocardiography is the most common imaging modality used to detect cardiac dysfunction before, during,

and after treatment (Fig. 10.5). Benefits of echocardiography include easy accessibility, portability, low cost, and no radiation exposure. Besides an assessment of LV systolic and diastolic function, it allows for assessment of the right ventricle, valvular dysfunction, pericardial diseases, and pulmonary hypertension.

Assessment of LVEF by three-dimensional echocardiography (3DE) is usually recommended if available in a given laboratory. For a two-dimensional (2DE) LVEF assessment, biplane Simpson's method using apical two- and four-chamber measurements is commonly used. A wall motion score index is also recommended as part of the LV function assessment. A conventional assessment of diastolic function is usually recommended, although diastolic parameters have not yet shown to be prognostic of CTRCD.[1]

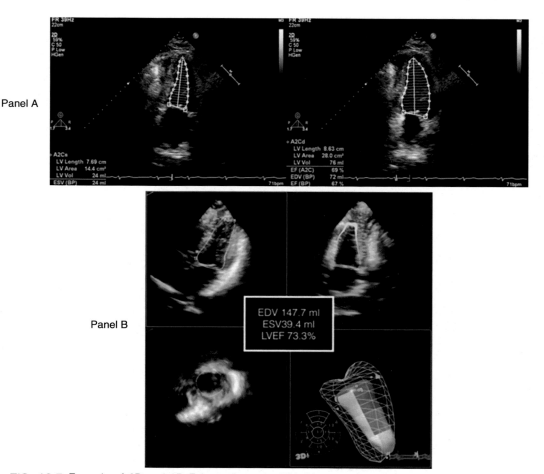

Panel A

Panel B

FIG. 10.5 Example of 2D and 3D Echocardiography With Measurement of the LVEF by the Modified Simpsons Biplanar Quantification Method With the Left Ventricular Endocardial Border Traced in End-Systole and End-Diastole to Create Disks Forming a Cylinder **(Panel A)** and 3D Dimensional Assessment. *LV*, left ventricular; *LVEF*, left ventricular ejection fraction. (Reproduced from Garg V, Vorobiof G. Echocardiography and alternative cardiac imaging strategies for long-term cardiotoxicity surveillance of cancer survivors treated with chemotherapy and/or radiation exposure. *Curr Oncol Rep.* 2016;18:52 with permission.)

DETECTION OF SUBCLINICAL CARDIOTOXICITY

Several studies have looked at subclinical markers that may help predict eventual reduction in LVEF in patients, and can be used to help identify patients at risk of developing cardiotoxicity, and help tailor their treatment before significant heart failure develops. These include changes in myocardial deformation (or strain imaging) as well as several serum biomarkers.

Strain Imaging

Newer markers of subclinical cardiotoxicity include assessment of myocardial deformation or stretch by using tissue-Doppler imaging (TDI) and speckle tracking (2D and 3D STE) strain measurements (Fig. 10.6). The strain (a measurement of total deformation during a cardiac cycle expressed as a percentage of its initial length) and strain rate (rate of change in deformation) can be measured in longitudinal, radial, and

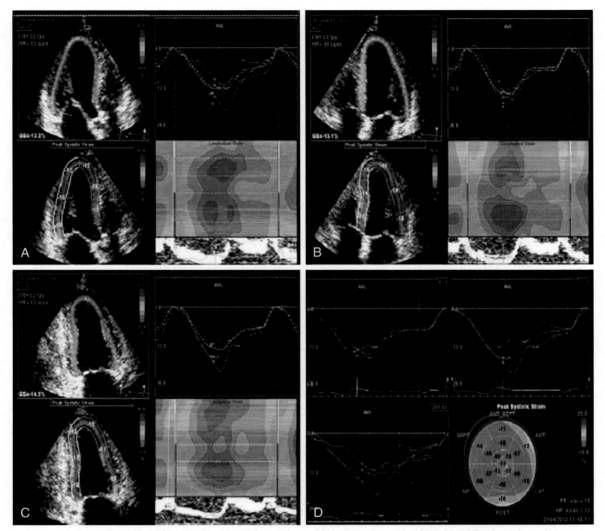

FIG. 10.6 Example of Speckle Tracking Echocardiographic Images Assessing Myocardial Strain. Images Are Obtained in the Apical Long Axis View **(Panel A)**, Four Chamber View **(Panel B)**, and Two Chamber View **(Panel C)** With Strain Curves and "Bull's Eye" Plot **(Panel D)** in a Patient With Breast Cancer Who Developed Left Ventricular Dysfunction After Doxorubicin and Trastuzumab Administration. Each Segment Has a Numeric and Color-Coded Strain Value, With Cardiac Dysfunction Presenting With Regional Abnormalities. (Reproduced from Plana JC, Galderisi M, Barac S, et al. Expert consensus for multimodality imaging evaluation of adult patients during and after cancer therapy: a report from the American Society of Echocardiography and the European Association of Cardiovascular Imaging. *J Am Soc Echocardiogr.* 2014;27:911–939 with permission.)

circumferential directions (Fig. 10.6). A 2D global systolic longitudinal strain (GLS) reduction of 9%–19% has been the most consistent and reliable measurement in studies suggestive of acute myocardial changes either during or immediately following anthracycline therapy.[45] When using TDI-based strain, a reduction of 9%–20% in the longitudinal strain rate of the basal intraventricular septum is suggestive of acute myocardial injury due to anthracycline use.[45] A fall in GLS of 10%–15% by STE has been correlated to the later

TABLE 10.5
Biomarkers and Trastuzumab-Induced Cardiotoxicity

Study	Biomarker	Timing	Chemotherapy	Outcomes	Correlation With Outcomes
Cardinale et al.[46]	Troponin I	Before and after each cycle	Trastuzumab	LVEF decrease >10% and below 50%	Positive
Fallah-Rad et al.[43]	Troponin T NT-proBNP	Baseline, and every 3 months for 1 year	Trastuzumab	LVEF decrease ≥10% and below 55% with signs/symptoms of CHF	Neutral
Morris et al.[47]	Troponin I	Baseline, every 2 wks, and 6, 9, and 18 months	Doxorubicin, cyclophosphamide, paclitaxel, trastuzumab, lapatinib	LVEF decrease >10% and below 55%, congestive heart failure	Negative
Sawaya et al.[48]	Troponin I NT-proBNP	Baseline, and 3 and 6 months during therapy	Anthracyclines, trastuzumab	LVEF decrease ≥5% and below 55% with symptoms of heart failure, an asymptomatic LVEF decrease of ≥10% to below 55%	Troponin: positive NTproBNP: negative
Ky et al.[49]	Troponin I NT-proBNP MPO	Baseline, and 3 and 6 months during therapy	Doxorubicin, trastuzumab	LVEF decrease ≥5% and below 55% with symptoms of heart failure, an asymptomatic LVEF decrease of ≥10% to below 55%	Troponin: positive NT-proBNP: negative MPO: positive
Putt et al.[50]	Troponin I NT-proBNP MPO GDF-15 PlGF	Baseline, and every 3 months for 15 months	Doxorubicin, trastuzumab	LVEF decrease ≥5% and below 55% with symptoms of heart failure, an asymptomatic LVEF decrease of ≥10% to below 55%	Troponin: negative NT-proBNP: negative MPO: positive GDF-15: positive PlGF: positive
Sandri et al.[51]	NT-proBNP	Baseline and after each cycle	High-dose chemotherapy	LVEF and diastolic parameters	Positive
Sawaya et al.[52]	Troponin I NT-proBNP	Baseline, and every 3 months for 15 months	Anthracyclines, taxanes, trastuzumab	LVEF decrease ≥5% and below 55% with symptoms of heart failure, an asymptomatic LVEF decrease of ≥10% to below 55%	Troponin: positive NTproBNP: negative
Grover et al.[53]	Troponin T	Baseline, and 1 and 4 months after therapy	Doxorubicin or epirubicin, trastuzumab	LV/RV structure and function on CMR	Negative
Zardavas et al.[54]	Troponin I and T	Baseline, week 13, 25, 52 month 18, 24, 30, 36, every unscheduled LVEF assessment	Trastuzumab	NYHA class III/IV symptoms, LVEF decrease >10% and below 50%, death due to cardiac cause	Positive

CHF, congestive heart failure; *CMR*, cardiac magnetic resonance imaging; *LVEF*, left ventricular ejection fraction; *MPO*, myeloperoxidase; *NT-proBNP*, N-terminal prohormone of brain natriuretic peptide.
Adapted from Shah KS, Yang EH, Maisel AS, Fonarow GC. The role of biomarkers in detection of cardio-toxicity. *Curr Oncol Rep.* 2017;19:42.

development of cardiotoxicity including both symptomatic and asymptomatic reduction in LVEF, whereas changes in global radial strain and global circumferential strain have not been found to be predictive.[45] Per the consensus statement by the American Society of Echocardiography released in 2014, a decrease in GLS >15% in patients with no significant change in LV function suggests subclinical LV dysfunction.[1]

Cardiac Biomarkers

Several studies have looked at multiple serum biomarkers at baseline, during, and post chemotherapy to evaluate their utility in signaling a risk of developing cardiotoxicity (Table 10.5). An elevation in troponin, a marker of myocardial injury, appears to correlate with development of cardiotoxicity. In one of the largest studies enrolling 703 patients with cancer and varying chemotherapy regimens, cardiac troponins were measured immediately after chemotherapy and 1 month later. Patients with increases in troponin ($\geq$0.08 ng/mL) early on or with persistently elevated levels had an increased risk of adverse cardiac events (cardiac death, acute pulmonary edema, heart failure, LVEF reduction by $\geq$25% or life-threatening arrhythmia) and increased severity of CTRCD.[57] Cardinale et al. also studied 251 breast cancer patients who underwent therapy, particularly with trastuzumab and measured troponin I (Tn-I) levels before and after each cycle. Patients with increased levels of troponin were noted to have more adverse cardiac events and low chance of recovery of systolic function.[46]

Myeloperoxidase (MPO), a peptide secreted by leukocytes and a prooxidant linked to atherogenesis, may be a useful biomarker of subclinical cardiotoxicity.[49,50] Ky et al.[49] looked at 8 biomarkers including Tn-I, high-sensitivity C-reactive protein, N-terminal prohormone brain natriuretic peptide (pro NT-BNP), growth differentiation factor, MPO, placental growth factor, soluble fms-like TKI, and galectin in 78 breast cancer patients undergoing treatment with doxorubicin and trastuzumab. A greater risk of cardiotoxicity was associated with early increases in Tn-I, MPO, and a combination of the two markers.[49]

Natriuretic peptides are commonly used as markers of myocardial stretch and pressure overload, and they have an important role in the diagnosis and management of heart failure. However, the few studies that have evaluated NT-proBNP use in trastuzumab have not found it to be a reliable predictor of subsequent CTRCD (Table 10.5).[58]

SURVEILLANCE OF TRASTUZUMAB CARDIOTOXICITY

According to the AHA/ACC guidelines on heart failure, an asymptomatic decline in LV function (AHA stage B) or a symptomatic decline (AHA stage C/D) is a progressive disorder that is associated with reduced mortality.[59] Given the significant event rate of both asymptomatic and symptomatic decline in LV function in the major trastuzumab trials (Table 10.3), the product label emulates clinical trial design and dictates the need and frequency of routine cardiac monitoring while undergoing therapy with trastuzumab. Early identification of cardiac dysfunction can lead to implementation of cardiac therapies at each AHA stage of heart failure that help reduce cardiovascular mortality.[59]

The frequency of this surveillance has come under scrutiny because of concerns that the clinical trial event rate of LV dysfunction is low in anthracycline-free regimens, TIC can be reversible without the use of medications, lack of evidence-based guidelines and prospective studies validating frequent testing, and concerns of rising healthcare costs.[60] However, clinical trials typically enroll younger and healthier subjects while often excluding patients with preexisting cardiac conditions and risk factors. Clinical trial data therefore likely significantly underestimate the real-world rate of symptomatic and asymptomatic LV dysfunction in patients treated with trastuzumab.[14] Based on the incidence of TIC in clinical trials and real-world TIC, several national and international societies have created guidelines based on expert consensus opinions, which will be reviewed below.

Prechemotherapy Surveillance

All major society guidelines agree that the first opportunity to offer surveillance for cardiotoxicity is before the onset of any cancer therapeutics. Similar to a preoperative evaluation, the American Society of Clinical Oncology (ASCO) strongly recommends that any patient with an active cardiac complaint or symptom should undergo further evaluation and referral to a cardiologist.[61]

Pretreatment assessment recommendations extend to asymptomatic patients who are about to receive cytotoxic chemotherapy (Fig. 10.7). The European Society of Medical Oncology (ESMO), ASCO, and the UK National Cancer Research Institute recommend a cardiac-focused medical history, physical examination, 12-lead ECG looking for arrhythmias and markers of LV structural damage, and a baseline measurement of LVEF for all patients with HER2-positive breast

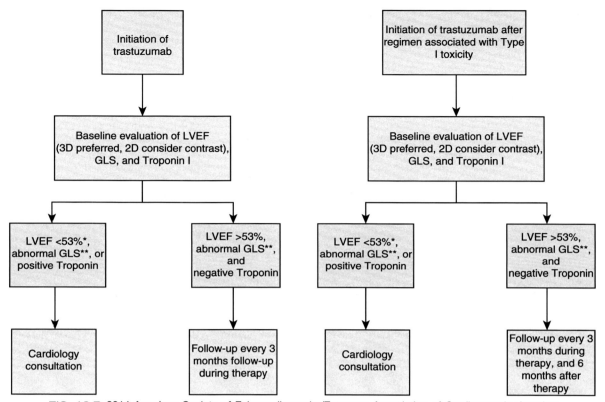

FIG. 10.7 2014 American Society of Echocardiography/European Association of Cardiovascular Imaging Expert Consensus of Multimodality Imaging of Adult Patients During and After Cancer Therapy in Regard to Monitoring of Cardiotoxicity Related to Trastuzumab (Type II Toxicity). *GLS*, global longitudinal strain; *LVEF*, left ventricular ejection fraction. *Consider confirming with cardiac MRI; **Normal values vary based on vendor, gender, and age. (Adapted from Figs. 14 and 15 from Plana JC, Galderisi M, Barac S, et al. Expert consensus for multimodality imaging evaluation of adult patients during and after cancer therapy: a report from the American Society of Echocardiography and the European Association of Cardiovascular Imaging. *J Am Soc Echocardiogr*. 2014;27:911–939 with permission.)

cancer.[61–63] Similar recommendations regarding baseline assessment of LVEF are mirrored by a joint statement by the American Society of Nuclear Cardiology (ASNC), the European Society of Cardiology (ESC), and the American Society of Echocardiography (ASE) with the European Association of Cardiovascular Imaging (EACVI).[1,64,65] Baseline assessment would allow clinicians to differentiate whether a subsequent decline in LVEF is due to cancer therapy versus preexisting LV dysfunction.

ESMO and ASCO use additional criteria based on the chemotherapy regimen and cardiac risk factors to identify high-risk individuals who would benefit from a baseline LVEF assessment. This includes high-dose anthracycline ($>/=250$ mg/m^2 doxorubicin, $>/=600$ mg/m^2 epirubicin), high-dose radiotherapy ($>/=30$ Gy where the heart is in the treatment field), low-dose anthracycline in combination with low-dose radiotherapy, low-dose anthracycline and two cardiac risk factors, therapy with trastuzumab alone and two cardiac risk factors, low-dose anthracycline followed by trastuzumab, age $>/=60$ years at cancer treatment, and/or known compromised cardiac function (such as lower limit of normal EF, history of myocardial infarction, or moderate or greater valvular heart disease).[61,63] The ASE/EACVI writing group use traditional cardiovascular risk factors such as age, gender, hypertension, hyperlipidemia, and family history of premature coronary artery disease to classify if a patient is high risk.[1] ASCO expands cardiac risk factors to also include smoking, diabetes, and obesity.[61] These traditional cardiac risk factors increase the risk of developing ischemic heart disease and other cardiomyopathies that may leave cardiac myocytes even more vulnerable to stress from cytotoxic chemotherapy.

Although most guidelines identify risk factors for TIC as a method to target routine cardiac surveillance, the Canadian Trastuzumab Working Group (CAN) recommends using certain risk factors as exclusion criteria from treatment with trastuzumab. Patients with existing heart failure or LVEF <50%, or both, should be excluded from receiving trastuzumab, unless their risk of disease recurrence is very high. They go on to recommend that patients with ischemic heart disease, valve dysfunction, or an LVEF at the lower limit of normal/mildly abnormal (EF 50%–55%) before trastuzumab therapy require special consideration. These recommendations are based on clinical trial data and may change as more real-world data are published (Table 10.2).[66]

Surveillance During Chemotherapy

After careful selection of patients into the adjuvant trastuzumab therapy pathway, all society guidelines consistently recommend routine surveillance of LVEF while on trastuzumab for 1 year (Table 10.6).[1,61–63,65,66] This recommendation originates from earlier clinical trials when anthracycline and trastuzumab were administered concurrently and the rate of symptomatic heart failure was up to 27%.[67] Subsequent adjuvant trials used strict cardiac monitoring and interruption of trastuzumab therapy based on changes in LVEF and saw a sharp decline in rate of severe heart failure (<1%).[21] Based on these trial designs and observations, different societies have developed surveillance protocols of LVEF during trastuzumab therapy and recommendations on adjustment of therapy based on the LVEF (Fig. 10.8). Frequent surveillance is used to identify early dysfunction of the heart so that cardiac medications can be initiated, which have been shown to aid in recovery of LVEF and prevent recurrent decline when trastuzumab is resumed.[26]

Patients should undergo routine surveillance for LV dysfunction before initiation of anthracycline and at the completion of its course and again 6 months after that. If patients are to receive more than 240 mg/m²

of doxorubicin or its equivalent, then an assessment of LVEF is needed before each additional dose of 50 mg/m². Once anthracycline is completed and/or before initiation of trastuzumab, a repeat LVEF assessment is recommended. This is repeated at 3-month intervals through the course of the therapy[52] and again at 6 months after completion of therapy. In addition, ESC and the NCRI agree that if a patient is at low risk for TIC during adjuvant therapy, LVEF assessment can be performed every 4 months (instead of 3 months).[62,65]

In regard to patients with metastatic disease who receive trastuzumab indefinitely, ESMO and ASCO agree that after baseline imaging, the frequency of cardiac imaging be determined by symptoms and/or clinical judgment. The NCRI recommends testing at baseline, 4 months, 8 months and then leaves further testing to the discretion of the physician.[61,63]

Postchemotherapy Surveillance

Once adjuvant cancer therapy is complete, ASCO and ESMO recommend a repeat echocardiogram between 6 and 12 months in higher risk patients, although this recommendation is directed primarily with patients with a history of anthracycline exposure. Beyond 1 year, there are no recommendations to support further testing.[1,63]

Surveillance With Biomarkers and Strain Imaging

In addition to assessment of LVEF, the ASE/EACVI recommends assessment of troponins and GLS at the same time LVEF surveillance is performed. ASE/EACVI/ESC recommend using an absolute change of >15% in GLS as well as a positive troponin as supportive indices of TIC to help aid in clinical decision-making regarding cessation of therapy.[1,65] Given TIC is not dose dependent and has a variable time of onset, measurement of troponin with every cycle of trastuzumab may be considered in high-risk patients.[49,68] The ASE/EACVI recommends using CMR as a confirmatory imaging modality when discontinuation of chemotherapy secondary to TIC is being considered. CAN and ASNC prefer MUGA over echocardiogram for routine surveillance because of its increased sensitivity in picking up a change in LVEF of 10%.[64,66] Whichever imaging modality is ultimately chosen, all guideline committees agree that using the same imaging modality, machine, operator, and calculation algorithms for each subsequent study is important[1,62] (Table 10.4). A general flow diagram for assessment of cardiotoxicity is shown in Figs. 10.7 and 10.8.

TABLE 10.6
Recommendations for Surveillance for Cardiac Dysfunction According to Major Societies

Society	Modality of Choice	Frequency of Monitoring
American Society of Clinical Oncology (ASCO)	1. Echocardiography: MUGA or MRI if echocardiography is not available, with MRI preferred over MUGA 2. Strain imaging and biomarkers (BNP, troponin) could be considered in conjunction with routine echocardiography	Frequency of surveillance should be determined by the provider based on patient's clinical characteristics
American Society of Echocardiography (ASE) and European Association of Cardiovascular Imaging (EACVI)	1. Echocardiography, ideally incorporating three-dimensional imaging and GLS 2. Consider measuring high-sensitivity troponin in conjunction with imaging	Every 3 months during therapy
European Society for Medical Oncology (ESMO)	1. Echocardiography or MUGA 2. May consider MRI as an alternative	Baseline, every 3, 6, 9, 12, and 18 months after initiation of treatment For patients with metastatic disease, obtain baseline measurement and only repeat if patient develops symptoms of HF
European Society of Cardiology (ESC)	1. Echocardiography including 3-dimensional assessment of LVEF and GLS 2. MUGA and MRI may be considered as alterantives	Baseline, every 3 months during therapy and once after completion
Canadian Cardiovascular Society (CCS)	1. Echocardiography including 3-dimensional imaging and strain, MUGA and MRI as alternatives 2. Consider concomitant measurement of biomarkers (BNP, troponin)	No specific recommendation
Trastuzumab labeling	1. Echocardiography or MUGA	Baseline (immediately preceding initiation of trastuzumab), every 3 months during or upon completion of therapy, and at every 6 months for at least 2 years following completion of therapy

BNP, B-type/brain natriuretic peptide; *GLS*, global longitudinal strain; *LVEF*, left ventricular ejection fraction; *MRI*, magnetic resonance imaging; *MUGA*, multigated acquisition.
Adapted from Florido R, Smith KL, Cuomo KK, Russell SD. Cardiotoxicity from human epidermal growth factor Receptor-2 (HER2) targeted therapies. *J Am Heart Assoc.* 2017;6.

PREVENTION AND TREATMENT STRATEGIES

Primary Prevention

It is unknown whether cardioactive therapies can prevent TIC. Few studies have evaluated therapies that may prevent the development of TIC (Table 10.7),

and of those, the majority included patients who were also treated with anthracyclines. The PRADA trial,[70] for example, included patients with breast cancer who were treated with anthracycline therapy and trastuzumab. Patients were started on candesartan (ACE-i) and metoprolol succinate (β-blocker) before

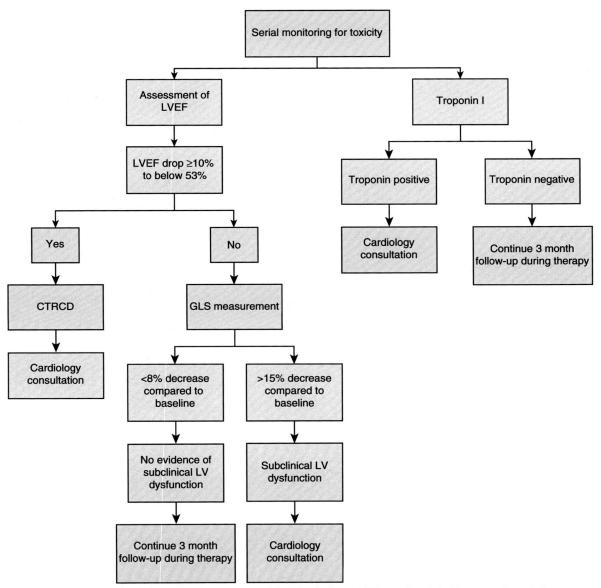

FIG. 10.8 Surveillance Algorithm From 2014 American Society of Echocardiography/European Association of Cardiovascular Imaging Expert Consensus of Multimodality Imaging of Adult Patients During and After Cancer Therapy in Regard to General Monitoring of Cardiotoxicity. *CTRCD*, cancer therapeutics-related cardiac dysfunction; *GLS*, global longitudinal strain; *LVEF*, left ventricular ejection fraction. (Adapted from Figs. 16 and 17 from Plana JC, Galderisi M, Barac S, et al. Expert consensus for multimodality imaging evaluation of adult patients during and after cancer therapy: a report from the American Society of Echocardiography and the European Association of Cardiovascular Imaging. *J Am Soc Echocardiogr.* 2014;27: 911–939.)

TABLE 10.7
Prevention and Treatment of Trastuzumab-Induced Cardiotoxicity

	Study Type	Chemotherapy	Cardiac Therapy	Design and Medication	Patients	Duration	Primary Outcome	Results
PRIMARY PREVENTION								
Gulati et al.[70]	RCT	FEC, taxanes, trastuzumab	ACEi, β-blocker	2 × 2 factorial: candesartan, metoprolol vs. placebo	120	10–61 weeks	LVEF on CMR	Candesartan protective against LVEF reduction, no benefit with metoprolol
Pituskin et al.[71]	RCT	Trastuzumab	β-blocker	Perindopril, bisoprolol, placebo 1:1:1	94	347–356 days	LV remodeling (change in LVEDV on CMR)	Perindopril and bisoprolol did not prevent LV remodeling; however, they independently predicted stable LVEF
Seicean et al.[72]	Observational	Athracyclines, trastuzumab	β-blocker	1:2 propensity matched β-blocker vs. no β-blocker	318	3.2 ± 2.0 years	HF event	Continuous β-blocker use was associated with lower risk of HF events
Seicean et al.[73]	Observational	Anthracyclines, trastuzumab	Statin	2:1 propensity matched statin vs. no statin	201	2.6 ± 1.7 years	New-onset HF	Statin group had lower risk of new-onset HF
Boekhout et al.[74]	RCT	Trastuzumab	ACEi	Candesartan vs. placebo	210	78 weeks	LVEF	No significant difference in cardiac events in the candesartan group
SECONDARY PREVENTION								
Negishi et al.[75]	Observational	Anthracyclines ± trastuzumab, trastuzumab alone	β-blocker	Patients with GLS reduction ≥11% after therapy (average 7 ± 7 mos), β-blockers vs. no β-blocker	52	6 months	GLS	β-blocker use was associated with improvement in GLS

ACEi, Angiotensin converting enzyme inhibitor; *CMR,* cardiac magnetic resonance imaging; *FEC,* 5-fluorouracil, epirubicin, cyclophosphamide; *GLS,* global longitudinal strain; *HF,* heart failure; *LV,* left ventricle; *LVEDV,* left ventricular end diastolic volume; *LVEF,* left ventricular ejection fraction; *RCT,* randomized controlled trial.
Adapted from Pun SC, Neilan TG. Cardioprotective interventions: where are we? J Am Coll Cardiol. 2016.

chemotherapy. They found that patients who were treated with candesartan had a lower incidence of reduction in LVEF; no benefit was seen with β-blockers. However a more recent RCT by Boekhout et al. did not show a benefit in cardiac events in patients treated with candesartan for 78 weeks.[74] The MANTICORE trial[71] specifically evaluated the benefit of β-blocker use during trastuzumab treatment only. In that study, β-blockers were effective at preventing decline in LVEF; however, they did not prevent LV remodeling as measured by the change in the LV end-diastolic volume index. Lipid lowering treatment with statin may also provide protection from development of heart failure. One observational study found that patients undergoing chemotherapy with anthracycline and/or trastuzumab who were treated with a statin had a lower incidence of heart failure than propensity-matched control patients.[73] Until larger randomized controlled trials are done and there are established guidelines, initiation of cardioactive medications before trastuzumab should be based on patient's cardiovascular risk factors as well as administration of other cardiotoxic agents such as anthracyclines.

Secondary Prevention

For patients who develop TIC, the consensus among different societies is to temporary withdraw trastuzumab therapy and allow for a drug holiday with reassessment of risks and benefits after several weeks.[58,76] One possible algorithm proposed by ESMO for deciding to withdraw therapy based on LVEF evaluation is shown in Fig. 10.9.[64] Whether cessation of therapy is in fact necessary after development of cardiotoxicity is currently under investigation.[77] The early trastuzumab studies showed that the majority of patients had cardiac recovery even with continuation of therapy.[15] For those patients with evidence of cardiac damage including asymptomatic or symptomatic LVEF drop ≥10% or ≤50%, have a relative change in GLS of ≥15%, or positive troponins, initiation of cardioactive medications should be considered. Only one trial has looked at using β-blockers in patients who have evidence of abnormal GLS after chemotherapy. Patients who had a drop in GLS ≥11% with chemotherapy and were subsequently treated with β-blockers had improvement in GLS compared with patients without β-blocker therapy.[75] For patients with sustained TIC,

ACC/AHA guideline–directed medical therapy for heart failure should be initiated by a cardiology specialist.[59] This includes initiation of an ACEi and β-blocker therapy.

Ultimately, larger studies with longer follow-up are needed to assess the optimal prevention and treatment strategies for patients undergoing chemotherapy with trastuzumab.

FUTURE AVENUES

Although there has been progress made in strategies aimed at potentially detecting and treating subclinical and clinical TIC, many of these studies are limited by small patient numbers, single institutional experience, and retrospective analyses of cardiotoxicity. As such, there remain a number of issues that require further investigation (Table 10.8). In addition, in many phase I/II trials analyzing the efficacy of anti-HER2 therapies, patients with preexisting cardiovascular risk factors and other comorbidities may be excluded, and thus the cardiotoxic impact of these therapies in "real-world" patients may be underestimated.

Given the recent increases in clinical trials examining the prevalence, detection, and treatment of chemotherapy-induced cardiotoxicity, the multidisciplinary field of cardio-oncology has gained international traction and interest among both fields of cardiovascular disease and hematology-oncology. One of the primary objectives of this field is to understand the mechanistic overlap between the effects of cancer treatments and cardiovascular disease, as well as to provide proactive clinical care and develop cardioprotective strategies to allow cancer patients to safely continue their treatment. Because of a theoretical higher risk of developing LV dysfunction in breast cancer patients with preexisting cardiovascular risk factors, which likely are present in older patients afflicted with breast cancer, cardio-oncology programs have evolved to assist patients, their oncology providers, and support staff with risk stratification of cardiotoxicity, initiation of cardioprotective therapy in selected patients, and provision of recommended strategies of short- and long-term surveillance of cardiotoxicity based on recent literature. The goal is to provide more consistent, streamlined avenues of care of cardioprotective therapies for patients at risk or those with cardiotoxicity to allow for the continuation of oncology treatments. Ongoing discussions with

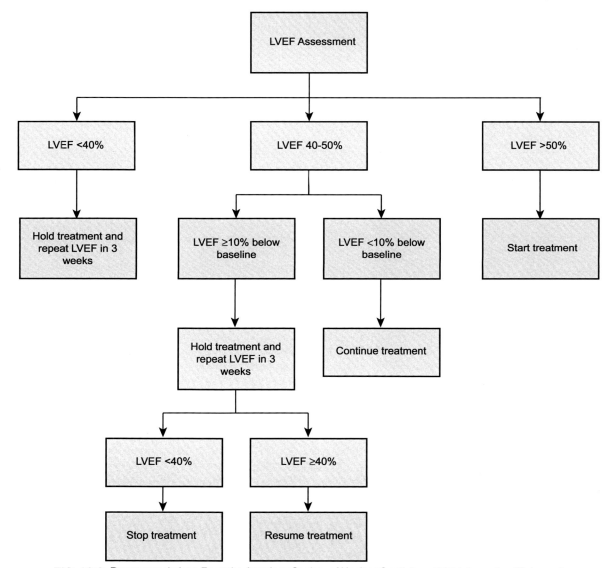

FIG. 10.9 Recommendations From the American Society of Nuclear Cardiology 2016 Information Statement for Altering Trastuzumab Therapy Based on Evaluation of Left Ventricular Ejection Fraction (LVEF). (Adapted from Russell RR, Alexander J, Jain D, et al. The role and clinical effectiveness of multimodality imaging in the management of cardiac complications of cancer and cancer therapy. *J Nucl Cardiol.* 2016;23:856–884.)

the patient's oncology team with the risks and benefits of continuing or changing treatment in patients who have experienced cardiotoxicity is critical for the patient to receive optimal oncologic and cardiovascular care.[78] However, further data and trials are needed to explore the impact on both cancer and cardiac outcomes in patients who receive cardio-oncology care in this nascent field.

Ongoing clinical trials are being designed and employed to further understand the natural course of

TABLE 10.8
Topics Requiring Further Investigation in Anti HER2-Related Cardiotoxicity

- Long-term cardiotoxicity surveillance in cancer survivors who have received anthracyclines and trastuzumab
- Cardiovascular and cancer outcomes, via establishment of national/international registries in cancer patients, who develop cardiotoxicity during trastuzumab treatment but continue chemotherapy with close cardiac monitoring and treatment
- Long-term cardiovascular outcomes in cancer survivors who develop cardiotoxicity during treatment with near complete recovery, or whose cardiac function does not recover with medical therapy
- Impact of cardio-oncology multidisciplinary care in cancer patients at risk for cardiotoxicity
- Role of pharmacologic/nonpharmacologic interventions during treatment in reducing risk of cardiotoxicity (i.e., exercise therapy, statin)
- Impact of prophylactic cardioprotective therapies (i.e., β-blockers, angiotensin converting enzyme inhibitors) in patients deemed to be high risk for cardiotoxicity before initiating anti-HER2 therapies
- Impact of early implementation of cardioprotective therapies with detection of subclinical cardiotoxicity (i.e., abnormal strain measurements with normal left ventricular function)
- Validation of risk prediction models that identify patients at highest risk for trastuzumab-induced cardiotoxicity

TIC and how interventional strategies can potentially reduce the risk of developing cardiotoxicity during treatment (Table 10.9). In regard to pharmacologic interventions, a prospective, multicenter, randomized, phase II placebo-controlled clinical trial cosponsored by the University of South Florida and the National Cancer Institute is evaluating the effects of an ACE-I (lisinopril) and β-blocker (carvedilol phosphate—extended release) on TIC with a target accrual of 468 patients (NCT01009918).[83] In patients who have experienced suspected TIC (LVEF ≥40% and 50%) while on treatment, the SAFE-HEaRt trial (NCT01904903) is looking at cardiac outcomes in this patient population with close cardiac monitoring and treatment with continued chemotherapy treatment.[77] While primarily

focused on anthracyline-based regimens in breast cancer treatment along with trastuzumab, the SAFE trial (NCT2236806) is a randomized phase III, four-arm, single-blind, placebo-controlled study aiming to look at the effects of bisoprolol, ramipril, or both drugs on subclinical cardiotoxicity by speckle tracking on TTE.[79] The STOP trial (NCT02674204) is a randomized, placebo-controlled trial analyzing the effects of statin usage (atorvastatin) on subclinical cardiotoxicity by cardiac MRI in patients being treated with trastuzumab.[80] The CARDAPAC study (NCT02433067) is a phase II multicenter randomized trial of 112 HER2 breast cancer patients undergoing adjuvant treatment with trastuzumab, which is looking at the impact of a 3-month supervised exercise program with moderate and high intensity activity on cardiotoxicity (defined as a decrease of LVEF under 50%, or an absolute drop of LVEF 10% at baseline and at 3 months).[86] In regard to patients also receiving radiation therapy, a study is being conducted looking at breathhold techniques during treatments to reduce cardiac toxicity, as demonstrated by cardiac MRI at 12 months (NCT02052102).[87] Finally, from an imaging perspective, a double-blinded, prospective observational study is being conducted comparing cardiac MRI with MUGA scans in patients receiving trastuzumab in regard to LVEF assessment and LV volumes, and also comparing serial biomarker levels with changes in cardiac structure and function.[82]

Although ongoing efforts on an international scale are providing invaluable insight into the incidence and historical course of TIC, continued challenges remain in determining the most optimal surveillance frequency for cardiotoxicity, as well as interventional strategies. As anti-HER2 treatments, traditional and newer agent, continue to extend into treatments of malignancies other than breast cancer, the importance of continuing these research efforts remain paramount. With the increase in multidisciplinary collaborations within the field of cardio-oncology and raised awareness and vigilance of TIC—in addition to overall cardiovascular risk stratification and modification in breast cancer patients—patients hopefully can continue potentially lifesaving treatments for their cancer with earlier detection and treatment of subclinical cardiotoxicity, with the aim of living their lives with significantly less cardiac and oncologic short- and long-term comorbidity and mortality (Fig. 10.10).[88]

TABLE 10.9
Current Clinical Trials Investigating Surveillance, Detection, and Treatment of Trastuzumab-Induced Cardiotoxicity

Trial Name or PI	Clinical Trials ID	Sponsor	Study Type	Population	Intervention	Target Enrollment	Start/ Completion Date	Cardiac Assessment
SAFE[79]	NCT02236806	Azienda Ospedaliero-Universitaria Careggi, Florene, Italy	Phase III/ randomized, placebo-controlled/drug prevention	Nonmetastatic primary invasive BC	Bisoprolol, ramipril, placebo	480	July 2015/ November 2017	Biomarkers (TnI, NT-pro-NP), TTE
STOP[80]	NCT02674204	Cedars-Sinai Medical Center, Los Angeles, CA, USA	Randomized, placebo-controlled/drug intervention	Stage 1–3 HER2 positive BC undergoing treatment with trastuzumab +/–AC	Atorvastatin, placebo	90	May 2016/ October 2019	CMR with global circumferential strain
Yu, et al.[81]	NCT02615054	Memorial Sloan Kettering Cancer Center, New York, NY, USA	Prospective observational/ imaging	Primary invasive BC >/=2 years with and without cardiotoxicity	TTE with speckle tracking, CPET	55	November 2015/ November 2018	TTE with speckle tracking, CPET
Brezden-Masley, et al.[82]	NCT01022086	St. Michael's Hospital, Toronto, Canada	Prospective observational/ imaging	Invasive HER2 positive BC, planned treatment with trastuzumab	CMR, biomarker testing	50	November 2009/ December 2019	CMR, biomarkers (BNP, TnI, TGF B1, PINP, PIIINP, CITP)
Guglin, et al.[83]	NCT01009918	University of South Florida, Tampa, FL, USA	Phase II/ prospective randomized, placebo-controlled/drug prevention	HER2 positive BC undergoing trastuzumab +/– pertuzumab	Lisinopril, carvedilol phosphate extended-release, placebo	468	March 2010/ July 2017	TTE or MUGA, biomarkers (BNP, TnI)
Yu, et al.[84]	NCT02177175	Memorial Sloan Kettering Cancer Center, New York, NY, USA	Phase II/ prospective randomized placebo-controlled/drug prevention/ imaging	Nonmetastatic primary invasive HER2-positive BC undergoing AC and anti-HER2 treatment	Carvedilol, placebo (intervention), TTE with speckle tracking (imaging)	82	June 2014/ June 2018	TTE with speckle tracking
OTT 15–05[85]	NCT02696707	Ottawa Hospital Research Institute, Ottawa, Canada	Prospective, randomized/ imaging surveillance	Early-stage HER2 positive BC with planned trastuzumab therapy	TTE or MUGA q3 months vs. q4 months	200	June 2016/ March 2018	TTE or MUGA

Continued

TABLE 10.9
Current Clinical Trials Investigating Surveillance, Detection, and Treatment of Trastuzumab-Induced Cardiotoxicity—cont'd

Trial Name or PI	Clinical Trials ID	Sponsor	Study Type	Population	Intervention	Target Enrollment	Start/ Completion Date	Cardiac Assessment
SAFE-HEaRt[77]	NCT01904903	Washington Heart Center, Washington DC, USA	Prospective, open label/ treatment	Stage 1–IV HER2-positive BC with LVEF>/ = 40% and <50% on TTE receiving anti-HER2 treatment	Serial TTEs, cardiac treatment with β-blockers and ACE-I during chemotherapy	30	August 2013/ August 2018	TTE with speckle tracking and biomarkers (TnI, hsTnT)
CARDAPAC[86]	NCT02433067	University of Franche-Comte, Doubs, France	Prospective open label/ intervention with exercise	Nonmetastatic HER2-positive BC undergoing trastuzumab monotherapy	Control arm: standard oncologic care Interventional arm: physical activity intervention 3X/week	117	April 2015/ April 2018	TTE, measurements of body composition, muscle function, metabolic/ hormonal/ inflammatory responses, quality of life
COBC	NCT02571894	Karolina University Hospital, Stockholm, Sweden	Prospective, randomized open label/ intervention	Newly diagnosed BC eligible for neoadjuvant/ adjuvant chemotherapy, +/- trastuzumab	Observational arm: standard oncologic care. Interventional arm: serial TTEs with speckle tracking and biomarkers (hesitant, BNP)	320	July 2014/ February 2019	Serial TTEs with speckle tracking and biomarkers (hs-TnT, BNP)
Joseph et al.	NCT02052102	AHS Cancer Control, Alberta, Canada	Prospective, open label/ intervention with radiation breathing techniques	Left-sided BC who is a candidate to adjuvant RT with prior history of AC/trastuzumab	Impact on cardiotoxicity of DIBH versus FB	63	October 2014/March 2017	Functional CMR and biomarker (BNP, PIIINP, CITP)

AC, anthracycline; ACE-I, angiotensin converting enzyme inhibitor; BC, breast cancer; BNP, B-type natriuretic peptide; CITP, carboxy-terminal telopeptide of collagen type 1; CMR, cardiac magnetic resonance imaging; CPET, cardiopulmonary exercise testing; DIBH, deep inspiration breathhold; FB, free breathing; HER2, human epidermal growth receptor factor 2; hsTnT, high-sensitivity troponin-T; LVEF, left ventricular ejection fraction; MUGA, mitigated acquisition scan; PI, principal investigator; PIIINP, amino-terminal propeptide of procollagen type III; PINP, amino-terminal propeptide of procollagen type I; RT, radiotherapy; TnI, troponin I; TTE, transthoracic echocardiography.

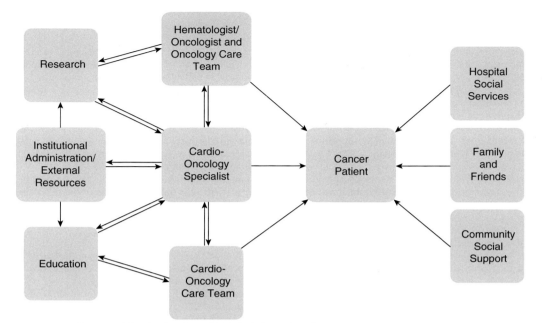

FIG. 10.10 Proposed Cardio-Oncology Multidisciplinary Care Team Model. (Reproduced from Okwuosa TM, Barac A. Buregoning cardio-oncology programs: challenges and opportunities for early career cardiologists/faculty directors. *J Am Coll Cardiol*. 2015;66:1193—1197 with permission.)

REFERENCES

1. Plana JC, Galderisi M, Barac A, et al. Expert consensus for multimodality imaging evaluation of adult patients during and after cancer therapy: a report from the American Society of Echocardiography and the European Association of Cardiovascular Imaging. *J Am Soc Echocardiogr*. 2014;27:911—939.
2. Jones LW, Haykowsky MJ, Swartz JJ, Douglas PS, Mackey JR. Early breast cancer therapy and cardiovascular injury. *J Am Coll Cardiol*. 2007;50:1435—1441.
3. Ewer MS, Lippman SM. Type II chemotherapy-related cardiac dysfunction: time to recognize a new entity. *J Clin Oncol*. 2005;23:2900—2902.
4. Lee KF, Simon H, Chen H, Bates B, Hung MC, Hauser C. Requirement for neuregulin receptor erbB2 in neural and cardiac development. *Nature*. 1995;378:394.
5. Gassmann M, Casagranda F, Orioli D, et al. Aberrant neural and cardiac development in mice lacking the ErbB4 neuregulin receptor. *Nature*. 1995;378:390.
6. Ozcelik C, Erdmann B, Pilz B, et al. Conditional mutation of the ErbB2 (HER2) receptor in cardiomyocytes leads to dilated cardiomyopathy. *Proc Natl Acad Sci*. 2002;99:8880.
7. Crone SA, Zhao YY, Fan L, et al. ErbB2 is essential in the prevention of dilated cardiomyopathy. *Nat Med*. 2002;8:459.
8. García-Rivello H, Taranda J, Said M, et al. Dilated cardiomyopathy in Erb-b4-deficient ventricular muscle. *Am J Physiol Heart Circ Physiol*. 2005;289:H1153—H1160.
9. Korte MA, de Vries EG, Lub-de Hooge MN, et al. 111Indium-trastuzumab visualises myocardial human epidermal growth factor receptor 2 expression shortly after anthracycline treatment but not during heart failure: a clue to uncover the mechanisms of trastuzumab-related cardiotoxicity. *Eur J Cancer*. 2007;43:2046.
10. Perik PJ, de Vries EG, Gietema JA, et al. Serum HER2 levels are increased in patients with chronic heart failure. *Eur J Heart Fail*. 2007;9:173.
11. Tocchetti CG, Ragone G, Coppola C, et al. Detection, monitoring, and management of trastuzumab-induced left ventricular dysfunction: an actual challenge. *Eur J Heart Fail*. 2012;14:130—137.
12. Moja L, Tagliabue L, Balduzzi S, et al. Trastuzumab containing regimens for early breast cancer. *Cochrane Database Syst Rev*. 2012;2012:4.
13. Slamon D, Eiermann W, Robert N, et al. Adjuvant trastuzumab in HER2-positive breast cancer. *N Engl J Med*. 2011; 365:1273—1283.
14. Bowles EJ, Wellman R, Feigelson HS, et al. Risk of heart failure in breast cancer patients after anthracycline and trastuzumab treatment: a retrospective cohort study. *J Natl Cancer Inst*. 2012;104:1293.
15. Suter TM, Cook-Bruns N, Barton C. Cardiotoxicity associated with trastuzumab (Herceptin) therapy in the treatment of metastatic breast cancer. *Breast*. 2004;13: 173—183.

16. Cobleigh MA, Vogel CL, Tripathy D, et al. Multinational study of the efficacy and safety of humanized anti-HER2 monoclonal antibody in women who have HER2-overexpressing metastatic breast cancer that has progressed after chemotherapy for metastatic disease. *J Clin Oncol.* 1999;17:2639–2648.

17. Romond EH, Jeong JH, Rastogi P, et al. Seven-year follow-up assessment of cardiac function in NSABP B-31, a randomized trial comparing doxorubicin and cyclophosphamide followed by paclitaxel (ACP) with ACP plus trastuzumab as adjuvant therapy for patients with node-positive, human epidermal gr. *J Clin Oncol.* 2012;30:3792.

18. Goldhar HA, Yan AT, Ko DT, et al. The temporal risk of heart failure associated with adjuvant trastuzumab in breast cancer patients: a population study. *J Natl Cancer Inst.* 2016:108.

19. Perez EA, Suman VJ, Davidson NE, et al. Cardiac safety analysis of doxorubicin and cyclophosphamide followed by paclitaxel with or without trastuzumab in the North Central Cancer Treatment Group N9831 adjuvant breast cancer trial. *J Clin Oncol.* 2008;26:1231.

20. Chen J, Long JB, Hurria A, Owusu C, Steingart RMGC. Incidence of heart failure or cardiomyopathy after adjuvant trastuzumab therapy for breast cancer. *J Am Coll Cardiol.* 2012;60:2504–2512.

21. Suter TM, Procter M, van Veldhuisen DJ, et al. Trastuzumab-associated cardiac adverse effects in the herceptin adjuvant trial. *J Clin Oncol.* 2007;25:3859–3865.

22. Guenancia C, Lefebvre A, Cardinale D, et al. Obesity as a risk factor for anthracyclines and trastuzumab cardiotoxicity in breast cancer: a systematic review and meta-analysis. *J Clin Oncol.* 2016;34:3157.

23. Cheraghi Z, Ayubi E, Doosti-Irani A. Obesity as a risk factor for anthracyclines and trastuzumab cardiotoxicity in breast cancer: methodologic issues to avoid misinterpretation in the meta-analysis. *J Clin Oncol.* 2017;35:923.

24. Seidman A, Hudis C, Pierri MK, et al. Cardiac dysfunction in the trastuzumab clinical trials experience. *J Clin Oncol.* 2002;20:1215.

25. Ezaz G, Long JB, Gross CP, Chen J. Risk prediction model for heart failure and cardiomyopathy after adjuvant trastuzumab therapy for breast cancer. *J Am Heart Assoc.* 2014:3.

26. Ewer MS, Vooletich MT, Durand JB, Woods ML, Davis JR, Valero V, Lenihan DJ. Reversibility of trastuzumab-related cardiotoxicity: new insights based on clinical course and response to medical treatment. *J Clin Oncol.* 2005;23:7820.

27. Krop IE, Suter TM, Dang CT, et al. Feasibility and cardiac safety of trastuzumab emtansine after anthracycline-based chemotherapy as (neo)adjuvant therapy for human epidermal growth factor receptor 2-positive early-stage breast cancer. *J Clin Oncol.* 2015;33:1136.

28. Krop IE, LoRusso P, Miller KD, et al. A phase II study of trastuzumab emtansine in patients with human epidermal growth factor receptor 2-positive metastatic breast cancer who were previously treated with trastuzumab, lapatinib, an anthracycline, a taxane, and capecitabine. *J Clin Oncol.* 2012;30:3234–3241.

29. Verma S, Miles D, Gianni L, et al. Trastuzumab emtansine for HER2-positive advanced breast cancer. *N Engl J Med.* 2013;368:2442.

30. Hurvitz SA, Dirix L, Kocsis J, et al. Phase II randomized study of trastuzumab emtansine versus trastuzumab plus docetaxel in patients with human epidermal growth factor receptor 2-positive metastatic breast cancer. *J Clin Oncol.* 2013;31:1157.

31. Baselga J, Gelmon KA, Verma S, et al. Phase II trial of pertuzumab and trastuzumab in patients with human epidermal growth factor receptor 2-positive metastatic breast cancer that progressed during prior trastuzumab therapy. *J Clin Oncol.* 2010;28:1138–1144.

32. Swain SM, Ewer MS, Cortés J, et al. Cardiac tolerability of pertuzumab plus trastuzumab plus docetaxel in patients with HER2-positive metastatic breast cancer in CLEOPATRA: a randomized, double-blind, placebo-controlled phase III study. *Oncologist.* 2013;18:257.

33. von Minckwitz G, Procter M, de Azambuja E. Ist for the ASC and I. Adjuvant pertuzumab and trastuzumab in early HER2-positive breast cancer. *N Engl J Med.* 2017:122–131.

34. Geyer CE, Forster J, Lindquist D, et al. Lapatinib plus capecitabine for HER2-positive advanced breast cancer. *N Engl J Med.* 2006;355:2733–2743.

35. Perez EA, Koehler M, Byrne J, Preston AJ, Rappold E, Ewer MS. Cardiac safety of lapatinib: pooled analysis of 3689 patients enrolled in clinical trials. *Mayo Clin Proc.* 2008;83:679–686.

36. Procter M, Suter TM, de Azambuja E, et al. Longer-term assessment of trastuzumab-related cardiac adverse events in the Herceptin Adjuvant (HERA) trial. *J Clin Oncol.* 2010;28:3422–3428.

37. Joensuu H, Bono P, Kataja V, et al. Fluorouracil, epirubicin, and cyclophosphamide with either docetaxel or vinorelbine, with or without trastuzumab, as adjuvant treatments of breast cancer: final results of the FinHer Trial. *J Clin Oncol.* 2009;27:5685–5692.

38. Blackwell KL, Burstein HJ, Storniolo AM, et al. Randomized study of Lapatinib alone or in combination with trastuzumab in women with ErbB2-positive, trastuzumab-refractory metastatic breast cancer. *J Clin Oncol.* 2010;28:1124.

39. Valachis A, Nearchou A, Polyzos NP, Lind P. Cardiac toxicity in breast cancer patients treated with dual HER2 blockade. *Int J Cancer.* 2013;133:2245–2252.

40. Harbeck N, Huang CS, Hurvitz S, et al. Afatinib plus vinorelbine versus trastuzumab plus vinorelbine in patients with HER2-overexpressing metastatic breast cancer who had progressed on one previous trastuzumab treatment (LUX-Breast 1): an open-label, randomised, phase 3 trial. *Lancet Oncol.* 2016;17:357–366.

41. Chan A, Delaloge S, Holmes FA, et al. Neratinib after trastuzumab-based adjuvant therapy in patients with HER2-positive breast cancer (ExteNET): a multicentre, randomised, double-blind, placebo-controlled, phase 3 trial. *Lancet Oncol.* 2016;17:367–377.

42. Fallah-Rad N, Lytwyn M, Fang T, Kirkpatrick I, Jassal D. Delayed contrast enhancement cardiac magnetic resonance imaging in trastuzumab induced cardiomyopathy. *J Cardiovasc Magn Reson.* 2008:10.

43. Fallah-Rad N1, Walker JR, Wassef A, et al. The utility of cardiac biomarkers, tissue velocity and strain imaging, and cardiac magnetic resonance imaging in predicting early left ventricular dysfunction in patients with human epidermal growth factor receptor II-positive breast cancer treated with adjuvant trastuzumab therapy. *J Am Coll Cardiol.* 2011;57:2263−2270.

44. Garg V, Vorobiof G. Echocardiography and alternative cardiac imaging strategies for long-term cardiotoxicity surveillance of cancer survivors treated with chemotherapy and/or radiation exposure. *Curr Oncol Rep.* 2016;18:52.

45. Thavendiranathan P, Poulin F, Lim KD, Plana JC, Woo A, Marwick TH. Use of myocardial strain imaging by echocardiography for the early detection of cardiotoxicity in patients during and after cancer chemotherapy: a systematic review. *J Am Coll Cardiol.* 2014;63:2751−2768.

46. Cardinale D, Colombo A, Torrisi R, et al. Trastuzumab-induced cardiotoxicity: clinical and prognostic implications of troponin I evaluation. *J Clin Oncol.* 2010;28:3910−3916.

47. Morris PG, Chen C, Steingart R, et al. Troponin I and C-reactive protein are commonly detected in patients with breast cancer treated with dose-dense chemotherapy incorporating trastuzumab and lapatinib. *Clin Cancer Res.* 2011;17:3490−3499.

48. Sawaya H, Sebag IA, Plana JC, et al. Early detection and prediction of cardiotoxicity in chemotherapy-treated patients. *Am J Cardiol.* 2011;107:1375−1380.

49. Ky B, Putt M, Sawaya H, et al. Early increases in multiple biomarkers predict subsequent cardiotoxicity in patients with breast cancer treated with doxorubicin, taxanes, and trastuzumab. *J Am Coll Cardiol.* 2014;63:809−816.

50. Putt M, Hahn VS, Januzzi JL, et al. Longitudinal changes in multiple biomarkers are associated with cardiotoxicity in breast cancer patients treated with doxorubicin, taxanes, and trastuzumab. *Clin Chem.* 2015;61:1164−1172.

51. Sandri MT, Salvatici M, Cardinale D, et al. N-terminal pro-B-type natriuretic peptide after high-dose chemotherapy: a marker predictive of cardiac dysfunction? *Clin Chem.* 2005;51:1405−1410.

52. Sawaya H, Sebag IA, Plana JC, et al. Assessment of echocardiography and biomarkers for the extended prediction of cardiotoxicity in patients treated with anthracyclines, taxanes, and trastuzumab. *Circ Cardiovasc Imaging.* 2012;5:596−603.

53. Grover S, Leong DP, Chakrabarty A, et al. Left and right ventricular effects of anthracycline and trastuzumab chemotherapy: a prospective study using novel cardiac imaging and biochemical markers. *Int J Cardiol.* 2013;168:5465−5467.

54. Zardavas D, Suter TM, Van Veldhuisen DJ, et al. Role of troponins I and T and N-Terminal prohormone of brain natriuretic peptide in monitoring cardiac safety of patients with early-stage human epidermal growth factor receptor 2-positive breast cancer receiving trastuzumab: a herceptin adjuvant study Ca. *J Clin Oncol.* 2017;35:878−884.

55. Shah KS, Yang EH, Maisel AS, Fonarow GC. The role of biomarkers in detection of cardio-toxicity. *Curr Oncol Rep.* 2017;19:42.

56. Khouri MG, Douglas PS, Mackey JR, et al. Cancer therapy-induced cardiac toxicity in early breast cancer: addressing the unresolved issues. *Circulation.* 2012;126:2749−2763.

57. Cardinale D, Sandri MT, Colombo A, et al. Prognostic value of troponin I in cardiac risk stratification of cancer patients undergoing high-dose chemotherapy. *Circulation.* 2004;109:2749−2754.

58. Florido R, Smith KL, Cuomo KK, Russell SD. Cardiotoxicity from human epidermal growth factor Receptor-2 (HER2) targeted therapies. *J Am Heart Assoc.* 2017:6.

59. Yancy CW, Jessup M, Bozkurt B, et al. 2013 ACCF/AHA guideline for the management of heart failure: a report of the American College of cardiology Foundation/American Heart Association Task Force on practice guidelines. *Circulation.* 2013;128:e240−327.

60. Guarneri V, Lenihan DJ, Valero V, et al. Long-term cardiac tolerability of trastuzumab in metastatic breast cancer: the M.D. Anderson Cancer Center experience. *J Clin Oncol.* 2006;24:4107−4115.

61. Armenian SH, Lacchetti C, Lenihan D. Prevention and monitoring of cardiac dysfunction in survivors of adult cancers: American Society of Clinical Oncology Clinical Practice Guideline summary. *J Oncol Pr.* 2017;13:270−275.

62. Jones AL, Barlow M, Barrett-Lee PJ, et al. Management of cardiac health in trastuzumab-treated patients with breast cancer: updated United Kingdom National Cancer Research Institute recommendations for monitoring. *Br J Cancer.* 2009;100:684−692.

63. Curigliano G, Cardinale D, Suter T, et al. Cardiovascular toxicity induced by chemotherapy, targeted agents and radiotherapy: ESMO Clinical Practice Guidelines. *Ann Oncol.* 2012;23:vii155−166.

64. Russell RR, Alexander J, Jain D, et al. The role and clinical effectiveness of multimodality imaging in the management of cardiac complications of cancer and cancer therapy. *J Nucl Cardiol.* 2016;23:856−884.

65. Zamorano JL, Lancellotti P, Rodriguez Muñoz D, et al. 2016 ESC position paper on cancer treatments and cardiovascular toxicity developed under the auspices of the ESC committee for practice guidelines: the task force for cancer treatments and cardiovascular toxicity of the European Society of Cardiology (ESC). *Eur Heart J.* 2016;37:2768−2801.

66. Mackey JR, Clemons M, Côté MA, et al. Cardiac management during adjuvant trastuzumab therapy: recommendations of the Canadian Trastuzumab Working Group. *Curr Oncol*. 2008;15:24–35.

67. Slamon DJ, Leyland-Jones B, Shak S, et al. Use of chemotherapy plus a monoclonal antibody against HER2 for metastatic breast cancer that overexpresses HER2. *N Engl J Med*. 2001;344:783.

68. Cardinale D, Colombo A, Lamantia G, et al. Anthracycline-induced cardiomyopathy: clinical relevance and response to pharmacologic therapy. *J Am Coll Cardiol*. 2010;55:213–220.

69. Pun SC, Neilan TG. Cardioprotective interventions: where are we? *J Am Coll Cardiol*. 2016.

70. Gulati G, Heck SL, Ree AH, et al. Prevention of cardiac dysfunction during adjuvant breast cancer therapy (PRADA): a 2 × 2 factorial, randomized, placebo-controlled, double-blind clinical trial of candesartan and metoprolol. *Eur Heart J*. 2016;37:1671–1680.

71. Pituskin E, Mackey JR, Koshman S, et al. Multidisciplinary approach to novel therapies in cardio-oncology research (MANTICORE 101-breast): a randomized trial for the prevention of trastuzumab-associated cardiotoxicity. *J Clin Oncol*. 2017;35:870–877.

72. Seicean S, Seicean A, Alan N, Plana JC, Budd GT, Marwick TH. Cardioprotective effect of β-adrenoceptor blockade in patients with breast cancer undergoing chemotherapy: follow-up study of heart failure. *Circ Heart Fail*. 2013;6:420426.

73. Seicean S, Seicean A, Plana JC, Budd GT, Marwick T. Effect of statin therapy on the risk for incident heart failure in patients with breast cancer receiving anthracycline chemotherapy: an observational clinical cohort study. *J Am Coll Cardiol*. 2012;60:2384–2390.

74. Boekhout AH, Gietema JA, Milojkovic Kerklaan B, et al. Angiotensin II-receptor inhibition with candesartan to prevent trastuzumab-related cardiotoxic effects in patients with early breast cancer: a randomized clinical trial. *JAMA Oncol*. 2016;2:1030–1037.

75. Negishi K, Negishi T, Haluska BA, Hare JL, Plana JCMT. Use of speckle strain to assess left ventricular responses to cardiotoxic chemotherapy and cardioprotection. *Eur Heart J Cardiovasc Imaging*. 2014;15:324–331.

76. Herrmann J, Lerman A, Sandhu NP, Villarraga HR, Mulvagh SL, Kohli M. Evaluation and management of patients with heart disease and cancer: cardio-oncology. *Mayo Clin Proc*. 2014;89:1287–1306.

77. Lynce F, Barac A, Tan MT, et al. Safe-heart: rationale and design of a pilot study investigating cardiac safety of HER2 targeted therapy in patients with HER2-positive breast cancer and reduced left ventricular function. *Oncologist*. 2017;22:518–525.

78. Okwuosa TM, Barac A. Buregoning cardio-oncology programs: challenges and opportunities for early career cardiologists/faculty directors. *J Am Coll Cardiol*. 2015;66:1193–1197.

79. Meattini I, Curigliano G, Terziani F, et al. SAFE trial: an ongoing randomized clinical study to assess the role of cardiotoxicity prevention in breast cancer patients treated with anthracyclines with or without trastuzumab. *Med Oncol*. 2017;34:75.

80. Goodman M. *STOP Heart Disease in Breast Cancer Survivors Trial*; 2017. Available at: https://clinicaltrials.gov/ct2/show/study/NCT02674204.

81. Yu A. *Assessment for Long-Term Cardiovascular Impairment Associated with Trastuzumab Cardiotoxicity in HER2-Positive Breast Cancer Survivors*; 2017. Available at: https://clinicaltrials.gov/ct2/show/NCT02615054.

82. Brezden-Masley CB. *Assessment of Cardiotoxicity by Cardiac Magnetic Resonance (CMR) in Breast Cancer Patients Receiving Trastuzumab*; 2017. Available at: https://clinicaltrials.gov/ct2/show/NCT01022086.

83. Guglin M, Munster P, Fink AKJ. Lisinopril or Coreg CR in reducing cardiotoxicity in women with breast cancer receiving trastuzumab: a rationale and design of a randomized clinical trial. *Am Heart J*. 2017;188:87–92.

84. Yu A. *Carvedilol for the Prevention of Anthracycline/Anti-HER2 Therapy Associated Cardiotoxicity Among Women with HER2-Positive Breast Cancer Using Myocardial Strain Imaging for Early Risk Stratification*; 2017. Available at: https://clinicaltrials.gov/ct2/show/NCT02177175.

85. Aseyey O. *An Integrated Consent Model Study to Compare Two. Standard of Care Schedules for Monitoringardiac Function in Patients Receiving Trastuzumab for Early Stage Breast Cancer (OTT 15–05)*; 2018. Available at: https://clinicaltrials.gov/ct2/show/NCT02696707.

86. Jacquinot Q, Meneveau N, Chatot M, et al. A phase 2 randomized trial to evaluate the impact of a supervised exercise program on cardiotoxicity at 3 months in patients with HER2 overexpressing breast cancer undergoing adjuvant treatment by trastuzumab: design of the CARDAPAC study. *BMC Cancer*. 2017;17:425.

87. Alberta ACC. *Study to See Whether Breath-Hold Techniques during RT Are Effective in Helping to Improve Sparing of the Heart*; 2017. Available at: https://clinicaltrials.gov/ct2/show/study/NCT02052102.

88. Mehta LS, Watson KE, Barac A, et al. AHA scientific statement: cardiovascular disease and breast cancer; where these entities intersect: a scientific statement from the American Heart Association. *Circulation*. 2018;137. https://doi.org/10.1161/CIR.0000000000000556.

CHAPTER 11

Noncardiac Toxicity of HER2-Targeted Therapy

AASHINI MASTER, DO

INTRODUCTION

Human epidermal growth factor receptor 2 (HER2) is a member of a family of tyrosine kinases that also include HER1 (epidermal growth factor receptor [EGFR]), HER3, and HER4. The HER family are involved in pathways that regulate proliferation, cell death, angiogenesis, and migration.[1] Approximately 15%–25% of breast cancers have HER2 overexpression,[2,3] which is historically associated with a poorer prognosis.[3,4] The development of targeted therapies that inhibit the HER family receptors has revolutionized the treatment of HER2-positive breast cancer. There are two broad categories of targeted therapies use in HER2-positive breast cancer: monoclonal antibodies and tyrosine kinase inhibitors (TKIs).[5] TKIs are less specific and have the potential to inhibit multiple targets simultaneously, resulting in more side effects.[6]

There are currently five US Food and Drug Administration–approved therapies for clinical use in HER2-positive breast cancer: trastuzumab, lapatinib, pertuzumab, ado-trastuzumab emtansine (T-DM1), and neratinib. Cardiotoxicity related to HER2-targeted therapies, particularly trastuzumab, is of particular concern and has been well described in the literature. Additional common side effects of anti-HER2 therapies include infusion-related reactions, rash, diarrhea, thrombocytopenia, and transaminitis. As trastuzumab only targets the HER2 receptor, a systematic review of side effects associated with anti-HER2 therapies indicated that trastuzumab monotherapy presents the most favorable side effect profile.[5] Some of the newer anti-HER2 agents target multiple receptors in the HER family, resulting in additional clinically significant side effects, including some grade 3. Side effects of anti-HER2 therapies can be difficult to ascertain as they are often given in combination with one another and standard chemotherapy. As such, as we review the noncardiac toxicities of the above anti-HER2 agents in this chapter, we will distinguish between side effects seen with monotherapy and commonly used combination therapies.

TRASTUZUMAB

Trastuzumab is a humanized monoclonal antibody that targets the extracellular domain of HER2.[7] It was the first humanized monoclonal antibody approved for the treatment of HER2-overexpressing metastatic breast cancer in 1998. Since this time, trastuzumab has been extensively investigated in the clinical setting, both as monotherapy in combination with standard chemotherapeutic agents and in combination with other anti-HER2 agents. Across trials, the most common adverse events observed included fevers, chills, pain, nausea, vomiting, and headache. These were mild to moderate in intensity and most commonly observed with the initial infusion.[8-13]

In a large phase II trial, 222 patients with HER2-overexpressing metastatic breast cancer that had progressed on chemotherapy were enrolled to receive trastuzumab monotherapy at weekly intervals. Patients received an initial loading dose of 4 mg/kg, followed by weekly administration of 2 mg/kg. Infusion was initially administered over 90 min and if tolerated well, subsequent infusions were given over 30 min.[10] The most common adverse events were fever (38%), chills (36%), pain (48%), asthenia (46%), nausea (36%), vomiting (28%), and headache (26%). Symptoms were successfully managed with interruption of the infusion and administration of acetaminophen, diphenhydramine, and/or meperidine. Symptoms usually did not recur with subsequent infusions. In a second phase II trial, 105 patients with previously untreated HER2-overexpressing metastatic breast cancer received trastuzumab monotherapy at 3-week intervals at an initial loading dose of 8 mg/kg followed by

6 mg/kg for subsequent doses over 90 min.[8] Similarly, the most common adverse events observed were rigors (18%), fever (15%), headache (10%), nausea (10%), and fatigue (10%). Fifty-four percent of patients had at least one symptom associated with their first infusion, which decreased to 29% with the second infusion and 20% with the third infusion. Three patients experienced serious infusion-related reaction, two of which were able to continue to receive trastuzumab.

In the pivotal phase III trial, 469 patients with HER2-overexpressing metastatic breast cancer were assigned to receive standard chemotherapy versus standard chemotherapy plus trastuzumab.[12] Infusion-related symptoms including chills and/or fevers were observed in 25% of patients, which resolved with slowing down of the infusion rate. Incidence of infection was higher in the trastuzumab plus chemotherapy arm compared with the chemotherapy arm (47% vs. 29%). Infections were mild to moderate and included upper respiratory tract infections, catheter-related infections, viral syndrome, and other infections. The addition of trastuzumab to chemotherapy also increased the frequency of leukopenia and anemia; however, grade 3 or 4 events were similar for anemia (2% in both arms) and only slightly increased for thrombocytopenia (11% in the chemotherapy plus trastuzumab arm vs. 9% in the chemotherapy alone arm).

In a phase III adjuvant trial (BCIRG-006), 3222 patients with HER2-amplified early-stage breast cancer received adjuvant doxorubicin and cyclophosphamide followed by docetaxel (AC-T), the same regimen plus 52 weeks of trastuzumab (trastuzumab beginning with the docetaxel, AC-TH) or docetaxel and carboplatin plus 52 weeks of trastuzumab (TCH).[14] Grade 3 or 4 adverse effects were similar between the AC-T and AC-TH groups with the exception of a slightly higher incidence of myalgia, neutropenia, and leukopenia in the trastuzumab arm. A significant difference favoring the TCH group, as compared with the AC-TH group, was noted for arthralgias, myalgias, hand-foot syndrome, stomatitis, vomiting, sensory neuropathy, and leukopenia. The AC-TH group experienced significantly less anemia and thrombocytopenia, compared with the TCH group (5.8% vs. 3.1% and 6.1% vs. 2.1%, respectively).

The rate of infusion-related reactions with trastuzumab is low, as such premedications are not recommended and initial infusion should be given over 90 min.[15] Management of infusion reactions includes decreasing the rate for mild to moderate reactions, interruption for dyspnea or hypotension, and discontinuation for severe or life-threatening reactions.

Supportive medications such as antihistamines, acetaminophen, and corticosteroids may be utilized to effectively manage symptoms for serious reactions. Postmarketing surveillance data, until March 2000, include 74 reports worldwide of serious infusion-related events from 25,000 patients treated with trastuzumab.[11] Sixty-five of the 74 patients responded well to supportive treatment and 33 of 39 were successfully rechallenged and continued to receive treatment with trastuzumab. Sixty-five percent of patients who experienced serious infusion-related reactions complained of respiratory symptoms, and nine patients (12%) died. All of these patients who died had preexisting, malignancy-related respiratory distress.

LAPATINIB

Lapatinib is an oral dual TKI of EGFR and HER2. Lapatinib has been shown to have activity in HER2-overexpressing metastatic breast cancer in several phase II and III clinical trials. The most common side effects observed are diarrhea and rash.[16]

In a phase I clinical trial, 67 patients with metastatic solid tumors were treated with lapatinib.[17] The most frequent adverse events were diarrhea (42%) and rash (acne, dermatitis acneiform) (31%), most of which were grade 1 or 2. Two patients experienced grade 3 diarrhea and one experienced grade 3 rash. The incidence of diarrhea was dose related, whereas the incidence of rash was not. Other less common side effects included nausea (13%) and fatigue (10%). No grade 4 toxicities was observed.

In a phase II study of lapatinib monotherapy in advanced or metastatic breast cancer, a dose of 1500 mg daily was generally well tolerated.[18] Consistent with prior lapatinib studies, the most common adverse events included diarrhea (59%), nausea (37%), and rash (32%). Grade 4 adverse events were noted in 6% of patients and 7% of patients required discontinuation because of side effects including nausea, diarrhea, abdominal pain, and increased bilirubin. Similarly, in another phase II trial of lapatinib monotherapy, the most common adverse events were rash (47%), diarrhea (46%), and nausea (31%).[19] Grade 3 rash and diarrhea were reported in 4% and 9% of patients, respectively. No grade 4 toxicities was observed.

Lapatinib is most commonly administered in combination with capecitabine or trastuzumab based on results of phase III trials, which revealed superior clinical outcomes compared with capecitabine alone or lapatinib alone, respectively. In a phase III trial of lapatinib plus trastuzumab versus lapatinib alone, the incidence of grade 1 and 2 diarrhea was higher in the combination therapy arm (60% for lapatinib plus trastuzumab vs. 48% for lapatinib).[20] The incidence of rash was higher in the monotherapy arm (39%) versus the combination therapy arm (22%), which was likely a result of a higher dose of lapatinib (1500 mg as monotherapy vs. 1000 mg in combination arm) in the monotherapy arm. Nausea and fatigue rates were similar between both arms. In the phase III trial comparing lapatinib plus capecitabine with capecitabine alone, all-grade diarrhea and rash were more common in the combination therapy arm versus the monotherapy arm (60% vs. 39% and 27% vs. 15%, respectively).[21] Incidence of grade 3 diarrhea and rash was low and similar between both arms. Grade 4 diarrhea did occur in two patients in the combination arm, which led to the discontinuation of lapatinib in these patients.

One hypothesis of the underlying mechanism of TKI-associated diarrhea relates to the role of HER receptors in intestinal ion transport, whereby HER dimerization leads to an inhibitory effect on chloride secretion and sodium absorption into the intestinal lumen. Inhibition of HER dimerization can then lead to an imbalance in the translumen ion and water transport, which results in diarrhea.[22]

Management of diarrhea is dependent on grade. For patients experiencing grade 1 or 2 diarrhea, recommendations include avoiding lactose, staying well hydrated, eating small frequent meals, and use of antidiarrheal agents such as loperamide.[16] Lapatinib should be held for grade 3 diarrhea or grade 1 or 2 diarrhea with complicating features such as abdominal cramping, fever, sepsis, neutropenia, and dehydration. Lapatinib

can be resumed at a lower dose when diarrhea improves to grade 1 or less. Lapatinib should be permanently discontinued for grade 4 diarrhea.[23]

The rash associated with lapatinib has been seen as a class effect of EGFR inhibitors including erlotinib, cetuximab, and gefitinib.[24] The rash is characterized by inflammatory papules and pustules most commonly seen on the face, chest, and back (Fig. 11.1). There are no clear evidence-based recommendations for management of lapatinib-associated rash; therefore we follow the same principles as for other EGFR inhibitors, which include clindamycin 1% gel, topical corticosteroids, oral antibiotics (tetracycline 250 mg four times daily or minocycline 100 mg two times daily), and colloidal oatmeal lotion.[16] Patients with extensive or persistent skin involvement should be referred to a dermatologist. A proposed algorithm for management of rash outlined in Fig. 11.2.

PERTUZUMAB

Pertuzumab is a humanized anti-HER2 monoclonal antibody that binds the extracellular subdomain II and impedes ligand-dependent heterodimerization, thereby inhibiting intracellular signaling.[25] Pertuzumab more effectively blocks HER2 heterodimerization with EGFR, HER3, and HER4.[26,27] By preventing HER2 heterodimerization with EGFR, pertuzumab causes similar side effects as EGFR antagonists, such as diarrhea and rash.[28,29] Most side effects are mild to moderate; however, increased rates of grade 3 neutropenia, febrile neutropenia, diarrhea, rash, and asthenia have been observed when pertuzumab is given in combination with chemotherapy.

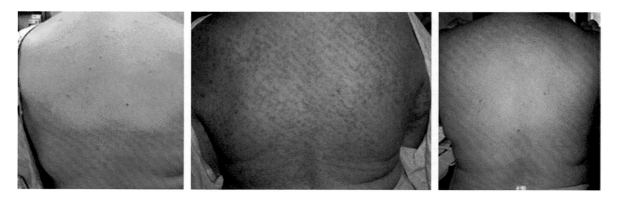

A   Grade 1   Grade 2   Grade 3

FIG. 11.1

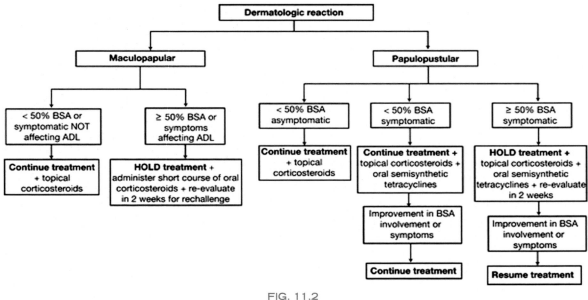

FIG. 11.2

The most common adverse event related to pertuzumab across trials is low-grade diarrhea. In the phase I study, most events were grade 1 and occasionally grade 2, with a 43% incidence of diarrhea. Twelve of 21 patients experienced at least one grade 3 or 4 adverse event; however, only 6 were thought to be related to study medication.[30] In a phase II metastatic breast cancer trial, 79 patients received pertuzumab monotherapy, with any grade diarrhea occurring in 51.2% of patients.[29] Again, the majority of cases were grade 1 or 2, with only 7.3% experiencing grade 3 events. In a phase II single-arm trial, 66 patients with metastatic disease were treated trastuzumab weekly (4 mg/kg loading dose and then 2 mg/kg every week) or every 3 weeks (8 mg/kg loading dose and then 6 mg/kg every 3 weeks) in combination with standard dose pertuzumab (840 mg loading dose, then 420 mg every 3 weeks).[31] Diarrhea was experienced by 64% of patients, regardless of trastuzumab dose, of which 3% was grade 3. No grade 4 diarrhea was reported.

Diarrheal events have been found to be higher among those receiving pertuzumab in combination with docetaxel. In the phase III CLEOPATRA trial, 808 patients with HER2-overexpressing metastatic breast cancer were assigned to trastuzumab and docetaxel with or without pertuzumab.[32] The most common event in both arms was diarrhea, with 66.8% of events in the pertuzumab arm versus 46.3% in the control arm. Subgroup analysis of CLEOPATRA suggested that patients ≥65 years and patients from Asia with metastatic breast cancer experience higher rates of diarrhea, including grade 3 diarrhea.[33,34] Diarrheal events were noted to be as high as 72.4% in the neoadjuvant TRYPHAENA trial among patients receiving docetaxel, carboplatin, trastuzumab, and pertuzumab.[35] Increased events were also noted in the neoadjuvant NeoSphere trial, ranging from 28% to 54% for pertuzumab-containing regimens, which the highest rates in the pertuzumab and docetaxel arm and lowest in the pertuzumab and trastuzumab arm.[36] No grade 4 diarrhea was observed in NeoSphere or TRYPHAENA. In the recently published adjuvant APHINITY trial, 1 year of pertuzumab was added to trastuzumab.[37] The incidence of diarrhea was one of the largest differences between treatment groups for all grades (71.2% with pertuzumab and 45.2% with placebo). Grade 3 diarrhea was observed in 9.8% of patients in the pertuzumab arm compared with 3.7% in the placebo arm.

Although diarrhea is a common side effect of pertuzumab, it is typically low grade, manageable, and less commonly observed with later cycles of therapy, regardless of docetaxel treatment. It is also important to note that no patients with early breast cancer discontinued any study drug because of diarrhea in the NeoSphere and TRYPHAENA trials, and in the metastatic setting,

2% in the pertuzumab arm of CLEOPATRA discontinued study drug versus 0.5% in the control arm.[38]

Grade 3 neutropenia and febrile neutropenia were higher in the pertuzumab containing arms in both the APHINITY and CLEOPATRA studies. Neutropenia increased from 15.7% to 16.3% in APHINITY and 45.8% to 48.9% in CLEOPATRA with the addition of pertuzumab. Grade 3 febrile neutropenia rated increased from 11.1% to 12.1% in APHINITY and 7.6% to 13.8% in CLEOPATRA, which was the only grade 3 adverse event to increase by >5%.

Pertuzumab significantly increases the risk of rash compared with controls. In a metaanalysis the incidence of all-grade and high-grade rash with pertuzumab were 24.6% and 1.1%, respectively.[39] In the phase I trial of pertuzumab, the incidence of rash was 43%. This was not acneiform and did not resemble the rash typical of EGFR inhibitors.[30] In the APHINITY study, rash occurred in 25.8% of patients receiving pertuzumab, which was similar to rates seen in the NeoSphere trial when given in combination with chemotherapy (26%−29%) and slightly lower than that observed in CLEOPATRA (33.7%). In the phase II single-arm study of pertuzumab plus trastuzumab, all-grade rash occurred in 26% of patients, suggesting that combination with chemotherapy does not significantly increase dermatologic side effects.

There is no evidence to guide the management of rash and diarrhea from pertuzumab. As toxicity is typically mild, diarrhea is usually managed successfully with loperamide. The management of rash is based on the same principles of the rash from lapatinib and other EGFR inhibitors, which includes the use of topical corticosteroids or antibiotics for mild cases and use of a tetracycline antibiotic for more severe cases (Fig. 11.2).[40]

TRASTZUMAB EMTANSINE

T-DM1 is an antibody drug conjugate, which combines the HER2-targeted properties of trastuzumab with the cytotoxic activity of the potent microtubule, DM1 (derivative of maytansine).[41] In the phase I dose escalation study the maximum tolerated dose was 3.6 mg/kg every 3 weeks based on the dose-limiting toxicity of grade 4 thrombocytopenia at 4.8 mg/kg. The other most commonly reported adverse events were elevated transaminases, fatigue, anemia, and nausea, all of which were grade 1 or 2 and reversible.[42]

Given the promising activity and mild, reversible toxicity, several phase II trials were conducted, which confirmed the side effect profile. Across multiple studies, all-grade fatigue was the most common side effect (49.3%−65.2%), followed by nausea (37.3%−50%), headache (21.8%−40.6%), increased AST (26.4%−43.5%), and thrombocytopenia (27.5%−38.2%). The most common grade 3 or 4 side effects were thrombocytopenia (7.2%−8%), increased AST (2.7%−8.7%), increased ALT (2.7%−10.1%), and fatigue (2.8%−4.5%).[43-45] Platelet counts typically nadir around day 8 and recover by day 15. Thrombocytopenia infrequently led to T-DM1 dose reduction and no patients discontinued because of a hemorrhagic event, which were rare.[45]

As thrombocytopenia is the dose-limiting toxicity of T-DM1, the mechanism by which it induces thrombocytopenia is of interest. When measured by platelet aggregometry, T-DM1 did not demonstrate a direct effect on platelet activation or aggregation but did markedly inhibit megakaryocyte differentiation via a cytotoxic effect.[46]

In the pivotal phase III EMILIA trial comparing lapatinib plus capecitabine with T-DM1, serious side effects were noted in 18% of patients in the lapatinib-capecitabine arm and 15.5% of patients in the T-DM1 arm. Again, the most commonly reported grade 3 or 4 events with T-DM1 were thrombocytopenia (12.9%), elevated AST (4.3%), and elevated ALT (2.9%).[47] Bleeding events were higher with T-DM1 (29.8% vs. 15.8% with lapatinib plus capecitabine); however, rates of grade 3 or 4 bleeding were low in both groups (1.4% and 0.8%, respectively). Both thrombocytopenia and transaminitis can be managed with appropriate dose modifications and rarely require T-DM1 discontinuation.[47]

NERATINIB

Neratinib is an irreversible oral pan-ErbB receptor TKI of EGFR (HER1), HER2, and HER4 targeting the intracellular domain, which leads to reduced phosphorylation and activation of downstream pathways.[48] It was approved in July 2017 for extended adjuvant treatment of patients with early-stage HER2-amplified breast cancer, following adjuvant trastuzumab therapy based on the ExteNET study.[49] Similar to other EGFR antagonists, diarrhea is the most commonly observed adverse event.

In the initial phase I trial, diarrhea of any grade was observed in 88% of patients. Additional frequent adverse events were nausea (64%), fatigue (63%), vomiting (50%), and anorexia (40%). Grade 3 diarrhea was observed in 32% of patients, with a median onset of diarrhea of 8.5 days.[50] In another phase I trial, neratinib was studied in combination with paclitaxel and trastuzumab.[51] Again, diarrhea occurred at a high frequency (19 out of 21 patients), with grade 3 diarrhea experienced by 38% of patients. Most patients experienced diarrhea within 1–3 days of initiating neratinib, with symptoms diminishing within 2 weeks.[51]

Multiple phase II trials were subsequently conducted in the metastatic HER2-overexpressing setting with neratinib monotherapy and combination therapy. In one open-label, phase II trial, 136 patients who had received prior trastuzumab and those who had not went on to receive neratinib.[52] The most common adverse events for neratinib included diarrhea (95%), nausea (36%), vomiting (31%) and fatigue (24%). Diarrhea was the only grade 3 or 4 adverse event occurring in more than 10% of patients and observed more often in patients who had received prior trastuzumab. The onset of diarrhea was 2–3 days, on average, lasted a median of 5–7 days per event, and improved in severity during multiple weeks of treatment.[52] In a second phase II study, 233 patients with locally advanced or metastatic HER2-overexpressing breast cancer were randomized to single-agent neratinib or to lapatinib plus capecitabine.[53] Diarrheal events were significantly higher in the neratinib arm (85% vs. 68%) and were also the most common grade 3 or 4 event in both arms. Median onset was 3 days in the neratinib arm with a median duration of 3 days and resolved in the majority of patients with either dose reduction (12%) or administration of antidiarrheal medications (79%). Neratinib was also studied in combination with capecitabine in a phase II dose escalation study.[54] In this study, incidence of diarrhea (88%), nausea (37%), vomiting (29%), and fatigue (18%) was consistent with phase II neratinib monotherapy trials.

In the pivotal phase III ExteNET trial, extended adjuvant neratinib was studied in early-stage HER2-positive breast cancer following adjuvant trastuzumab-based therapy.[49] A total of 2840 patients were randomized to receive neratinib or placebo for 12 months. Adverse events including diarrhea, nausea, fatigue, and vomiting were most common, as observed in phase II trials. Grade 3 diarrhea occurred in 40% of patients, arose in the first month, and led to dose reductions in 26% and discontinuation in 17% of patients.

Diarrheal prophylaxis with loperamide is recommended with the first dose of neratinib and continuing for the first two cycles. In patients with loperamide-refractory diarrhea, additional antidiarrheal agents, dose reductions, or interruptions may be required.[55] A loperamide prophylaxis guideline can be seen in Table 11.1. For grade 2 diarrhea lasting 5 or more days or grade 3 diarrhea lasting longer than 2 days,

TABLE 11.1
Loperamide Prophylaxis

Time of Neratinib	Dose	Frequency
Weeks 1–2 (days 1–14)	4 mg	TID
Weeks 3–8 (days 15–56)	4 mg	BID
Weeks 9–52 (days 57–365)	4 mg	As needed (not to exceed 16 mg per day)

neratinib should be held and supportive measures initiated. If diarrhea resolves to grade 0–1 in 1 week or less, neratinib can be resumed at the same dose. If diarrhea resolved to grade 0–1 in more than 1 week, neratinib should be resumed at a reduced dose. For grade 4 diarrhea or diarrhea that recurs at grade 2 at the lowest dose (120 mg daily), neratinib should be permanently discontinued.[55] An ongoing phase II clinical trial (CONTROL, NCT02400476) will address whether adding oral budesonide or colestipol to loperamide prophylaxis will help mitigate this side effect.

CONCLUSIONS

The development of anti–HER2-targeted therapies has dramatically improved prognosis for patients with HER2-positive breast cancer. As prognosis improves, patients are receiving these therapeutic agents for prolonged periods. Although these therapies are typically well tolerated, it is important to be knowledgeable about the distinct side effect profiles of each agent and management principles to prevent interruption or early cessation of treatment and maintain quality of life.

REFERENCES

1. Nagy P, Jenei A, Damjanovich S, Jovin TM, Szolosi J. Complexity of signal transduction mediated by ErbB2: clues to the potential of receptor-targeted cancer therapy. *Pathol Oncol Res.* 1999;5(4):255–271.
2. Hynes NE. Amplification and overexpression of the erbB-2 gene in human tumors: its involvement in tumor development, significance as a prognostic factor, and potential as a target for cancer therapy. *Semin Cancer Biol.* 1993;4(1): 19–26.
3. Slamon DJ, Clark GM, Wong SG, Levin WJ, Ullrich A, McGuire WL. Human breast cancer: correlation of relapse and survival with amplification of the HER-2/neu oncogene. *Science.* 1987;235(4785):177–182.

4. Slamon DJ, Godolphin W, Jones LA, et al. Studies of the HER-2/neu proto-oncogene in human breast and ovarian cancer. *Science*. 1989;244(4905):707−712.

5. Sodergren SC, Copson E, White A, et al. Systematic review of the side effects associated with anti-HER2-targeted therapies used in the treatment of breast cancer, on behalf of the EORTC quality of life group. *Target Oncol*. 2016; 11(3):277−292.

6. Widakowich C, de Castro Jr G, de Azambuja E, Dinh P, Awada A. Review: side effects of approved molecular targeted therapies in solid cancers. *Oncologist*. 2007;12(12): 1443−1455.

7. Carter P, Presta L, Gorman CM, et al. Humanization of an anti-p185HER2 antibody for human cancer therapy. *Proc Natl Acad Sci USA*. 1992;89(10):4285−4289.

8. Baselga J, Carbonell X, Castaneda-Soto NJ, et al. Phase II study of efficacy, safety, and pharmacokinetics of trastuzumab monotherapy administered on a 3-weekly schedule. *J Clin Oncol*. 2005;23(10):2162−2171.

9. Boekhout AH, Beijnen JH, Schellens JH. *Trastuzumab Oncol*. 2011;16(6):800−810.

10. Cobleigh MA, Vogel CL, Tripathy D, et al. Multinational study of the efficacy and safety of humanized anti-HER2 monoclonal antibody in women who have HER2-overexpressing metastatic breast cancer that has progressed after chemotherapy for metastatic disease. *J Clin Oncol*. 1999;17(9):2639−2648.

11. Cook-Bruns N. Retrospective analysis of the safety of Herceptin immunotherapy in metastatic breast cancer. *Oncology*. 2001;61(suppl 2):58−66.

12. Slamon DJ, Leyland-Jones B, Shak S, et al. Use of chemotherapy plus a monoclonal antibody against HER2 for metastatic breast cancer that overexpresses HER2. *N Engl J Med*. 2001;344(11):783−792.

13. Vogel CL, Cobleigh MA, Tripathy D, et al. Efficacy and safety of trastuzumab as a single agent in first-line treatment of HER2-overexpressing metastatic breast cancer. *J Clin Oncol*. 2002;20(3):719−726.

14. Slamon D, Eiermann W, Robert N, et al. Adjuvant trastuzumab in HER2-positive breast cancer. *N Engl J Med*. 2011; 365(14):1273−1283.

15. *Trastuzumab*. San Francisco, CA: Genentech; 2017 [package insert].

16. Moy B, Goss PE. Lapatinib-associated toxicity and practical management recommendations. *Oncologist*. 2007;12(7): 756−765.

17. Burris 3rd HA, Hurwitz HI, Dees EC, et al. Phase I safety, pharmacokinetics, and clinical activity study of lapatinib (GW572016), a reversible dual inhibitor of epidermal growth factor receptor tyrosine kinases, in heavily pre-treated patients with metastatic carcinomas. *J Clin Oncol*. 2005;23(23):5305−5313.

18. Burstein HJ, Storniolo AM, Franco S, et al. A phase II study of lapatinib monotherapy in chemotherapy-refractory HER2-positive and HER2-negative advanced or metastatic breast cancer. *Ann Oncol*. 2008;19(6):1068−1074.

19. Blackwell KL, Pegram MD, Tan-Chiu E, et al. Single-agent lapatinib for HER2-overexpressing advanced or metastatic breast cancer that progressed on first- or second-line trastuzumab-containing regimens. *Ann Oncol*. 2009; 20(6):1026−1031.

20. Blackwell KL, Burstein HJ, Storniolo AM, et al. Randomized study of Lapatinib alone or in combination with trastuzumab in women with ErbB2-positive, trastuzumab-refractory metastatic breast cancer. *J Clin Oncol*. 2010; 28(7):1124−1130.

21. Geyer CE, Forster J, Lindquist D, et al. Lapatinib plus capecitabine for HER2-positive advanced breast cancer. *N Engl J Med*. 2006;355(26):2733−2743.

22. Van Sebille YZ, Gibson RJ, Wardill HR, Bowen JM. ErbB small molecule tyrosine kinase inhibitor (TKI) induced diarrhoea: chloride secretion as a mechanistic hypothesis. *Cancer Treat Rev*. 2015;41(7):646−652.

23. *Lapatinib*. Research Triangle Park, NC: GlaxoSmithKline; 2015 [package insert].

24. Shah NT, Kris MG, Pao W, et al. Practical management of patients with non-small-cell lung cancer treated with gefitinib. *J Clin Oncol*. 2005;23(1):165−174.

25. Franklin MC, Carey KD, Vajdos FF, Leahy DJ, de Vos AM, Sliwkowski MX. Insights into ErbB signaling from the structure of the ErbB2-pertuzumab complex. *Cancer Cell*. 2004;5(4):317−328.

26. Agus DB, Akita RW, Fox WD, et al. Targeting ligand-activated ErbB2 signaling inhibits breast and prostate tumor growth. *Cancer Cell*. 2002;2(2):127−137.

27. Badache A, Hynes NE. A new therapeutic antibody masks ErbB2 to its partners. *Cancer Cell*. 2004;5(4):299−301.

28. Cortes J, Fumoleau P, Bianchi GV, et al. Pertuzumab monotherapy after trastuzumab-based treatment and subsequent reintroduction of trastuzumab: activity and tolerability in patients with advanced human epidermal growth factor receptor 2-positive breast cancer. *J Clin Oncol*. 2012;30(14):1594−1600.

29. Gianni L, Llado A, Bianchi G, et al. Open-label, phase II, multicenter, randomized study of the efficacy and safety of two dose levels of Pertuzumab, a human epidermal growth factor receptor 2 dimerization inhibitor, in patients with human epidermal growth factor receptor 2-negative metastatic breast cancer. *J Clin Oncol*. 2010;28(7): 1131−1137.

30. Agus DB, Gordon MS, Taylor C, et al. Phase I clinical study of pertuzumab, a novel HER dimerization inhibitor, in patients with advanced cancer. *J Clin Oncol*. 2005;23(11): 2534−2543.

31. Baselga J, Gelmon KA, Verma S, et al. Phase II trial of pertuzumab and trastuzumab in patients with human epidermal growth factor receptor 2-positive metastatic breast cancer that progressed during prior trastuzumab therapy. *J Clin Oncol*. 2010;28(7):1138−1144.

32. Baselga J, Cortes J, Kim SB, et al. Pertuzumab plus trastuzumab plus docetaxel for metastatic breast cancer. *N Engl J Med*. 2012;366(2):109−119.

33. Miles D, Baselga J, Amadori D, et al. Treatment of older patients with HER2-positive metastatic breast cancer with pertuzumab, trastuzumab, and docetaxel: subgroup analyses from a randomized, double-blind, placebo-controlled phase III trial (CLEOPATRA). *Breast Cancer Res Treat.* 2013;142(1):89–99.
34. Swain SM, Im YH, Im SA, et al. Safety profile of Pertuzumab with Trastuzumab and Docetaxel in patients from Asia with human epidermal growth factor receptor 2-positive metastatic breast cancer: results from the phase III trial CLEOPATRA. *Oncologist.* 2014;19(7):693–701.
35. Schneeweiss A, Chia S, Hickish T, et al. Pertuzumab plus trastuzumab in combination with standard neoadjuvant anthracycline-containing and anthracycline-free chemotherapy regimens in patients with HER2-positive early breast cancer: a randomized phase II cardiac safety study (TRYPHAENA). *Ann Oncol.* 2013;24(9):2278–2284.
36. Gianni L, Pienkowski T, Im YH, et al. Efficacy and safety of neoadjuvant pertuzumab and trastuzumab in women with locally advanced, inflammatory, or early HER2-positive breast cancer (NeoSphere): a randomised multicentre, open-label, phase 2 trial. *Lancet Oncol.* 2012;13(1):25–32.
37. von Minckwitz G, Procter M, de Azambuja E, et al. Adjuvant pertuzumab and trastuzumab in early HER2-positive breast cancer. *N Engl J Med.* 2017;377(2):122–131.
38. Swain SM, Schneeweiss A, Gianni L, et al. Incidence and management of diarrhea in patients with HER2-positive breast cancer treated with pertuzumab. *Ann Oncol.* 2017;28(4):761–768.
39. Drucker AM, Wu S, Dang CT, Lacouture ME. Risk of rash with the anti-HER2 dimerization antibody pertuzumab: a meta-analysis. *Breast Cancer Res Treat.* 2012;135(2):347–354.
40. Lacouture ME, Anadkat MJ, Bensadoun RJ, et al. Clinical practice guidelines for the prevention and treatment of EGFR inhibitor-associated dermatologic toxicities. *Support Care Cancer.* 2011;19(8):1079–1095.
41. Remillard S, Rebhun LI, Howie GA, Kupchan SM. Antimitotic activity of the potent tumor inhibitor maytansine. *Science.* 1975;189(4207):1002–1005.
42. Krop IE, Beeram M, Modi S, et al. Phase I study of trastuzumab-DM1, an HER2 antibody-drug conjugate, given every 3 weeks to patients with HER2-positive metastatic breast cancer. *J Clin Oncol.* 2010;28(16):2698–2704.
43. Burris 3rd HA, Rugo HS, Vukelja SJ, et al. Phase II study of the antibody drug conjugate trastuzumab-DM1 for the treatment of human epidermal growth factor receptor 2 (HER2)-positive breast cancer after prior HER2-directed therapy. *J Clin Oncol.* 2011;29(4):398–405.
44. Hurvitz SA, Dirix L, Kocsis J, et al. Phase II randomized study of trastuzumab emtansine versus trastuzumab plus docetaxel in patients with human epidermal growth factor receptor 2-positive metastatic breast cancer. *J Clin Oncol.* 2013;31(9):1157–1163.
45. Krop IE, LoRusso P, Miller KD, et al. A phase II study of trastuzumab emtansine in patients with human epidermal growth factor receptor 2-positive metastatic breast cancer who were previously treated with trastuzumab, lapatinib, an anthracycline, a taxane, and capecitabine. *J Clin Oncol.* 2012;30(26):3234–3241.
46. Uppal H, Doudement E, Mahapatra K, et al. Potential mechanisms for thrombocytopenia development with trastuzumab emtansine (T-DM1). *Clin Cancer Res.* 2015;21(1):123–133.
47. Verma S, Miles D, Gianni L, et al. Trastuzumab emtansine for HER2-positive advanced breast cancer. *N Engl J Med.* 2012;367(19):1783–1791.
48. Rabindran SK, Discafani CM, Rosfjord EC, et al. Antitumor activity of HKI-272, an orally active, irreversible inhibitor of the HER-2 tyrosine kinase. *Cancer Res.* 2004;64(11):3958–3965.
49. Chan A, Buyse M, Yao B. Neratinib after trastuzumab in patients with HER2-positive breast cancer - author's reply. *Lancet Oncol.* 2016;17(5):e176–e177.
50. Wong KK, Fracasso PM, Bukowski RM, et al. A phase I study with neratinib (HKI-272), an irreversible pan ErbB receptor tyrosine kinase inhibitor, in patients with solid tumors. *Clin Cancer Res.* 2009;15(7):2552–2558.
51. Jankowitz RC, Abraham J, Tan AR, et al. Safety and efficacy of neratinib in combination with weekly paclitaxel and trastuzumab in women with metastatic HER2positive breast cancer: an NSABP Foundation Research Program phase I study. *Cancer Chemother Pharmacol.* 2013;72(6):1205–1212.
52. Burstein HJ, Sun Y, Dirix LY, et al. Neratinib, an irreversible ErbB receptor tyrosine kinase inhibitor, in patients with advanced ErbB2-positive breast cancer. *J Clin Oncol.* 2010;28(8):1301–1307.
53. Martin M, Bonneterre J, Geyer Jr CE, et al. A phase two randomised trial of neratinib monotherapy versus lapatinib plus capecitabine combination therapy in patients with HER2+ advanced breast cancer. *Eur J Cancer.* 2013;49(18):3763–3772.
54. Saura C, Garcia-Saenz JA, Xu B, et al. Safety and efficacy of neratinib in combination with capecitabine in patients with metastatic human epidermal growth factor receptor 2-positive breast cancer. *J Clin Oncol.* 2014;32(32):3626–3633.
55. *Neratinib.* Los Angeles, CA: puma Biotechnology; 2017 [package insert].

CHAPTER 12

Novel Non–HER2-targeted Therapies in HER2+ Breast Cancer

MARINA N. SHARIFI, MD, PHD • RUTH M. O'REGAN, MD

INTRODUCTION

While the treatment of HER2-positive (HER2+) breast cancer has benefited greatly from the development of therapies directly targeting the HER2 receptor and its downstream signaling, de novo and acquired resistance to HER2-targeted therapies remains a problem.[1] Almost a quarter of patients receiving adjuvant trastuzumab with chemotherapy for operable HER2+ disease experienced disease recurrence within the follow-up period of 10 years in a combined analysis of the B-31 and N9831 trials.[2] In the metastatic setting, patients with HER2+ disease receiving dual HER2-targeted therapy with trastuzumab and pertuzumab had an impressive median overall survival (OS) of 5 years in the CLEOPATRA trial, but median disease-free survival (DFS) was only 18.7 months, and disease progression occurred within the first year in 40%.[3] The elucidation of mechanisms of resistance to HER2-targeted therapies and the search for additional molecular targets in HER2+ tumors remain active areas of investigation. As a consequence, a number of additional targeted therapies are being studied in HER2+ disease.

The HER2 receptor is a member of the ERBB family of receptor tyrosine kinases (RTKs), which becomes active on homodimerization or heterodimerization with another ERBB family member (HER1/EGFR, HER3, or HER4). This leads to activation of key signaling pathways that promote cell proliferation and survival, including the PI3K/AKT/mTOR and Ras/MAPK pathways.[4] Preclinical and clinical studies have suggested several major categories of mechanisms that lead to resistance to HER2-targeted therapies[5–7] (Fig. 12.1), which we will review briefly as they inform the preclinical rationale for many non–HER2-targeted therapies we will discuss.

HER2 signaling can be reactivated at the membrane receptor level through alterations in HER2 itself, compensatory changes in activity of ERBB family members such as EGFR, or increased ligand production. Bypass signaling involving non-ERBB membrane receptors including MET, Eph2A, insulin-like growth factor 1 receptor (IGF-1R), FGFR, and estrogen receptor (ER) can activate the same pro-proliferative and pro-survival pathways as intact HER2. ER signaling is a particularly crucial resistance mechanism and is discussed elsewhere in this volume. Another major mechanism of resistance involves mutations in downstream signaling components in the PI3K/AKT pathway, which lead to constitutive pathway activation without ongoing HER2 input. Defects in cell cycle regulation such as activating mutations in the cyclin/cyclin-dependent kinase (CDK)/Rb pathway and defects in the apoptosis machinery eliminate the need for upstream pathway activity. Finally, there is significant evidence suggesting that the antitumor effect of anti-HER2 antibodies is partly due to the stimulation of host antibody-dependent cell-mediated cytotoxicity, which implicates modulation of host immunity in resistance.

CDK4/6 INHIBITORS

Dysregulation of the cell cycle to allow uncontrolled proliferation is one of the core changes acquired by tumor cells.[8] CDKs are the gatekeepers of cell cycle regulation, and pro-proliferative signaling through HER2 and other growth factor pathways converges on activation of CDKs to drive proliferation, whether in a physiologic setting or co-opted by a tumor cell. Regulatory subunits known as cyclins control CDK activity and thus progression through the cell cycle. Activating mutations in cyclins and CDKs and the loss of function mutations in CDK inhibitors such as the INK4 proteins and the Cip/Kip family proteins are found in a wide variety of cancers,[9] including breast. This has led to considerable interest in CDK inhibition as a therapeutic strategy

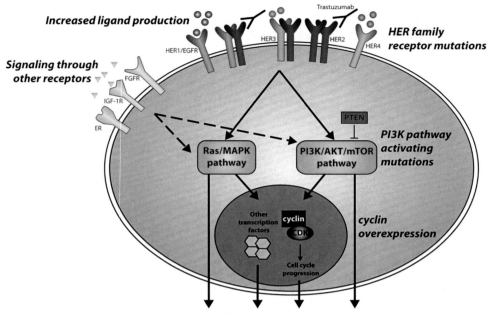

FIG. 12.1 Mechanisms of trastuzumab resistance. Intrinsic and acquired resistance to anti-HER2 therapy can occur at the cell surface receptor tyrosine kinase (RTK) level via increased ligand production, mutations in the HER/ErbB family receptors, or bypass signaling through other growth factor receptors such as estrogen receptor (ER), insulin-like growth factor receptor 1 (IGF-1R), and fibroblast growth factor receptor (FGFR), among others. Downstream activating mutations in the phosphatidylinositol-3 (PI3) kinase pathway such as activating *PIK3CA* mutations and loss of the inhibitor PTEN can render tumor cells independent of RTKs altogether, as can mutations in the cell proliferation machinery itself, such as cyclin D overexpression.

and the development of the CDK4/6 selective oral small molecule inhibitors palbociclib, ribociclib, and abemaciclib.

Preclinical Data for Targeting CDKs in HER2+ Breast Cancer

Abnormal activation of the cyclin D/CDK4 complex is found in 50%–70% of human breast cancers, with the most common alteration being cyclin D1 overexpression, particularly in luminal B and HER2+ tumors.[10] In the case of luminal B disease, CDK inhibition has found significant success in the clinic. Palbociclib was approved as first-line therapy for advanced hormone receptor–positive (HR+) HER2-negative breast cancer in 2015 based on the significant improvement in progression-free survival (PFS) for palbociclib with letrozole compared with letrozole alone in the phase III PALOMA trials.[11] Ribociclib was approved for the same indication after similar results were seen for ribociclib with letrazole in the phase III MONALEESA trial.[12] In the phase III MONARCH 2 trial,

abemaciclib similarly increased PFS in combination with fulvestrant in advanced HR+ HER-negative breast cancer that had progressed on endocrine therapy,[13] an indication for which it is now FDA approved, while the recently completed MONARCH 3 phase III trial of abemaciclib with letrozole as first-line therapy has demonstrated results similar to those reported with palbociclib and ribociclib as first-line therapy.[14]

A large body of preclinical evidence supports a similar role for CDK inhibition in HER2+ disease. The CDK4/6 activating function of cyclin D1 is required for HER2-driven tumorigenesis.[15,16] Inactivation of cyclin D1 or treatment with CDK4/6 inhibitor palbociclib halted tumor growth and triggered tumor cell senescence in established HER2-driven mouse mammary tumors,[17] demonstrating that CDK4/6 activity is required not only for tumor initiation but also for ongoing growth and proliferation of HER2-driven breast cancer, and thus that CDK4/6 inhibition might have activity against HER2+ cancers in the clinic. Indeed, palbociclib induced growth arrest in HER2-amplified human breast cancer cell lines in vitro, an effect which was synergistic with trastuzumab treatment.[18] More recently, cyclin D1 overexpression has been demonstrated as a mechanism of acquired resistance to HER2-directed therapy in both an inducible HER2-driven mouse mammary tumor model and in HER2+ human breast cancer cell lines, the latter of which were shown to be resensitized to HER2-directed therapy with CDK4/6 inhibitor abemaciclib.[19]

Taken together, there is strong preclinical mechanistic evidence for CDK4/6 inhibition in treating HER2+ breast cancer and in particular in the face of resistance to HER2-directed therapy. However, CDK4/6 inhibition leads principally to growth arrest rather than cell death, which has several therapeutic implications. First, there is a theoretical concern that in causing a growth arrest, CDK4/6 inhibitors could induce resistance to cytotoxic chemotherapies, which rely on cell proliferation for their efficacy and thus may not produce optimal benefit when combined. Second, unless combined with an additional therapy such as HER2-targeted therapy, CDK4/6 inhibitors would be expected to halt progression and lead to stable disease but not necessarily tumor regression.

Clinical Studies of CDK Inhibitors in HER2+ Breast Cancer

Phase I and II clinical trials testing CDK inhibition in HER2+ breast cancer are ongoing (Table 12.1). Most of these target locally advanced or metastatic disease that has failed prior HER2-directed therapy and are primarily in combination with HER2-directed therapy (trastuzumab, pertuzumab, or T-DM1) or taxanes. Several specifically target HR+ HER2+ disease given the success of palbociclib in HR+ HER2-negative disease and include hormonal therapy as well. PATINA is a phase III clinical trial for metastatic HR+ HER2+ disease, in which patients initially receive 4—8 cycles of induction therapy, followed by anti-HER2 therapy (trastuzumab and pertuzumab), endocrine therapy (letrozole, anastrozole, exemestane, or fulvestrant), and either palbociclib or placebo until disease progression, with a primary endpoint of PFS assessed over 24 months. There are also several ongoing phase II trials in the neoadjuvant setting, one that exploits the relatively good safety profile of palbociclib to offer it as stand-alone neoadjuvant therapy for early-stage breast cancer in patients who are not candidates for other neoadjuvant therapy (NCT02008734) and two that add palbociclib to standard-of-care neoadjuvant therapy for HR+ HER2+ disease (NCT02907918; NCT02530424).

Side Effect Profile

Although phase I trials utilizing CDK4/6 inhibitors in HER2+ disease are still underway, dose-limiting toxicities can be inferred from the trials in HR+ disease, where palbociclib was found to be very well tolerated. The primary dose-limiting toxicity is myelosuppression, particularly neutropenia, and is readily reversible.[20]

PI3K PATHWAY INHIBITORS

The PI3K/AKT/mTOR pathway translates activation of membrane receptors such as ERBB2 into coordination of cell growth, proliferation, survival, and metabolism[21] (Fig. 12.2). Class I PI3Ks are lipid kinases comprised of a p85 regulatory subunit and one of the four catalytic subunits (p110α, β, γ, or δ). Signaling from growth factor RTKs including ERBB/HER2, FGFR, and IGF-1R activates the p110 subunit to phosphorylate phosphatidylinositol 4,5 bisphosphate (PIP_2) to phosphatidylinositol 3,4,5-triphosphate (PIP_3), which then acts with the mTOR/Rictor (mTORC2) complex to activate serine/threonine kinase AKT. AKT in turn regulates multiple key functions required for coordinating cell metabolism and cell growth/proliferation. It promotes cell cycle entry, inhibits apoptosis, and activates the mTOR/Raptor (mTORC1) complex to promote mRNA translation and protein synthesis for cell growth, as well as modulating angiogenesis, cell metabolism, and cell migration. Upstream PI3K pathway activation is regulated by PTEN and INPP4B, which dephosphorylate PIP_3 to inhibit PI3K signaling. Aberrant activation of the PI3K pathway plays a well-established role in tumor growth. Mutations in this pathway are found in 30%—50% of breast cancers, most commonly activating mutations in the PIK3CA gene that encodes the p110 catalytic subunit of the class I PI3K itself or loss of function of PI3K pathway inhibitors PTEN or INPP4B.[10]

Preclinical Data for Targeting the PI3K/mTOR Pathway in HER2+ Breast Cancer

HER2 induces PI3K pathway activation via activation of HER3, and this pathway appears to be an important mediator of the oncogenicity of HER2, as the PI3K catalytic subunit p110α is required for HER2-mediated tumorigenesis in a genetic mouse model.[22] There is extensive preclinical evidence demonstrating that trastuzumab inhibits PI3K pathway activation and conversely that activating mutations in the PI3K pathway confer trastuzumab resistance. Trastuzumab activates PI3K inhibitor PTEN[23] and inhibits PI3K/AKT pathway function in breast cancer cell lines, while constitutively active AKT induces trastuzumab

TABLE 12.1
Selected Ongoing Trials With CDK Inhibitors

Identifier	Phase	Setting	Design	Outcomes
PALBOCICLIB				
NCT01976169	Ib	Trastuzumab-refractory HER2+ MBC	Palbociclib with T-DM1; recruiting	MTD, ORR
NCT03054363	Ib/II	First- or second-line HR+ HER2+ MBC	Palbociclib with tucatinib (small molecule HER2 inhibitor) and letrozole; not yet recruiting	AEs, PFS
NCT02530424 (NA-PHER2)	II	Neoadjuvant ER+ HER2+	Palbociclib with H, Pt, and fulvestrant; ongoing	pCR
NCT02907918 (PALTAN)	II	Neoadjuvant ER+ HER2+	Palbociclib with H and letrozole; recruiting	pCR, AEs
NCT02448420 (PATRICIA)	II	Heavily pretreated HER2+ MBC	Cohort A: palbociclib with H in ER-/HER2+	6-month PFS
			Cohort B: palbociclib with H +/− letrozole in ER+ HER2+; recruiting	
NCT02774681	II	HER2+ CNS metastases	Palbociclib with H; recruiting	CNS ORR
NCT02947685 (PATINA)	III	HR+ HER2+ MBC	H, Pt, and endocrine therapy +/− palbociclib after completion of standard anti-HER2 and chemotherapy; recruiting	PFS, OS, ORR
ABEMACICLIB				
NCT02057133	I	Metastatic pretreated HER2+	Abemaciclib with H; recruiting	AEs, PFS
NCT02675231 (monarcHER)	II	H/T-DM1- refractory HR+ HER2+ MBC	Abemaciclib with H +/− fulvestrant versus standard-of-care H with chemotherapy; recruiting	PFS, OS, ORR
NCT02308020	II	HR+ HER2+ CNS metastases	Abemaciclib with H; recruiting	CNS ORR
RIBOCICLIB				
NCT02657343	Ib/II	HER2+ MBC	Cohort A: ribociclib with T-DM1 after prior H/taxane	MTD, CBR, ORR, PFS
			Cohort B: ribociclib with trastuzumab after prior H, Pt, and T-DM1 (in any setting); recruiting	

AE, adverse event; *CBR*, clinical benefit rate (complete remission + partial response + stable disease for >6 months); *CDK*, cyclin D kinase; *CNS*, central nervous system; *H*, trastuzumab; *HR*, hormone receptor; *MBC*, advanced/metastatic breast cancer; *MTD*, maximum tolerated dose; *ORR*, overall response rate (complete remission + partial response); *OS*, overall survival; *pCR*, pathologic complete response; *PFS*, progression-free survival; *Pt*, pertuzumab; *T-DM1*, trastuzumab emtansine.

resistance in these cells.[24] PTEN loss and activating PIK3CA mutations have been identified in an RNAi screen in vitro as predictors of trastuzumab resistance.[25] Importantly, pan-PI3K inhibitor treatment rescues trastuzumab resistance due to PTEN loss[23] and has been shown to sensitize a panel of intrinsically trastuzumab-resistant breast cancer cell lines to trastuzumab.[26]

The mTORC1 complex is a key downstream effector in the PI3K pathway for which multiple small molecule

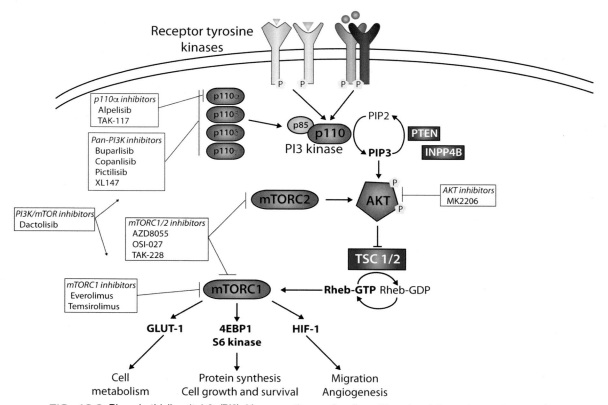

FIG. 12.2 Phosphatidylinositol-3 (PI3) kinase pathway signaling. Phosphorylation of receptor tyrosine kinases such as HER2 leads to activation of one of the four p110 catalytic subunits (α, β, γ, or δ) of the class I PI3 kinases via the p85 regulatory subunit. The activated p110 subunit then phosphorylates PIP_2 to phosphatidylinositol 3,4,5-triphosphate (PIP_3). PIP_3 acts with mammalian target of rapamycin complex (mTORC) 2 to activate serine/threonine kinase AKT; this step is negatively regulated by the proteins PTEN and INPP4B, which dephosphorylate PIP3. AKT in turn inhibits TSC1/2 (tuberous sclerosis proteins 1 and 2) to promote accumulation of the active guanosine-5′-triphosphate (GTP)—bound form of the small g-protein Rheb (Ras homolog enriched in brain), which in turn activates mTORC1. mTORC1 then activates a number of downstream effectors to promote pro-tumorigenic functions including protein synthesis, cell growth and survival, cell migration, and angiogenesis.

inhibitors are available. Interestingly, activating PIK3CA mutations, but not PTEN loss, were associated with sensitivity to mTOR inhibitor everolimus in a panel of breast cancer cell lines,[27] while dual treatment with trastuzumab and mTORC1 inhibitor RAD001 was more effective at inducing HER2+ tumor regression in a genetic mouse model than either treatment alone.[28] Unfortunately, in preclinical models, mTORC1 inhibition has been shown to stimulate a feedback loop through both mTORC2 and PI3Ks, which activates upstream signaling, including AKT.[29] This can be mitigated through use of dual mTORC1/mTORC2 inhibitors and even more effectively through a newer class of dual PI3K/mTOR inhibitors, which have shown efficacy in vitro and in mouse models in overcoming de novo and acquired trastuzumab and lapatinib resistance in HER2+ breast cancer cells.[30,31]

Finally, several mTOR and PI3K inhibitors, including mTOR inhibitors everolimus, temsirolimus, PI3K inhibitors buparlisib, PX-885 and SAR245408, and dual PI3K/mTOR inhibitors BEZ234, SAR245409, and GNE-317, have demonstrated ability to cross the blood-brain barrier and in preclinical models have had some efficacy toward central nervous system (CNS) metastases, an area of great unmet need in the treatment of advanced disease.[32]

PI3K Pathway Activation and Resistance to HER2-Directed Therapies in the Clinic

HER2+ cancers frequently have PIK3CA mutations (39%), PTEN loss (19%), and INPP4B loss (30%),[10] and the preclinical work above suggests a role for pharmacologic inhibition of PI3K or mTOR in mitigating trastuzumab resistance, perhaps particularly in the setting of these mutations. In the CLEOPATRA trial comparing pertuzumab with placebo in addition to trastuzumab and docetaxel in a large cohort of patients with metastatic HER2+ disease, PIK3CA mutations were associated with shorter PFS across the board, although the increased benefit of pertuzumab was maintained in the PIK3CA mutant group.[33] PIK3CA mutations and PTEN loss were also associated with shorter PFS in the lapatinib plus capecitabine arm of the EMILIA trial for metastatic HER2+ disease, although intriguingly not in the trastuzumab emtansine arm.[34] Interestingly, the association is less clear in earlier-stage HER2+ disease. In the NeoALTTO trial of neoadjuvant lapatinib and trastuzumab, PIK3CA mutations were associated with a decreased rate of pathologic complete response (pCR) in all treatment arms, but analysis of the N9831 adjuvant trastuzumab trial found no association between PTEN loss and either overall DFS or trastuzumab response,[35] while that of the NSABP B-31 trial found similar results for PIK3CA mutation status.[36]

Clinical Studies of PI3K Pathway Inhibitors
mTOR and dual inhibitors

mTORC1 inhibitors have been used clinically as immunosuppressants in the transplant setting since the early 2000s and were therefore among the first-studied PI3K pathway inhibitors in solid tumors. The mTORC1 inhibitors temsirolimus and everolimus (RAD001) are already FDA approved for some oncologic indications, while ridaforolimus is in phase III clinical trials. In HR+ HER2-negative advanced breast cancer, where the PI3K pathway has been shown to mediate resistance to endocrine therapy, the combination of everolimus plus exemestane showed significant PFS benefit over exemestane alone in postmenopausal women with disease progression while on a nonsteroidal aromatase inhibitor (AI) in the BOLERO-2 trial,[37] an indication for which it is now FDA approved. In contrast, temsirolimus did not show any PFS benefit in combination with letrozole in the first-line setting for advanced disease in the HORIZON trial.[38]

In HER2+ disease, phase I/II trials in trastuzumab-resistant advanced disease demonstrated tolerability of combining everolimus with trastuzumab and taxanes or vinca alkaloids, as well as encouraging clinical responses. The BOLERO-3 trial[39] was a randomized, double-blind, phase III trial that evaluated this combination in women with HER2+ trastuzumab-resistant advanced disease and prior taxane therapy. Patients received trastuzumab, vinorelbine, and either placebo or oral everolimus at a dose of 5 mg/day as established in a prior phase 1 study (notably lower than the 10 mg/day that is tolerated in combination with trastuzumab and paclitaxel). At final analysis with a median follow-up of 20.2 months, there was a small but statistically significant improvement in the primary outcome of median PFS with everolimus at 7 months versus 5.78 months for placebo, although no significant increase in overall response rate (ORR) was noted. Interestingly, exploratory subgroup analysis demonstrated a more significant benefit in the HR-negative than the HR-positive subpopulation. While OS data are still pending, the increase in median PFS does provide proof of principle in the clinical setting that inhibition of the PI3K pathway at the level of mTOR can at least partially overcome trastuzumab resistance in pretreated patients. However, addition of everolimus was associated with a significant increase in severe adverse events (AEs) (42% for everolimus group vs. 20% for placebo), a caveat to the clinical use of this combination.

As first-line therapy for advanced disease, the BOLERO-1[40] randomized, double-blind, phase III trial evaluated the addition of everolimus at 10 mg daily to trastuzumab and paclitaxel in women with advanced HER2+ disease with no previous systemic therapy for advanced disease and no trastuzumab or chemotherapy for 12 months prior to randomization. At final analysis, the primary outcome of median PFS was not significantly different between the everolimus group (14.95 months) and placebo (14.49 months). There was a trend toward increased PFS in the prespecified HR-negative subpopulation with a median PFS of 20.27 months for the everolimus group compared with 13.08 months with placebo, but this did not reach protocol-specified significance. In terms of tolerability, there was an increase in serious AEs in the everolimus group (36%) versus the placebo group (15%), as well as 17 (4%) on-treatment AE-related deaths in the everolimus group with none in the placebo group.

While everolimus was associated with only a small increase in PFS in trastuzumab-resistant advanced disease and possibly none at all in the first-line setting in unselected populations, there is a signal suggesting that there may be a more significant clinical response in HR-negative HER2+ patients, which may in turn outweigh the increased risk of AEs. In addition, a combined retrospective exploratory analysis of molecular subtypes in BOLERO-1 and BOLERO-3 to identify subgroups with PIK3CA mutations, PTEN loss of expression, or hyperactive PI3K pathway (any of PTEN loss, PIK3CA mutation, or AKT activating mutation) identified a statistically significant PFS benefit in the PI3K pathway-activated subgroup by all three definitions with HR ranging from 0.54 to 0.67 in contrast to the subgroup without such mutations.[41] While as described above, newer anti—HER2-directed therapies such as T-DM1 and pertuzumab seem to improve outcomes irrespective of PI3K pathway status, and in patients who are resistant to these therapies there may still be benefit in investigating mTOR inhibition in selected populations such as HR-negative or known PI3K pathway-activated disease that may derive clinically significant benefit. In addition, this work highlights the heterogeneity of disease even within the category of HER2+ breast cancer and the importance of biomarker-directed enrollment for trials of targeted therapies such as these.

Earlier phase trials of everolimus and temsirolimus with small molecule HER2 inhibitors are ongoing (Table 12.2), and a newer mTORC1 inhibitor ridaforolimus has been evaluated in a phase IIb trial in combination with trastuzumab in 34 patients with HER2+ trastuzumab-resistant metastatic breast cancer (mBC).[42] This combination was associated with partial response in 15% and stable disease in 41% with a median PFS of 5.4 months. Finally, given preclinical data suggesting that everolimus and other mTOR and PI3K inhibitors can cross the blood-brain barrier, several ongoing phase I/II trials are evaluating everolimus in HER2+ breast cancer with CNS metastases (Table 12.2). Given the incidence of adverse effects and equivocal efficacy in the advanced disease setting, there has been little interest in exploring mTORC1 inhibitors for adjuvant or neoadjuvant treatment.

While the clinical efficacy of mTORC1 inhibitors has been disappointing, preclinical data suggest that their efficacy may be limited due to feedback activation of AKT, which in preclinical models can be overcome through dual inhibition of mTORC1/2 or PI3K/mTOR (Figure 12.2). Dual MTORC1/2 inhibitors including AZD8055, TAK-228 (INK-128, MLN0128), and OSI-027 are in phase I/II trials in multiple solid tumor types, including several phase II trials in estrogen receptor—positive (ER+) HER2-negative breast cancer and triple-negative breast cancer (TNBC) with TAK-228 (Table 12.2), but no trials are yet evaluating these in HER2+ disease. Dual PI3K/mTOR inhibitors currently

in clinical trials in solid tumors include BEZ235 (dactolisib) and XL765 (voxtalisib). BEZ235 is in phase I/II trials in advanced HR+ HER2-negative and HER2+ disease (Table 12.2). XL765 is in a phase I/II trial in HR+ HER2-negative breast cancer, but has not yet been studied in the HER2+ setting.

AKT inhibitors
The AKT inhibitor MK2206 has been evaluated in several phase I/II clinical trials in HER2+ breast cancer. A phase I trial in advanced HER-overexpressing tumors including breast demonstrated tolerability of MK2206 plus trastuzumab in 31 patients, including 27 with advanced HER2+ breast cancer, with 1 partial and 1 complete response and 4 patients with stable disease.[43] A phase II trial of MK2206 for patients with advanced cancer with known PIK3CA, AKT, or PTEN mutations was completed with 8 of the 21 patients with objective responses and a median PFS of 5.8 months (NCT01277757). Additional phase I trials of MK2206 plus paclitaxel and plus lapatinib have been completed (Table 12.2).

PI3K inhibitors
Inhibitors of the class I PI3 kinases themselves, including the pan-class I PI3K inhibitors buparlisib (BKM120), copanlisib (BAY80-6946), XL147, and pictilisib (GDC-0941), as well as p110α selective inhibitors alpelisib (BYL719) and TAK-117, are in clinical development, although none has yet been FDA approved. In the breast cancer setting, buparlisib has been the most extensively studied of the pan-class I PI3K inhibitors, primarily in hormone-refractory HR+ HER2-negative breast cancer, where it is currently in phase III trials in combination with fulvestrant (BELLE-2 NCT01610284; BELLE-3 NCT01633060). In HER2+ breast cancer, it has been studied in phase I/II trials in both the neoadjuvant and advanced disease setting. The NeoPHOEBE trial was a phase II, randomized, placebo-controlled trial of buparlisib versus placebo in addition to trastuzumab and paclitaxel as neoadjuvant therapy for HER2+ breast cancer. It was terminated early because of increased rates of liver toxicity in the buparlisib arm, and there was no difference in primary outcome of pCR in the 50 patients enrolled before termination, though a trend toward increased ORR in the ER+ HER2+ subset.[44] In contrast, in advanced trastuzumab-resistant HER2+ disease, the combination of buparlisib plus lapatinib was relatively well tolerated in the PIKHER2 phase IB trial, and a clinical response was noted in 7 of the 24 patients with 1 remission and 6 instances of stable disease for at least 24 weeks.[45]

TABLE 12.2
Selected Ongoing Trials With PI3K Pathway Inhibitors

Target	Compound	Identifier	Setting/Design
Pan PI3K	BKM120 (buparlisib)	NCT01132664	Phase Ib/II: BKM120 plus H in H-refractory HER2+ breast cancer; terminated
		NCT01285466	Phase Ib: BKM120, paclitaxel and H in H-refractory HER2+ MBC; completed
		NCT01300962	Phase I: BKM120 with capecitabine and H or L in H-refractory HER2+ MBC; ongoing
	XL147 (SAR245408)	NCT01042925	Phase I: XL147 plus H with or without paclitaxel in H-refractory HER2+ MBC; completed
	BAY80-6946 (copanlisib)	NCT02705859	Phase Ib/II: BAY80-6946 plus H in pretreated recurrent or metastatic HER2+ breast cancer; recruiting
	GDC-0941 (pictilisib)	NCT00928330	Phase Ib: GDC-0941 plus H or T-DM1 in H-refractory HER2+ MBC; completed
Selective p110α	BYL719 (alpelisib)	NCT02038010	Phase I: BYL719 plus T-DM1 in H-refractory HER2+ MBC; ongoing
		NCT02167854	Phase I: BYL719 plus anti-HER3 antibody LJM716 and H in H-refractory HER2+ MBC with PIK3CA mutation; recruiting
	TAK-117 (MLN1117)	NCT01449370	Phase I; dose escalation of TAK-117 in advanced solid malignancies; completed
		NCT01899053	Phase Ib: TAK-117 with TAK-228 (mTORC1/2 inhibitor) in advanced solid malignancies; completed
AKT	MK2206	NCT01263145	Phase I: MK2206 with paclitaxel in MBC; completed
		NCT01245205	Phase I: MK2206 plus L in advanced HER2+ breast cancer; completed
PI3K/mTOR	BEZ235 (dactolisib)	NCT01285466	Phase Ib: dose escalation of BEZ235, paclitaxel and H in treatment-refractory HER2+ MBC; completed
		NCT01471847	Phase Ib/II: BEZ235 plus H compared to L plus capecitabine in advanced H-refractory HER2+ disease; completed
mTORC1	Everolimus	NCT01283789	Phase II: everolimus plus L in HER2+ MBC; ongoing
		NCT01783756	Phase Ib/II: everolimus plus L and capecitabine for HER2+ CNS metastases; ongoing
		NCT01305941	Phase II: everolimus plus weekly vinorelbine and H for HER2+ CNS metastases; ongoing
	Temsirolimus	NCT01111825	Phase I/II: IV temsirolimus plus neratinib in HER2+ or TN MBC; completed
mTORC1/2	AZD8055	NCT00973076	Phase I: advanced solid malignancies; completed
		NCT00731263	Phase I/II: advanced solid malignancies; completed
	OSI-027	NCT00698243	Phase I: advanced solid malignancy or lymphoma; completed
	TAK-228 (INK-128, MLN0128)	NCT02719691	Phase Ib: TAK-228 plus alisertib (aurora A inhibitor) in TN MBC and other advanced solid malignancies; recruiting.
		NCT01351350	Phase I: TAK-228 plus paclitaxel in advanced solid malignancies with addition of H for HER2+ disease; completed

CNS, central nervous system; *H*, trastuzumab; *HR*, hormone receptor; *L*, lapatinib; *MBC*, advanced/metastatic breast cancer; *mTOR*, mammalian target of rapamycin; *mTORC1/2*, mammalian target of rapamycin complex 1/2; *PI3K*, phosphoinositide 3-kinase; *PIK3CA*, phosphatidylinositol-4,5-bisphosphate 3-kinase catalytic subunit alpha; *Pt*, pertuzumab; *T-DM1*, trastuzumab emtansine; *TN*, triple negative.

The combination of buparlisib plus trastuzumab in advanced disease was also well tolerated in a phase IB trial and had some preliminary evidence of clinical benefit with 2 partial responses and 7 patients with stable disease for at least 6 weeks out of 17 treated patients.[46] Phase I trials in advanced HER2+ disease are also evaluating combinations of buparlisib with paclitaxel/trastuzumab, capecitabine/trastuzumab, and capecitabine/lapatinib, as well as combinations of the newer pan-PI3K inhibitors copanlisib, pictilisib, and XL147 with trastuzumab or T-DM1 (Table 12.2).

Inhibitors selective for the p110α PI3K catalytic subunit are also in phase I/II trials in advanced solid malignancies. Only one of these agents, alpelisib (BYL719), is being studied specifically in HER2+ breast cancer. Alpelisib is in phase I trials in combination with T-DM1 or trastuzumab in advanced trastuzumab-resistant HER2+ breast cancer (Table 12.2). A phase I dose escalation study of p110α inhibitor TAK-117 (MNS1117) alone has been completed, as well as several phase I/Ib trials assessing tolerability of TAK-117 with mTORC1/2 inhibitor TAK-228 in advanced solid malignancies, while a phase II trial in metastatic TNBC evaluating efficacy of TAK-228 plus TAK-117 followed by cisplatin and nab-paclitaxel is currently recruiting (Table 12.2). As yet there are no trials specifically in HER2+ breast cancer.

Side Effect Profile
The toxicities of mTOR inhibitors are well understood and include stomatitis, rash, myelosuppression, and metabolic effects (hyperlipidemia and hyperglycemia). While these are mostly grade 1–2, both the BOLERO-1 and BOLERO-3 trials did report a significant increase in overall and severe AEs in the everolimus group, with most common events being stomatitis, cytopenias, diarrhea, and alopecia. In BOLERO-3, serious AEs were noted in 42% of the everolimus group compared with 20% of the placebo group, with the most frequently reported serious AEs in the everolimus group being febrile neutropenia (10%), pyrexia (5%), anemia (4%), and stomatitis (3%). Stomatitis is a frequently dose-limiting toxicity, with optimal mitigation strategies currently under study. A less common but serious and often asymptomatic toxicity is noninfectious pneumonitis (occurring in 5%–10%), which can be life-threatening if not promptly identified and treated with steroids. Given the metabolic side effects, hyperglycemia and hyperlipidemia should be optimized prior to initiation of mTOR inhibitor therapy. The AKT inhibitor MK2206 has had similar toxicities in phase I trials, including fatigue, rash, hyperglycemia,

and nausea.[43] For pan-PI3K inhibitors such as buparlisib, common AEs include diarrhea, nausea, rashes, transaminase elevation, and hyperglycemia. Notably, buparlisib is associated with mood changes such as depression, anxiety, and even psychosis in as many as 25%–50% of patients,[44,45] possibly because of its ability to cross the blood-brain barrier. These psychiatric AEs can be successfully managed with dose reduction and antidepressant medication.[46] For selective p110α inhibitors, preliminary results from an early phase I study of BYL719 in advanced solid malignancies (NCT01387321) reported a similar AE profile including rash (50%), diarrhea (42%), and hyperglycemia (38%).

ANTIANGIOGENIC AGENTS
Angiogenesis is a crucial function required to support the nutrient and oxygen needs of growing tumors and to facilitate tumor cell dissemination and metastasis.[8] It is a complex and highly regulated process driven by the balance between pro- and antiangiogenic factors in a given microenvironment. Transcriptional activator hypoxia-inducible factor 1 is a key regulator of tumor-associated angiogenesis that is activated in response to hypoxia and oncogenic signaling. One of its major downstream targets is the vascular endothelial growth factor (VEGF) family of soluble protein ligands, pro-angiogenic factors that bind to VEGF RTKs (VEGFR1-3) on vascular endothelial cells to stimulate new blood vessel formation. In addition to VEGF, fibroblast growth factors (FGF), platelet-derived growth factors (PDGF), and transforming growth factors also contribute to pro-angiogenic signaling in the tumor microenvironment.[47] The sustained activation of angiogenesis in the tumor microenvironment creates distorted and leaky vessels and inconsistent blood flow, facilitating tumor cell dissemination and metastasis and impairing drug delivery to the tumor bed.[8] Inhibition of VEGF has consequently been extensively studied as a therapeutic strategy, and in 2003, the monoclonal anti-VEGF antibody bevacizumab was the first agent to receive FDA approval for use in metastatic colon cancer. Applications for bevacizumab have since expanded to multiple other tumor types, while several additional classes of VEGF inhibitors have been developed, and in some cases approved, in different solid tumors. This includes the soluble decoy VEGF receptor ziv-aflibercept, monoclonal anti-VEGFR2 antibody ramucirumab, and multiple small molecule RTK inhibitors such as axitinib, pazopanib, regorafenib, sorafenib, and sunitinib, which inhibit not only VEGFRs but also FGFRs and PDGFRs.

Preclinical Data Supporting the Use of Antiangiogenic Agents in HER2+ Breast Cancer

There is significant preclinical evidence supporting a role for HER2 signaling in promoting angiogenesis through regulation of VEGF expression. Activation of HER2 signaling induces VEGF mRNA expression via PI3K pathway activation in human breast cancer cell lines[48] VEGF overexpression is associated with HER2 overexpression in primary tumor tissue in several large cohorts of breast cancer patients.[49,50] Trastuzumab downregulates VEGF expression in HER2-overexpressing breast cancer cell lines in vitro and in xenograft models, and combining anti-HER2 therapy with VEGF inhibition has synergistic effects on tumor cell proliferation in vitro, as well as tumor growth and angiogenesis in xenografts.[48,51]

Clinical Studies of Antiangiogenic Agents in HER2+ Breast Cancer
Bevacizumab in advanced disease

There have been a number of phase II/III trials evaluating the addition of bevacizumab to chemotherapy and trastuzumab in HER2+ metastatic disease. A phase II trial evaluating bevacizumab plus capecitabine and trastuzumab as first-line therapy for metastatic disease was promising, demonstrating a 73% ORR with 14.4 month PFS, though with 44% of participants experiencing a grade 3–4 AE.[52] Two small phase II trials of bevacizumab plus docetaxel and trastuzumab as first- or second-line treatment of HER2+ advanced/metastatic disease were also somewhat promising, which demonstrated good tolerability of the combination as well as a 50%–80% ORR and a PFS of 13–14 months.[53,54] Unfortunately, a subsequent large phase III trial of this combination of trastuzumab and bevacizumab with a taxane, the AVAREL study, did not demonstrate a statistically significant increase in PFS in the bevacizumab group, though the addition of bevacizumab to trastuzumab/taxane was overall well tolerated, with an increased incidence of grade 3–4 hypertension seen in the bevacizumab group (a well-established AE with bevacizumab) but no new safety signals and no increase in other cardiac events.[55] There was a nonsignificant 3-month increase in PFS in the bevacizumab group, which may reflect an as-yet undefined subpopulation with some clinical benefit. The study included an exploratory analysis on a subgroup of 162 patients willing to undergo biomarker analysis via plasma VEGF-A level, and while the hazard ratio for bevacizumab treatment was fairly similar in high versus low VEGF-A subgroups (0.70 vs. 0.83, both nonsignificant), the median PFS in the high VEGF-A group was 16.6 months with bevacizumab versus 8.5 months without compared to a median PFS in the low VEGF-A group of 16.5 months with bevacizumab versus 13.6 months without, suggesting the possibility of a more significant clinical benefit in the VEGF-A high subpopulation,[55] which merits further investigation. The phase III ECOG 1105 trial evaluating the addition of bevacizumab to paclitaxel plus carboplatin plus trastuzumab was terminated early due to slow accrual. For the 96 (out of planned 489) patients enrolled, the combination was fairly well tolerated with no increase in grade 3–4 AEs in the bevacizumab arm, but there was no evidence of clinical activity with no difference in PFS between the bevacizumab and placebo arms.[56]

There has been some interest in using bevacizumab as a chemotherapy-sparing agent, and a phase II trial of bevacizumab plus trastuzumab alone as first-line therapy for 50 patients with metastatic or locally recurrent disease did demonstrate clinical activity with an ORR 48%, a median PFS of 9.2 months, and an OS of 43.8 months. The combination was fairly well tolerated with the most common AE being hypertension (60% with grade 3–4 in 36%), one grade 4 cardiac AE, and one grade 5 AE (perforated ulcer resulting in death) observed.[57] A more recent phase II trial randomized 84 patients with metastatic disease to receive first-line therapy with either bevacizumab plus trastuzumab and paclitaxel (upfront chemotherapy) or bevacizumab plus trastuzumab alone with addition of paclitaxel on disease progression (delayed chemotherapy). PFS of 1 year was somewhat lower in the delayed chemotherapy arm (62.2%) versus the upfront chemotherapy arm (74.4%), the caveat being that the study was not designed to compare the two arms but rather to assess efficacy of each separately. Interestingly, median PFS was similar in the upfront and delayed chemotherapy arms (19.8 and 19.6 months, respectively), though median PFS prior to addition of paclitaxel in the delayed chemotherapy arm was 10.2 months.[58]

Bevacizumab has also been combined with lapatinib in several early-phase trials. A phase II trial of bevacizumab plus lapatinib demonstrated a 13% ORR and a 6-month median PFS in a heavily pretreated population (median of three prior chemotherapy regimens in the metastatic setting). The combination was reasonably well tolerated, with AEs leading to treatment discontinuation in 10%.[59] However, given the consistent lack of clinical benefit in combining bevacizumab with trastuzumab, it seems unlikely that the combination with lapatinib would lead to a significantly different clinical outcome.

Overall, there is no evidence to suggest a benefit for bevacizumab in unselected patients in the metastatic setting, and certainly given the advent of newer HER2-directed therapies such as pertuzumab, which are safer and more efficacious, this is not an avenue of study likely to be fruitful. There may still be an as-yet defined role for bevacizumab in selected populations, such as patients with high-serum VEGF-A levels or in patients who wish to defer cytotoxic chemotherapy (though bevacizumab comes with significant toxicities of its own), but these potential clinical applications would require additional clinical investigation. Given that HER2 signaling is likely a major driver of pro-angiogenic signaling and increased VEGF activity in HER2+ breast tumors, it may be that anti-HER2 treatment provides such a significant reduction in VEGF activity in this setting that adding a second anti-VEGF agent becomes redundant. However, newer tyrosine kinase inhibitors (TKIs) that act not only on VEGF receptors but also on PDGF and FGF receptors may have a greater clinical effect in this context.

Ziv-aflibercept and ramucirumab

The soluble VEGF decoy receptor ziv-aflibercept and the anti-VEGFR2 antibody ramucirumab have FDA approval as non—first-line therapy for metastatic colon cancer, and in the case of ramucirumab, gastric and gastroesophageal junction adenocarcinoma, and non—small-cell lung cancer, neither has been extensively studied in breast cancer. A phase II trial of monotherapy with aflibercept in 21 patients with pretreated mBC included 4 patients with HER2+ disease, but only 1 patient achieved even a partial response, and 16 of the 21 patients experienced at least a grade 3 AE, of which the most common was hypertension; the study was terminated.[60] The lack of clinical response is not surprising as many antiangiogenic therapies have minimal effect as single agents, but given the high rate of toxicities and the negative results with bevacizumab in this disease setting, aflibercept seems an unlikely candidate for further investigation. There have been no trials of ramucirumab in HER2+ breast cancer.

Antiangiogenic Tyrosine Kinase Inhibitors

Sorafenib, sunitinib, and pazopanib are all in early-phase trials in HER2+ breast cancer with variable results, whereas axitinib and regorafenib have not yet been studied in this setting. A phase II trial of sorafenib monotherapy in patients with mBC with prior anthracycline or taxane exposure included three HER2+ patients but had no partial or complete responses and was terminated.[61] Sorafenib with capecitabine has been

evaluated in a phase I trial in advanced breast cancer, which has been completed but without available results (NCT01640665), and a phase I study now recruiting combines whole-brain radiation therapy with sorafenib for breast cancer CNS metastases (NCT01724606).

A phase II trial of sunitinib monotherapy in mBC pretreated with an anthracycline or taxane included 12 HER2+ patients, of whom 3 had partial responses.[62] A phase I trial of sunitinib with docetaxel and trastuzumab as first-line therapy for locally recurrent or metastatic HER2+ breast cancer demonstrated an ORR of 73% and a median PFS of 15 months, which is comparable with trials of trastuzumab plus chemotherapy alone.[63] There was a high rate of temporary treatment discontinuations and dose reductions (84%) with the most frequent AEs resulting in treatment modification being neutropenia, asthenia, and transaminase elevation.[63] A larger phase II trial of sunitinib with trastuzumab in HER2+ metastatic disease as first- or second-line therapy did not demonstrate much clinical efficacy, with an ORR of 37% and a median PFS of 6.4 months at 24 months of follow-up, and had a high rate of significant AEs with 80% of patients requiring temporary treatment discontinuation or dose reduction due to AEs and 30% requiring permanent discontinuation of one of the study drugs.[64] Forty percent of patients experienced decreases in left ventricular ejection fraction (LVEF), 10% of patients had symptomatic LVEF decreases, and there was one death from cardiogenic shock.[64] There are currently no actively recruiting or ongoing studies with sunitinib in HER2+ breast cancer, unsurprising given the poor toxicity profile without evidence of clinical benefit in the completed studies above.

Two randomized phase II trials have examined the combination of pazopanib with lapatinib in advanced HER2+ breast cancer. The first was comprised of two fairly large cohorts of patients (n = 76, n = 88) with relapsed inflammatory HER2+ breast cancer, the first comparing lapatinib plus high-dose pazopanib to lapatinib alone and the second, added after demonstration of unacceptable rates of high-grade diarrhea with high-dose pazopanib, comparing lapatinib plus low-dose pazopanib to lapatinib or pazopanib alone.[65] In the high-dose pazopanib cohort, ORR for the combination was 45% compared with 29% with lapatinib alone, with similar median PFS (3.5 months for the combination and 4 months for lapatinib alone). There was a striking increase in grade ≥3 AEs in the combination arm, occurring in 71% of the combination arm patients versus 24% of the patients on the lapatinib monotherapy arm. Similar results were found in the low-dose pazopanib cohort, with an ORR for the combination of 58% compared with 47% for lapatinib alone and 31% for pazopanib alone, with no difference in median PFS between lapatinib and the combination (both 4 months). Grade ≥3 AEs were again significantly higher in the arms receiving pazopanib, with 17% for lapatinib alone compared with 50% for combination and 46% for pazopanib, as were treatment discontinuations (0%, 24%, and 23%, respectively). The second trial had a similar design, with one cohort of patients randomized to lapatinib with or without low-dose pazopanib and a second cohort of patients all receiving lapatinib and high-dose pazopanib.[66] There was no difference in the primary outcome of 12 week progressive disease rate between the combination (36.2%) and lapatinib monotherapy (38.9%) arms of the first cohort, though there was a trend toward a difference in the 12-week response rate (36.2% in the combination vs. 22.2% for monotherapy). The high-dose pazopanib cohort had a 12-week response rate of 33%, similar to that of the low-dose pazopanib group. As with the previous study, there was a striking increase in grade ≥3 AEs going from lapatinib alone (22%) to low-dose pazopanib combination (42%) to high-dose pazopanib combination (60%), with the most common grade ≥ 3 event being diarrhea, which occurred in 40% of the high-dose pazopanib cohort patients. There was a similar trend in AEs resulting in treatment discontinuation from lapatinib alone (4%) to low-dose pazopanib combination (17%) to high-dose pazopanib combination (30%). There is also a phase I trial evaluating the combination of lapatinib plus pazopanib plus paclitaxel in advanced cancer including breast, for which results are not yet available.

Taken together, early phase trials with both sunitinib and pazopanib have been disappointing, demonstrating a tolerable but fairly significant toxicity profile without much indication of clinical benefit in advanced disease. There are no trials evaluating either agent in earlier-stage disease. In the metastatic setting, it may be that the combination of these agents with anti-HER2 antibodies would be better tolerated than with a second TKI. As with bevacizumab, a better understanding of the molecular or clinical characteristics that predict sensitivity to these agents may also be required to define the patient population in which they would have clinical utility. Given the spectrum of other more effective and better-tolerated therapies recently established and emerging for HER2+ breast cancer, however, none of the antiangiogenic agents has much clinical promise in the metastatic setting.

Adjuvant/Neoadjuvant Trials

Several phase II trials have examined adjuvant bevacizumab in node-positive and high-risk node-negative HER2+ disease as an agent mechanistically well suited to target residual/micrometastatic disease. A phase II trial evaluating efficacy of adjuvant docetaxel, trastuzumab, and bevacizumab in 29 patients with pN2 or pN3 disease reported 5-year DFS and OS rates of 89.7% and 100%, quite high for patients with high-risk disease, without a concerning increase in AEs.[67] The BETH trial, a multicenter, phase III, randomized, open-label trial, evaluating the addition of bevacizumab to either six cycles of docetaxel, carboplatin, and trastuzumab followed by trastuzumab in a cohort of ~3000 patients or to three cycles of trastuzumab and docetaxel followed by three cycles of 5-fluorouracil, epirubicin, and cyclophosphamide followed by trastuzumab in a smaller cohort of ~280 patients, was terminated at 38 months due to an unacceptable increase in the rate of grade 3–4 AEs in the bevacizumab arm, at which time the DFS in all arms was around 92% with no added benefit with the addition of bevacizumab to either treatment regimen.[68] The lack of measurable clinical benefit in combination with significant toxicity makes bevacizumab a less appealing agent for further study in the adjuvant setting, particularly given other emerging novel treatment options with fewer associated toxicities.

Unfortunately results have been similar in the neoadjuvant setting, with most phase II trials demonstrating an increase in AEs, particularly postoperative complications, without a benefit in terms of pCR with the addition of bevacizumab to chemotherapy. These include a phase II trial adding bevacizumab to neoadjuvant nab-paclitaxel, carboplatin, and trastuzumab followed by adjuvant trastuzumab plus bevacizumab in which the rate of pCR was 56% (not significantly improved over typical rates with chemotherapy with trastuzumab) but with postoperative wound healing complications in 35% of participants such that 20 of the 29 participants were unable to complete adjuvant therapy per protocol.[69] A phase II trial evaluating four cycles of neoadjuvant epirubicin plus cyclophosphamide followed by four cycles of neoadjuvant docetaxel, trastuzumab, and bevacizumab followed by adjuvant trastuzumab plus bevacizumab likewise demonstrated a pCR of 46% with a 15% rate of postoperative complications.[67] A phase II trial restricted to inflammatory HER2+ breast cancer, which typically carries a poorer prognosis, evaluated neoadjuvant treatment with four cycles of fluorouracil, epirubicin, cyclophosphamide, and bevacizumab followed by four cycles of docetaxel, trastuzumab, and bevacizumab, with a pCR of 63.5%, again similar to pCR rates observed for trastuzumab plus chemotherapy without bevacizumab in the neoadjuvant setting. There is also an ongoing European phase II study (NCT01690325) evaluating the addition of bevacizumab to neoadjuvant docetaxel and trastuzumab (data not yet available). The only phase II trial demonstrating clinical benefit for neoadjuvant bevacizumab is the AVATAXHER trial, in which patients with HER2+ early-stage disease who were predicted nonresponders by positron emission tomography (PET-CT) after two cycles of neoadjuvant trastuzumab plus docetaxel were randomized to either add bevacizumab or to continue on trastuzumab plus docetaxel alone.[70] Compared with a pCR of 53% in PET-predicted responders, the PET nonresponders who did not receive bevacizumab had a pCR of 24%, whereas nonresponders who received bevacizumab had a pCR of 44%, suggestive of clinical benefit in this selected subgroup.

As with bevacizumab in advanced HER2+ breast cancer, there is fairly clear evidence that there is no clinical benefit, and indeed some excess toxicity, in unselected patients in the adjuvant/neoadjuvant setting. Although there is a suggestion that there may be subpopulations of patients in which bevacizumab is effective in this setting, given the advances in other well-tolerated targeted therapies, this would be unlikely to be of significant clinical utility.

Side Effect Profile
The toxicities of bevacizumab are well understood, including hypertension (common), proteinuria, minor and major bleeding, thromboembolism, gastrointestinal perforation, and impaired wound healing. The antiangiogenic TKIs do cause some hypertension but overall have a profile similar to other classes of TKIs. Frequent toxicities reported in a phase II trial of sunitinib alone for mBC included fatigue (67%), nausea (63%), diarrhea (58%), mucositis (47%), and transient cytopenias, with the most common grade 3 toxicities being fatigue (14%), nausea (8%), dyspnea (9%), and hand-foot syndrome (9%) and no grade 4 toxicities.[62] Toxicities reported with pazopanib similarly include diarrhea (46%), transaminase elevations (23%), fatigue (23%), hypertension (23%), and neutropenia (23%).[65]

DUAL HER2/EGFR INHIBITORS
HER2 must dimerize with other HER family members such as EGFR (HER1), HER3, and HER4 to stimulate downstream pro-proliferative signaling. Signaling through these other family members can maintain downstream pathway activation in the setting of HER2 inhibition, which has led to the development of several TKIs with activity across multiple HER family members. The earliest of these, lapatinib, is a reversible dual EGFR/HER2 inhibitor that has been FDA approved for advanced/metastatic disease in combination with capecitabine or letrozole, whereas two newer agents, afatinib, an irreversible EGFR/HER2 inhibitor, and neratinib, an irreversible EGFR/HER2/HER4 inhibitor, are in clinical development.

Preclinical Data Supporting Dual/Pan HER Family Inhibitors
HER2-overexpressing human breast cancer cells with acquired trastuzumab resistance have been shown to upregulate EGFR expression and to have high levels of EGFR phosphorylation and EGFR/HER2 heterodimerization, sensitizing them to EGFR inhibitors and the dual EGFR/HER2 inhibitor lapatinib in vitro and in xenografts.[71] Conversely, it has been found that overexpression of EGFR in HER2-overexpressing human breast cancer cell lines is sufficient to induce trastuzumab resistance.[72] With these data in mind, it is unsurprising that treating HER2-overexpressing human breast cancer cells with the combination of lapatinib and anti-HER2 antibodies results in greater inhibition of tumor growth in xenografts than single agents.[73] Preclinical work has been supported by a post hoc correlation of EGFR expression with clinical outcomes of the HER2+ breast cancer patients enrolled in the NCCTG N9831 phase III Alliance trial evaluating the safety and efficacy of adding concurrent or sequential trastuzumab to adjuvant anthracycline and taxane-based chemotherapy. Patients with low EGFR expression had better outcomes in the trastuzumab arms versus chemotherapy alone, whereas those with high EGFR expression did not benefit from the addition of trastuzumab to chemotherapy, presumably because of inherent resistance to trastuzumab.[74]

Multi-HER Inhibitors in Advanced Disease
Lapatinib, a reversible HER2/EGFR inhibitor, was the first to be developed and has shown significant activity in combination with chemotherapy in advanced disease. In the EGF 100151 trial, an open-label, randomized phase III trial in patients with HER2+ advanced or mBC with progression on trastuzumab and chemotherapy, the combination of lapatinib plus capecitabine nearly doubled median PFS from 4.4 to 8.4 months compared with capecitabine alone, although without

a statistically significant increase in OS, possibly due to high crossover from the monotherapy to the combination arm.[75] The combination of lapatinib and capecitabine consequently received FDA approval for treatment of trastuzumab-resistant HER2+ mBC. However, the antibody drug conjugate trastuzumab emtansine (T-DM1) has since been shown in a large, multicenter, randomized, open-label phase III trial to be superior to lapatinib plus capecitabine in this setting and with lower incidence of significant toxicities.[76] In the first-line metastatic setting, the randomized, open-label, phase III MA.31 trial compared lapatinib or trastuzumab in combination with taxane-based chemotherapy in HER2+ mBC patients and found that lapatinib was inferior to trastuzumab in terms of PFS and also associated with increased toxicity.[77] At this time, therefore, lapatinib with capecitabine remains a third-line or later agent for metastatic HER2+ disease behind taxane-based chemotherapy combined with trastuzumab and T-DM1. This is discussed in more detail in Chapters 3 and 4.

Given significant preclinical evidence of an added benefit of the combination of trastuzumab and lapatinib over single-agent trastuzumab, several phase I/II trials have evaluated the combination of trastuzumab plus lapatinib with different chemotherapy backbones in the first- and second-line metastatic setting. A phase Ib dose escalation trial of lapatinib, trastuzumab, and docetaxel as first-line therapy for metastatic HER2+ breast cancer patients (n = 53) found that the combination had some clinical activity with an ORR of 31% and was well tolerated, with the most common toxicities being neutropenia (42%, grade 3–4 in 38%), diarrhea (87%, grade 3–4 in 15%), nausea (72%), alopecia (70%), and rash (51%).[78] A small phase II safety study of lapatinib, trastuzumab, and paclitaxel, again in the first-line metastatic setting, found that dehydration secondary to diarrhea was a dose-limiting toxicity requiring reduction of the lapatinib dose from 1000 to 750 mg/day (and the addition of prophylactic antimotility agent loperamide) without compromising in efficacy. Similar ORRs were seen in patients enrolled in 1000 mg/day cohorts (cohort 1, n = 29, ORR 79%; cohort 2, n = 14, ORR 71%) and 750 mg/day cohorts (cohort 3, n = 20, ORR 71%).[79] Additional trials evaluating dual anti-HER2 therapy with trastuzumab and lapatinib plus chemotherapy are ongoing (Table 12.3), but the success of dual HER2 blockade with trastuzumab plus pertuzumab in the first-line metastatic setting has dramatically altered the landscape of dual anti-HER2 therapy since the lapatinib trials were initiated.

There has also been interest in combining lapatinib with trastuzumab without chemotherapy in the metastatic setting, which was shown to increase median OS by 4.5 months versus lapatinib alone in heavily pretreated HER2+ mBC patients in the EGF104900 study without an increase in cardiac AEs,[80] making this a chemotherapy-sparing option for refractory disease. In the first-line metastatic setting, this combination also showed clinical activity with an ORR of 50% and a median PFS of 7.4 months,[81] an improvement over previously reported response rates with trastuzumab monotherapy.[82] With the striking success of the newer anti-HER2 therapies pertuzumab and T-DM1, the combination of lapatinib and trastuzumab does not currently have scope for clinical use outside of a clinical trial, but these data do provide proof of principle that lapatinib may be useful as part of a chemotherapy-sparing regimen utilizing multiple anti–HER2-directed agents. Indeed, ongoing trials are evaluating lapatinib in combination with newer anti-HER2 therapies and other targeted therapies in the metastatic setting and may help clarify its place in the armamentarium of anti–HER2-directed therapies (Table 12.3).

Finally, several phase II trials have shown benefit for lapatinib in the setting of HER2+ CNS metastases, a setting with limited treatment options. Lapatinib plus capecitabine showed clinical efficacy in previously untreated HER2+ CNS metastases in the single-arm phase II LANDSCAPE trial with a CNS ORR of 66%, a promising result somewhat dampened by a high incidence (49%) of grade 3–4 toxicities.[83] A phase II study of lapatinib monotherapy in patients who developed CNS progression while on trastuzumab, however, saw a no clinical activity with monotherapy and a much lower rate of CNS ORR (20%) in a subset of patients who were enrolled in a lapatinib plus capecitabine extension on progression.[84] Nonetheless, ongoing trials continue to evaluate a role for lapatinib in CNS disease (Table 12.3).

The newer, irreversible pan HER family TKIs neratinib and afatinib have shown robust preclinical efficacy in trastuzumab-resistant HER2-overexpressing cell lines and are now in phase I, II, and III clinical trials in HER2+ breast cancer, with neratinib being recently approved in the adjuvant setting (see below). Neratinib initially demonstrated surprisingly good clinical activity as a single agent. In a phase II trial in HER2+ mBC patients, neratinib monotherapy had an ORR of 56% for trastuzumab-naïve and 24% for trastuzumab-refractory patients with median PFS of 9 and 5 months, respectively.[85] Efficacy in the trastuzumab-naïve group compared favorably to historical results with

TABLE 12.3
Selected Trials With HER Family Inhibitors

Identifier	Phase	Setting	Design	Outcomes
LAPATINIB				
NCT00429299 (CHER-LOB)[99]	II	Neoadjuvant	Paclitaxel with H, L, or H + L followed by FEC with H, L or H + L in HER2+ breast cancer; completed	pCR (ypT0/is ypN0): H 25% L 26.3% H + L 46.7% (significant vs. H)
NCT00769470 (TRIO US B07)[100]	II	Neoadjuvant	Docetaxel + carboplatin with H, L, or H + L in HER2+ breast cancer; completed	pCR (ypT0 ypN0) H 42% L 25% H + L 52% (not significant vs. H)
NCT00524303 (LPT 109096)[101]	II	Neoadjuvant	FEC followed by paclitaxel with H, L, or H + L in HER2+ breast cancer; completed	pCR (ypT0/is ypN0) H 54% L 45% H + L 74% Significance not reported
NCT00548184 (TBCR006)[102]	II	Neoadjuvant	H + L (with letrozole if ER+) in HER2+ breast cancer; completed	pCR (ypY0 ypN0) All 22% ER+ 21% ER– 36%
NCT00999804 (TBCR023)[103]	II	Neoadjuvant	H + L (with letrozole if ER+) for 12 or 24 weeks in HER2+ breast cancer; completed	pCR (ypY0 ypN0) All—24 weeks 24.2% ER+ 33.2% ER– 8.7% All—12 weeks 12.2% ER+ 8.7% ER– 20%
NCT02073487	II	Neoadjuvant	T-DM1 + L followed by abraxane versus H + pertuzumab + paclitaxel in HER2+ breast cancer; recruiting	pCR
NCT00367471	I	Metastatic	Carboplatin, paclitaxel, H and L in HER2+ breast cancer; ongoing	AEs, PFS
NCT02073916 (STELA)	Ib/II	Metastatic heavily pretreated	T-DM1 with L followed by abraxane in treatment-refractory (≥2 prior therapies) HER2+ breast cancer; recruiting	MTD for T-DM1
NCT02238509	II	Metastatic heavily pretreated	H with L or H with chemotherapy (any) in heavily pretreated (including H and L) HER2+ breast cancer; recruiting	CBR
NCT01160211	III	Metastatic HR+	Aromatase inhibitor with H, L or both in postmenopausal HR+ HER2+ H-refractory (one prior trastuzumab regimen) breast cancer; ongoing	PFS, OS

Continued

TABLE 12.3
Selected Trials With HER Family Inhibitors—cont'd

Identifier	Phase	Setting	Design	Outcomes
NCT01873833	II	Metastatic H-refractory	Capecitabine, cyclophosphamide, H and L in H-refractory HER2+ breast cancer; recruiting	PFS
NCT00444535	II	Advanced	L with bevacizumab in HER2+ breast cancer, no prior treatment in metastatic setting required; ongoing	12 week PFS, ORR
NCT01400962	I	Metastatic H-refractory	L or H or no anti-HER2 therapy with capecitabine and buparlisib (PI3K) dose escalation in H-refractory HER2+ breast cancer; ongoing	MTD for buparlisib, ORR
NCT01283789	II	Metastatic H-refractory	L with everolimus (mTOR) in H-refractory HER2+ breast cancer; ongoing	6-month ORR
NCT00684983	II	Advanced H-refractory	L and capecitabine with or without cixutumumab (IGF-1R) in H-refractory HER2+ breast cancer; ongoing	PFS, OS
NCT02650752	I	CNS metastases	Intermittent high-dose L dose escalation with capecitabine in HER2+ breast cancer with CNS mets; recruiting	MTD for lapatinib
NCT01783756	Ib/II	CNS metastases	L with capecitabine and everolimus in HER2+ breast cancer with H-refractory CNS mets; ongoing	CNS ORR
NCT01622868	II	CNS metastases	L or no systemic therapy with whole-brain radiation therapy or SRS in HER2+ breast cancer with CNS mets; recruiting	CR rate in measurable brain metastases
NERATINIB (HKI-272)				
NCT00398567[87]	I/II	Advanced H-refractory	H with N dose escalation in H-refractory HER2+ breast cancer; ongoing	ORR 27% No dose-limiting toxicities noted
NCT01423123[88]	I	Advanced H-refractory	H with N dose escalation and paclitaxel in H-refractory HER2+ breast cancer; completed	Grade 3–4 AEs: diarrhea 38%, dehydration 14%, electrolyte abnormalities 19%, fatigue 19% ORR: 38%
NCT00445458[141]	I/II	Advanced H-refractory	N dose escalation with paclitaxel in H-refractory HER2+ breast cancer (any solid tumor in phase I; ongoing	Grade 3–4 AEs: diarrhea 29%, peripheral neuropathy 3%, neutropenia 20%, leukopenia 18% ORR (0–1 prior regimens without lapatinib): 71% ORR (2–3 prior regimens, lapatinib allowed): 77%

TABLE 12.3
Selected Trials With HER Family Inhibitors—cont'd

Identifier	Phase	Setting	Design	Outcomes
NCT00706030[91]	I/II	Metastatic H-refractory	N with vinorelbine in H-refractory HER2+ breast cancer (any HER2+ solid tumor in phase I); ongoing	ORR (no prior lapatinib): 41% ORR (prior lapatinib): 8%
NCT02236000 (NSABP FB-10)	Ib/II	Metastatic H-refractory	N dose escalation with T-DM1 in H-refractory HER2+ breast cancer; recruiting	MTD, ORR
NCT01111825[142]	I/II	Metastatic H-refractory	N with temsirolimus dose escalation in H-refractory HER2+ breast cancer; completed	Grade 3–4 AEs: diarrhea (24%), mucositis (12%), hyperglycemia (8%). ORR: 40%
NCT03065387	I	Advanced	N with everolimus, palbociclib, or trametinib in advanced solid tumor with EGFR, HER2, HER3 or HER4 mutations or EGFR or HER 2 amplification; not yet recruiting	MTD, ORR
NCT03101748	Ib/II	Cohort A: advanced	Cohort A: N dose escalation with H, Pt and paclitaxel in advanced HER2+ breast cancer	Cohort A: MTD, PFS
		Cohort B: neoadjuvant	Cohort B: N dose escalation with H, Pt and paclitaxel followed by AC in locally advanced inflammatory breast cancer; not yet recruiting	Cohort B: MTD, pCR
NCT03289039	II	Advanced H-refractory	N with or without fulvestrant in advanced H-refractory ER+/HER2+ breast cancer; not yet recruiting	PFS, ORR, OS
NCT02673398	II	Metastatic H-refractory	N monotherapy in H-refractory HER2+ breast cancer in patients 60 and older; recruiting	Percent grade ≥2 AEs, adherence, ORR, PFS, OS
NCT01494662 (TBCRC 022)[92,93]	II	CNS metastases	Cohort 1: N monotherapy in HER2+ breast cancer with new or progressive CNS disease	Cohort 1: CNS ORR 8%
			Cohort 2: N before/after resection in HER2+ breast cancer with operable CNS disease	Cohort 3A: CNS ORR 49%
			Cohort 3: N with capecitabine in lapatinib-naïve (3A) or exposed (3B) HER2+ breast cancer with measurable CNS disease; ongoing	
NCT01808573 (NALA)	III	Advanced heavily pretreated	L or N with capecitabine in H-refractory (≥2 HER2 regimens) HER2+ breast cancer; ongoing	PFS, OS

AC, doxorubicin/cyclophosphamide; *AE*, adverse event; *CBR*, clinical benefit rate (complete remission + partial response + stable disease for >6 months); *CNS*, central nervous system; *EGFR*, epidermal growth factor receptor; *ER*, estrogen receptor; *FEC*, 5-fluorouracil, epirubicin, cyclophosphamide; *H*, trastuzumab; *HR*, hormone receptor; *IGF-1R*, insulin-like growth factor 1 receptor; *L*, lapatinib; *MBC*, advanced/metastatic breast cancer; *MTD*, maximum tolerated dose; *mTOR*, mammalian target of rapamycin; *N*, neratinib; *ORR*, overall response rate (complete remission + partial response); *OS*, overall survival; *pCR*, pathologic complete response; *PFS*, progression-free survival; *PI3K*, phosphoinositide 3-kinase; *Pt*, pertuzumab; *T-DM1*, trastuzumab emtansine.

single-agent trastuzumab or lapatinib. As with lapatinib, diarrhea was a dose-limiting toxicity, occurring in 93% of participants with grade 3–4 in 21% (disproportionately in the patients with prior trastuzumab exposure), but diarrhea typically improved with time, and almost all patients were able to remain on treatment with antidiarrheal medication and dose modifications. There was no evidence of cardiotoxicity.

Based on these promising early results, a phase II noninferiority trial compared single-agent neratinib with lapatinib plus capecitabine for trastuzumab-refractory HER2+ mBC.[86] Neratinib was better tolerated than lapatinib with capecitabine and again showed single-agent activity, with an ORR of 29% for neratinib versus 47% for lapatinib plus capecitabine and a median PFS of 4.53 months for neratinib versus 6.83 months for lapatinib plus capecitabine, but failed to conclusively demonstrate either inferiority or noninferiority based on the prespecified statistical thresholds. Given these results, several additional phase I/II trials evaluated the safety and efficacy of neratinib in combination with chemotherapy in trastuzumab-refractory advanced HER2+ breast cancer[87–89] (Table 12.3). Neratinib plus capecitabine was well tolerated in a single-arm phase I/II study and demonstrated good clinical activity with an ORR of 64% and median PFS of 9 months for patients without prior lapatinib exposure,[90] laying the groundwork for the currently ongoing NALA trial (NCT01808573), a phase III randomized trial comparing neratinib plus capecitabine with lapatinib plus capecitabine (Table 12.3). Neratinib plus paclitaxel was well tolerated in the phase I stage and ultimately compared with trastuzumab plus paclitaxel in the large phase II randomized NEfERT-T trial as first-line therapy for advanced HER2+ breast cancer. In this trial of over 400 women, participants with advanced or metastatic HER2+ breast cancer without prior treatment in the metastatic setting were randomized to receive neratinib or trastuzumab in combination with paclitaxel.[91] The study was designed to assess superiority of neratinib to trastuzumab but failed to meet this target, with an identical median PFS of 12.9 months in both arms and an ORR of 74.8% in the neratinib versus 77.6% in the trastuzumab arm. Neratinib does have some CNS penetration in preclinical models, and intriguingly, there was a significant difference in the prespecified secondary endpoint of CNS progression, which occurred in only 8.3% of participants in the neratinib arm versus 17.43% in the trastuzumab arm. Unfortunately, this was confounded by a significantly higher rate of CNS metastasis at baseline in the trastuzumab arm, though the difference in

CNS efficacy between neratinib and trastuzumab remained significant even after adjusting for this imbalance. A single-arm phase II trial specifically evaluating the activity of single-agent neratinib in HER2+ CNS disease failed to demonstrate clinical activity,[92] but the combination of neratinib with capecitabine in lapatinib-naïve patients preliminarily showed a CNS ORR of 49%.[93] In addition, ongoing trials are evaluating neratinib monotherapy in older patients, as well as neratinib in combination with anti-HER2 therapies, other novel targeted therapies, and other chemotherapy backbones (Table 12.3).

Overall, these trials support significant clinical activity of neratinib in the metastatic setting, with the results of the NALA trial pending to establish neratinib as a second- or third-line treatment and the NEfERT-T trial providing preliminary evidence suggesting that it could become an option for first-line therapy, although further trials are needed to evaluate neratinib in the context of the current standard-of-care dual anti–HER2-targeted therapy with pertuzumab and trastuzumab. Finally, the NEfERT-T trial also hinted at possible activity in the setting of CNS disease, a finding that certainly warrants further evaluation given the great need for effective CNS-penetrating therapy.

Afatinib monotherapy is approved for treatment of EGFR mutant NSCLC but has had significantly less clinical success in breast cancer. An early phase II trial of single-agent afatinib in heavily pretreated trastuzumab-refractory HER2+ mBC demonstrated some clinical activity with an ORR of 11% but a median PFS of 3 months.[94] Beyond monotherapy, phase I trials in advanced solid tumors demonstrated tolerability of afatinib plus vinorelbine. This combination was compared with trastuzumab plus vinorelbine in HER2+ mBC after progression on one line of trastuzumab-based treatment in the adjuvant or metastatic setting in the open-label, randomized phase III LUX-Breast 1 trial.[95] Toxicities were significantly higher in the afatinib arm, and ultimately the study was stopped early based on a risk-benefit assessment by the independent data monitoring committee, who felt that afatinib arm was unlikely to meet predefined superiority criteria. Patients in the afatinib arm who wished to stay on study were required to switch treatment to trastuzumab plus vinorelbine, afatinib monotherapy, or vinorelbine monotherapy or to receive treatment outside the trial, which significantly limits the originally planned comparison. However, at a median follow-up of 9.3 months, median PFS was 5.5 months in the afatinib arm and 5.6 months in the trastuzumab arm with an ORR of 46% versus 47%, respectively. Common grade ≥ 3 toxicities were neutropenia and diarrhea. Serious AEs disproportionately affected the afatinib arm (36% vs. 26% with trastuzumab), and permanent treatment discontinuations occurred in 15% versus 7% for afatinib and trastuzumab, respectively. Given the suggestion of possible benefit of neratinib in CNS disease, an open-label, randomized phase II trial called LUX-Breast 3 evaluated afatinib monotherapy versus afatinib in addition to vinorelbine versus investigator's choice in HER2+ CNS metastases that had progressed while on trastuzumab or lapatinib[96] but found no increase in patient benefit for either afatinib arm, as well as poor tolerance of afatinib-containing regimens. Finally, the LUX-Breast 2 phase II trial evaluating afatinib monotherapy followed by the addition of either vinorelbine or paclitaxel on progression for patients with HER2+ mBC that failed/progressed on neoadjuvant or adjuvant HER2-targeted treatment with trastuzumab and/or lapatinib (NCT01271725) was recently completed, with no results yet available. Afatinib's increased toxicity profile compared with the other drugs in this class and lack of clinical benefit in a large phase III trial make it a much less appealing candidate for further development in the metastatic setting than neratinib.

Of the three multi-HER TKIs either approved or under study in the advanced/metastatic setting, lapatinib's role is fairly well established but is being overtaken by newer and more effective multi-HER inhibitors such as pertuzumab and possibly neratinib. Neratinib has shown some very promising clinical activity, but its place in the armamentarium of treatment options for advanced disease remains to be defined, whether in the hierarchy of non—first-line options, as an addition to pertuzumab or trastuzumab in first-line dual anti-HER2 therapy or chemotherapy-sparing regimens, or in the setting of CNS disease, roles where lapatinib may also find some clinical use. Finally, afatinib's utility has been limited by more significant toxicities and lack of demonstrated clinical efficacy and so seems less likely to find a role in treatment of advanced HER2+ breast cancer.

Multi-HER Inhibitors in Adjuvant/Neoadjuvant Therapy

In the adjuvant setting, the randomized, open-label, phase III ALTTO (Adjuvant Lapatinib and/or Trastuzumab Treatment Optimization) trial had four arms: lapatinib monotherapy (closed early), trastuzumab monotherapy, lapatinib plus trastuzumab, and trastuzumab followed by lapatinib. This trial failed to demonstrate any benefit in DFS from dual therapy, with DFS rates at median 4.5 years of follow-up at

86% for trastuzumab, 87% for trastuzumab followed by lapatinib, and 88% for the combination of trastuzumab with lapatinib.[97] There was a significant increase in grade ≥3 toxicities in the lapatinib-containing arms. Of note, several significant changes to the study protocol—including discontinuation of the lapatinib monotherapy arm due to inferior results compared with the trastuzumab arm, with lapatinib patients being offered trastuzumab instead—are likely to have significantly reduced the statistical power of the study, possibly obscuring a significant improvement in the combination arm.

In the neoadjuvant setting, the randomized phase III GeparQuinto trial compared trastuzumab and lapatinib head to head in combination with chemotherapy, specifically epirubicin (an anthracycline) and cyclophosphamide with trastuzumab or lapatinib followed by docetaxel with trastuzumab or lapatinib.[98] For their primary outcome of pCR (ypT0 ypN0), pCR was 30.3% in the trastuzumab group versus 22.7% in the lapatinib group, which met the predefined threshold for statistical significance for inferiority of lapatinib, an effect that was sustained across several less-stringent definitions of pCR in their prespecified secondary analyses.

Although lapatinib monotherapy was demonstrated to be inferior to trastuzumab in GeparQuinto, multiple phase II trials evaluating trastuzumab plus lapatinib with different chemotherapy backbones and without chemotherapy did find evidence of benefit with combination therapy,[99–103] (Table 12.3) and only one of the three phase III studies evaluating the combination found a statistically significant benefit to dual therapy, the NeoALTTO trial. This randomized, open-label, phase III trial compared the combination of lapatinib plus trastuzumab (L+T) with either alone (L or T), with 6 weeks of anti-HER2 therapy (L+T, L, or T) followed by the addition of paclitaxel for 12 weeks, and then continuation of the HER2-targeted regimen for 1 year after surgery.[104] There was an increase in the pCR in the dual therapy group of 51.3% for dual therapy versus 29.5% for trastuzumab alone versus 24.7% for lapatinib alone that met the prespecified significance threshold. The phase III randomized trials NSABP 41 and CALGB 40601 also evaluated dual anti-HER2/EGFR therapy compared with monotherapy with different chemotherapy backbones, but while both demonstrated a trend toward increased pCR in the dual therapy arm, neither achieved statistical significance. In NSABP 41, patients received four cycles of doxorubicin/cyclophosphamide without anti-HER2 therapy followed by four cycles of paclitaxel in combination with trastuzumab, lapatinib, or both, followed by anti-HER2 therapy (L+T, L, or T) until surgery.[105] pCR was 52.5% for trastuzumab, 53.2% for lapatinib, and 62% for the combination, with similar nonsignificant results for HR+ and HR-negative subgroups. In CALGB 40601, patients received paclitaxel with trastuzumab, lapatinib, or both.[106] The lapatinib-only arm was closed early based on accumulating evidence for the inferiority of lapatinib monotherapy compared with trastuzumab, but the enrollment targets were revised in the remaining arms to retain statistical power. pCR was 46% for trastuzumab, 32% for lapatinib, and 56% for the combination. Interestingly, a significant increase in pCR with combination therapy versus trastuzumab was observed in the HR-negative subgroup in a prespecified secondary analysis, with no such difference in the HR+ subgroup. In all of these studies, there was an increase in toxicities in the lapatinib arms very similar to that seen in the ALTTO trial, with frequent dose reductions of lapatinib required.

There are many possible reasons for the differences between the results of these three studies, including timing of anti-HER2 therapy, choice of chemotherapy backbone, and patient population (particularly given the significantly lower monotherapy pCR rate in Neo-ALTTO compared with the other two studies), but as highlighted by the results of the CALGB 40601 study, it also seems likely that intratumor heterogeneity may be a significant contributor. In the end, however, the success of the novel anti-HER2 antibody pertuzumab in combination with trastuzumab and neratinib has eclipsed lapatinib's possible role in early-stage disease.

Given the clinical activity of neratinib in the metastatic setting in HER2+ breast cancer, there has been considerable interest in evaluating a role for neratinib in adjuvant and neoadjuvant treatment. The ExteNET study was a large, randomized, double-blind, phase III trial designed to evaluate the efficacy of extending adjuvant treatment with neratinib after completion of adjuvant trastuzumab therapy in HER2+ breast cancer. In this trial, nearly 3000 participants who had completed neoadjuvant and adjuvant trastuzumab therapy up to 1−2 years prior to enrollment were randomized to receive either neratinib or placebo for 12 months (with hormone therapy if HR+), with a primary outcome of DFS at 2 years.[107] The trial protocol did go through some significant changes due to three changes in ownership of the drug, including an early amendment restricting recruitment to patients with node-positive disease, as well as cessation of enrollment at 2842 of 3850 originally planned participants.

However, the primary outcome of DFS at 2 years was increased in the neratinib group at 93.9% versus 91.6% in the placebo arm, with a statistically significant HR of 0.67 ($P = .009$). Follow-up is ongoing (planned for 5 years), so final DFS and OS data are not yet mature. Interestingly, in contrast to neoadjuvant trials with both lapatinib (CALGB 40601 as above) and neratinib (NSABP FG-7 below) in which TKI benefit was enriched in HR-negative tumors, a prespecified secondary analysis according to HR status showed that the majority of the benefit with neratinib in this trial was in HR+ disease with a DFS HR of 0.51, whereas in HR-negative patients the HR was 0.93 and nonsignificant. Based on the results of the ExteNET trial, neratinib received FDA approval as extension adjuvant therapy, though an OS benefit remains to be seen.

In the neoadjuvant setting, the NSABP FB-7 randomized phase II trial compared paclitaxel with neratinib, trastuzumab, or both together followed by doxorubicin and cyclophosphamide in a cohort of 126 patients with HER2+ breast cancer.[108] With this regimen, pCR (ypT0 pyN0) was significantly increased in the combination arm (50% vs. 33% with neratinib vs. 38% with trastuzumab), although the benefit was concentrated in HR-negative subgroup with no difference between arms in the HR+ subgroup. Neratinib was also included in the I-SPY 2 phase II trial,[109] a neoadjuvant trial implementing a unique randomization algorithm known as adaptive randomization that uses biomarker assessments to allocate patients to multiple different experimental therapy groups in combination with chemotherapy versus a control chemotherapy-only arm. The goal of this design is to identify biomarker signatures that are associated with efficacy for specific experimental agents using prespecified efficacy thresholds for the biomarker signatures, which can then be used as the basis for enrollment in phase III trials for those agents. In this trial, neratinib crossed the prespecified threshold for the HER2+ HR-negative signature, based on which a phase III confirmatory trial (I-SPY 3) is planned. Overall, neratinib is emerging as a significant player in the neoadjuvant and adjuvant setting, though its scope of benefit remains unclear, particularly with reference to HR status. Based on current clinical data, it does seem that HR status significantly impacts neratinib's clinical efficacy, but the discrepancies between current neoadjuvant and adjuvant data remain to be resolved, whether through mechanistic preclinical studies or as additional clinical data from larger trials become available.

Afatinib has also been investigated in the neoadjuvant setting in several small phase II trials, the largest of which was a single-arm study with 65 participants evaluating dual anti-HER2/EGFR therapy with trastuzumab plus afatinib along with chemotherapy.[110] In this trial, patients received 6 weeks of afatinib and trastuzumab followed by addition of paclitaxel to anti-HER2/EGFR therapy for 12 weeks followed by 12 weeks of epirubicin, cyclophosphamide, and trastuzumab before surgery. They observed a pCR (ypT0/is ypN0) rate of 49.2%, with again a discrepancy between HR-negative (pCR 63%) and HR+ (pCR 43%) tumors. This pCR is on the lower end of what has been reported in neoadjuvant trials of dual anti-HER2 blockade with other therapies, which range from 50% to 60%, and did not meet the trial's goal of pCR rate of 70% to demonstrate likely superiority over other anti-HER2 agents, consistent with afatinib's poorer performance compared with other anti-HER2 therapies in the metastatic setting.

Of the HER family TKIs, neratinib has shown the most promise in the adjuvant/neoadjuvant setting and is already FDA approved for extension of anti-HER2 adjuvant therapy after completion of trastuzumab. A phase III trial with neratinib in the neoadjuvant setting is ongoing. Neratinib is the most likely member of this class to have a significant role in treatment of early HER2+ breast cancer going forward. An important consideration in the early-disease setting appears to be HR status, with a strong and consistent signal in the neoadjuvant setting indicating that benefit with HER family TKIs is concentrated in the subgroup of HR-negative tumors. It remains to be seen how this is to be reconciled with the benefit seen in HR+ tumors in the adjuvant setting in the ExteNET trial.

Side Effect Profile

Toxicities for all three agents are fairly similar and are typical for small molecule TKIs, including diarrhea, nausea/vomiting, rash, and fatigue. Cardiotoxicity is rare and does not occur in excess in combination with trastuzumab. In the large trial of lapatinib plus capecitabine for treatment-refractory advanced disease,[111] toxicities that were increased in the lapatinib arm included diarrhea (60%), rash (27%), nausea/vomiting (44%), and palmar-plantar erythrodysesthesia (49%). Common toxicities for neratinib monotherapy in the initial phase I trial included diarrhea (84%), nausea (55%), asthenia (45%), and rash (10%),[112] which is fairly similar to what has been seen subsequently for both monotherapy and combination therapy. The prominent early diarrhea seen with neratinib has proven relatively amenable to prophylactic or as-needed antidiarrheal agents, with a clinical trial currently ongoing to assess the efficacy of intensive

loperamide prophylaxis in patients receiving adjuvant neratinib (NCT02400476). For afatinib, diarrhea is again the most significant toxicity, occurring in 90% of patients in the phase II monotherapy trial, as well as rash (66%), fatigue (41%), nausea/vomiting (39%), and stomatitis (36%).[94]

OTHER GROWTH FACTOR PATHWAYS

Beyond the ErbB/HER family of receptors themselves, many other cell surface RTKs have been implicated in trastuzumab resistance in HER2+ breast cancer, including IGF-1R, c-MET, fibroblast growth factor receptor 2 (FGFR2), ephrin receptor 2A (Eph2A), and AXL.[7] Although all of these have been extensively studied in the preclinical setting, only inhibitors of IGF-1R, c-MET, and FGFR2 are currently being evaluated in clinical trials, so these three receptors will be the focus of this section.

PreClinical Data for IGF-1R, FGFR, and c-MET in Anti-HER2 Inhibitor Resistance

Binding of insulin-like growth factor 1 to its receptor IGF-1R leads to activation of the same downstream effectors as ErbB family receptors, including the Ras/MAPK and PI3K/AKT pathways. Perhaps unsurprisingly, IGF-1R overexpression can induce trastuzumab resistance in breast cancer cells in vitro.[113] In addition, IGF-1R can also directly heterodimerize with HER2 and HER3, and presence of these complexes is associated with trastuzumab resistance in human breast cancer cell lines in vitro, while inhibition of IGF-1R or disruption of this dimerization restores trastuzumab sensitivity in resistant cell lines.[114] Interestingly, pertuzumab, which binds to HER2's dimerization domain, only moderately disrupts the interaction with IGF-1R in trastuzumab-resistant breast cancer cell lines in vitro.[114] In tissue microarrays of 4000 tumor tissue samples in patients with stage I—III breast cancer, high IGF-1R protein expression by immunohistochemistry was associated with worse prognosis, specifically in the HER2+ subset.[115] Biomarker analysis in a trial of 40 patients receiving neoadjuvant trastuzumab plus vinorelbine found that IGF-1R protein expression was associated with worse pathologic response, with a response rate of 50% in the group with IGF-1R membrane expression versus 97% without ($P = .001$),[116] supporting the in vitro data and suggesting a role for IGF-1R in trastuzumab resistance.

The c-MET RTK and its ligand hepatocyte growth factor (HGF) have also been implicated in trastuzumab resistance. Like IGF-1R and ErbB family receptors, c-MET activates the Ras/MAPK and PI3K pathways. c-MET has been shown to be upregulated in response to trastuzumab in HER2-overexpressing breast cancer cells. Activation of c-MET by HGF in HER2-overexpressing breast cancer cells induces trastuzumab resistance, and inhibition of c-MET increased trastuzumab sensitivity in these cell lines.[117] In addition, the c-MET inhibitor foretinib acted synergistically with lapatinib in a panel of human tumor cell lines with both c-MET and HER2 amplification, including several breast cancer cell lines.[118] In a group of 130 HER2+ metastatic breast tumors treated with trastuzumab, c-MET and HGF copy number gain were both associated with trastuzumab failure,[119] while high c-MET protein expression was associated with shorter PFS in patients treated with lapatinib.[118] Taken together, these data support a role for c-MET in trastuzumab resistance in a subset of HER2+ tumors and the possibility that inhibition of c-MET along with HER2 may be beneficial in these patients.

FGFR2 is an RTK that, on ligand binding, activates AKT and downstream signaling, as well as the Ras/MAPK pathway. A recent study has identified FGFR2 overexpression as the mechanism of acquired anti-HER2 therapy resistance. In this work, HER2+ xenografts with acquired resistance to dual anti-HER2/EGFR blockade with lapatinib plus trastuzumab were found to have activated FGFR signaling as evidenced by an increased copy number of multiple FGFRs and increased FGFR phosphorylation; treatment with FGFR inhibitors was sufficient to overcome the dual blockade resistance.[120] This study also found that FGFR1 overexpression was associated with shorter PFS in HER2+ early breast cancers treated with adjuvant trastuzumab in the FinHer trial and with lower pCR rates in HER2+ early breast cancer treated with anti-HER2 therapy in the NeoALTTO trial, providing fairly strong circumstantial evidence for a role for FGFR signaling in HER2 therapy resistance, at least in a subset of patients.

ErbB family receptor signaling does not exist in a vacuum, and as these preclinical data highlight, tumor cells are notoriously able to adapt to circumvent targeted inhibition of individual signaling pathways. Significant clinical gains have been made with the evolution of targeted ErbB receptor therapies from HER2 to HER family–directed therapy. Moving forward, molecularly directed targeting of additional upstream RTKs such as those described here may help prevent or treat resistance to HER family therapy.

Clinical Trials

Several monoclonal anti–IGF-1R antibodies are currently in clinical development in solid tumors, including IMC-A12 (cixutumumab), R1507 (teprotumumab), MK-0646 (dalotuzumab), AMG-479 (ganitumab), and CP-751,871 (figitumumab), but results of early-phase trials have been disappointing. A systematic review of clinical trials evaluating these agents in breast, colorectal, lung, pancreatic, and ovarian cancer, including several large phase III trials in pancreatic and lung cancer, found that only 1 out of 17 published trials demonstrated any clinical activity.[121] Given the preclinical evidence supporting a particular dependence of at least a subset of HER2+ breast cancers on IGF-1R signaling, it may be that these agents could still find some success in HER2+ disease, and indeed a phase II trial (NCT00684983) evaluating cixutumumab with lapatinib and capecitabine in trastuzumab-refractory HER2+ mBC is currently ongoing. Additional relevant ongoing trials of anti–IGF-1R antibodies are listed in Table 12.4, including several that seek to validate a biological effect of these inhibitors on IGF-1R expression.

For c-MET, both small molecule TKIs and several anti–c-MET antibodies are in clinical trials or clinical use in solid tumors. Relevant TKIs include the competitive c-MET inhibitor ARQ197 (tivantinib), the dual inhibitor crizotinib, which inhibits both anaplastic lymphoma kinase (ALK) and c-MET and is approved for use in ALK-positive NSCLC, and the more broadly acting TKIs XL184 (cabozantinib) and (XL880) foretinib, which both inhibit a spectrum of RTKs including c-MET, VEGFR2, and AXL, among others.[122] Onartuzumab is a monoclonal anti–c-MET antibody, and AMG102 (rilotumumab) is humanized monoclonal antibody that neutralizes c-MET's ligand HGF.[122] These inhibitors have met with significant success in NSCLC and have demonstrated synergy with EGFR-directed TKIs in this setting.[122] On the other hand, c-MET inhibitors have shown minimal clinical effect in upper GI tract cancers, which also commonly overexpress c-MET.[123] In breast cancer, several of these inhibitors have been studied in phase II trials in metastatic TNBC, including tivantinib, foretinib, and cabozantinib monotherapy, as well as the addition of onartuzumab to the combination of bevacizumab and paclitaxel, without clear evidence of clinical activity. However, TNBC represents a markedly different molecular entity to HER2+ breast cancer, and it is difficult to infer from these results how these inhibitors might perform in HER2+ disease. On the other hand, the minimal

TABLE 12.4
Selected Trials With Other Growth Factor Inhibitors

Target	Compound	Identifier	Setting	Outcomes
IGF-1R	IMC-A12 (cixutumumab)	NCT00684983	Phase II: Lapatinib plus capecitabine with or without IMC-A12 in advanced HER2+ trastuzumab-refractory breast cancer; ongoing	PFS, OS
		NCT00699491	Phase I/II: IMC-A12 with temsirolimus in mBC including HER2+; ongoing	MTD, ORR, AEs
	AMG-479 (ganitumab)	NCT01708161	Phase Ib/II: Alpelisib with AMG-479 in advanced ovarian or HR+ breast cancer with PIK3CA mutation; completed	Incidence of DLT; ORR
	R1507 (teprotumumab)	NCT00882674	Phase I: R1507 given as a single dose 1 week prior to surgery in operable HER2+ breast cancer; completed	IGF-1R expression in surgical breast tumor specimen versus pretreatment biopsy
	MK-0646 (dalotuzumab)	NCT00759785	Phase I: MK-0646 as a single dose with pre- and postdose biopsy in operable TN or ER+/luminal B breast cancer; completed	Change in growth factor gene expression signature and IGF-1R expression pre- versus posttreatment
c-MET	XL184 (cabozitinib)	NCT02260531	Phase II: XL184 with trastuzumab in HER2+ breast cancer with new or progressive CNS metastases (study also includes cabozitinib alone in HR+/HER2 and TN CNS metastases); recruiting	CNS ORR
FGFR	Lucatinib (FGFR/VEGFR inhibitor)	NCT02202746	Phase II: Lucatinib monotherapy in patients with mBC including HER2+, stratified by FGFR pathway activation; ongoing	PFS, ORR
	INCB054828 (selective FGFR1-3 inhibitor)	NCT02393248	Phase I/II: Dose escalation (part 1) followed by dose expansion (part 2) followed by combination therapy (part 3) in advanced solid tumors including breast; trastuzumab combination therapy will be included in part 3	MTD, ORR

AE, adverse event; *CNS*, central nervous system; *DCIS*, ductal carcinoma in situ; *DFS*, disease-free survival; *DLT*, dose-limiting toxicity; *ER*, estrogen receptor; *FGFR*, fibroblast growth factor receptor; *H*, trastuzumab; *HR*, hormone receptor; *IGF-1R*, insulin-like growth factor 1 receptor; *MBC*, advanced/metastatic breast cancer; *MTD*, maximum tolerated dose; *ORR*, overall response rate (complete remission + partial response); *OS*, overall survival; *pCR*, pathologic complete response; *PFS*, progression-free survival; *PIK3CA*, phosphatidylinositol-4,5-bisphosphate 3-kinase catalytic subunit alpha; *Pt*, pertuzumab; *T-DM1*, trastuzumab emtansine; *TN*, triple-negative.

effect these agents have had in upper GI tract cancers, which often overexpress HER2, does speak against a possible clinical benefit in the HER2+ setting. A single clinical trial of a c-MET inhibitor in HER2+ breast cancer, specifically in patients with CNS metastases, is currently recruiting (Table 12.4).

There are a multitude of anti-FGFR therapies in clinical trials in solid tumors, although as yet none has received FDA approval.[124] These include TKIs selective for FGFR family members such as AZD4547, TAS120, BGJ398, and JNJ-42756493 (erdafitinib) and broad-spectrum TKIs including dovitinib (which also inhibits

VEGFR3, FLT3, and c-KIT), orantinib and nintedanib (which also inhibit VEGFRs and PDGFRs), and brivanib and lucitanib (which also inhibit VEGFRs). Notably, different TKIs have different activity against FGFR family members themselves. There is also a ligand trap and several anti-FGFR antibodies under development. In breast cancer, a number of phase I/II trials are ongoing or have been completed evaluating many of these agents in HER2-negative breast cancer as single agents and in combination with chemotherapy or endocrine therapy. In a phase II trial of postmenopausal patients who progressed on endocrine therapy and who were randomized to fulvestrant with either dovitinib or placebo, the median PFS was doubled from 5.5 to 10.9 months in the dovitinib arm in a prespecified FGF pathway–amplified subgroup, though not in the study population as a whole.[125] AZD4547 has also shown clinical activity in the phase I/II setting in combination with aromatase inhibitors in ER+ mBC that progressed on aromatase inhibitor monotherapy.[126] Other FGFR inhibitors with early signs of clinical activity in the phase I setting in HER2-negative breast cancer include lucitanib, BGJ398, and JNJ-42756493. A common theme that has emerged from successful trials with FGF pathway inhibitors across tumor types is the utilization of FGF pathway activation as an enrollment criterion.[127] Selected ongoing trials relevant to the HER2+ breast cancer setting are listed in Table 12.4.

Overall, inhibitors of IGF-1R, c-MET, and FGFR have shown variable clinical success thus far, with the only FDA approval for any of these agents the c-MET/ALK inhibitor crizotinib in ALK-positive NSCLC, which was based more on its activity toward ALK than c-MET. As a class, the IGF-1R inhibitors have had very minimal clinical activity across a variety of solid tumors, including HER2-negative breast cancer, though biomarkers of pathway activation have not been used to stratify or limit patient selection in the majority of these studies, and HER2+ tumors may also represent a subset of tumors biologically more likely to respond, with an initial phase II trial of IGF-1R inhibitor cixutumumab currently underway in refractory HER2+ breast cancer. c-MET inhibitors have thus far not been successful in breast cancer but have only been investigated in the TNBC setting; there is an ongoing trial in HER2+ CNS disease. Finally, FGFR inhibitors have shown early signs of success in ER+ HER-negative breast cancer, in part perhaps because of higher utilization of FGF pathway activation to identify patients more likely to respond to therapy. There are as yet no FGFR inhibitor trials specifically targeting HER2+ breast cancer, but this would likely be a fruitful area of future clinical investigation.

Side Effect Profile

With IGF-1R inhibitors, common toxicities include fatigue, rashes, diarrhea, nausea/vomiting, hyperglycemia, anorexia, and stomatitis, as well as thrombocytopenia and anemia.[128] Overall, however, they are well tolerated. A review combining AE data from 15 individual studies reported the four most common grade ≥3 AEs to be fatigue (4.9%), thrombocytopenia (3.5%), neutropenia (2.8%), and hyperglycemia (2.7%).[128] For c-MET inhibitors, the antibody inhibitor onartuzumab is associated with peripheral edema, alopecia, fatigue, nausea, and diarrhea and in combination with paclitaxel had a fairly high rate of grade ≥3 AEs at 50%.[129] Common cabozantinib toxicities include fatigue, nausea/vomiting, diarrhea, anorexia, and palmar-plantar erythrodysesthesia, though grade ≥3 AEs occur less frequently, with the most common being palmar-plantar erythrodysesthesia in 13% and fatigue in 11%.[130] Other c-MET TKIs are also well tolerated with a similar spectrum of AEs. Finally, for FGFR inhibitors, common toxicities associated with dovitinib include diarrhea, nausea/vomiting, asthenia, and headaches, with the most frequent grade ≥3 AEs including hypertension (in 20%), diarrhea (14.9%), transaminase elevations (15%), and fatigue (13%).[125]

IMMUNOTHERAPY

Strategies that augment host antitumor responses have been associated with growing clinical success across many solid tumor types, including breast cancer. These strategies attempt to leverage host adaptive immunity not only for acute control of the tumor but also to establish a durable response with the goal of prolonged control of micrometastatic disease and take two basic approaches. Cancer vaccines seek to prime and expand tumor-specific T cells to stimulate a cellular and humoral immune response for both immediate immune clearance of tumor and the formation of immunologic memory for durable disease control. However, tumors are adept at evading adaptive immune responses, which has made the development of effective vaccines challenging. A major evasive mechanism utilized by solid tumors is the misappropriation of immune checkpoint pathways. Physiologically, immune checkpoint pathways are crucial to maintain the immune system's tolerance of self-antigens, thereby preventing autoimmune disorders. Mechanistically, immune checkpoint pathways are cell surface receptor/ligand interactions that negatively regulate adaptive immune responses. In the tumor microenvironment, increased expression of immune checkpoint ligands such as PD-L1 and PD-L2 leads to extinction of antitumor T cell responses. This can be counteracted with immune checkpoint blockade, specifically with monoclonal antibodies that inhibit the CTLA-4 and PD-1 immune checkpoint receptors, as well as antibodies against the PD-L1 and PD-L2 ligands. Immune checkpoint inhibitors have found significant clinical success in a number of different solid tumor types, with durable responses in a subset of patients with melanoma and lung cancer. Studies are ongoing in many other types of tumors, including breast cancer. In the context of HER2+ disease, an often underappreciated component of the antitumor responses induced by anti-HER2 antibodies such as trastuzumab and pertuzumab occurs through engagement of the host immune system to activate antibody-dependent cell-mediated cytotoxicity against HER2-expressing tumor cells, suggesting that this could be a particularly successful setting for the deployment of both tumor vaccines and checkpoint blockade.

Preclinical Data Supporting Immunotherapy in HER2+ Disease

In preclinical mouse models, anti—CTLA-4 and PD-1 antibodies synergize with anti-HER2 antibodies, while in a secondary analysis of the NeoSphere neoadjuvant trial of docetaxel, pertuzumab, and trastuzumab, high PD-L1 expression was associated with lower rates of pCR and markers of immune activation with higher rates of pCR.[131] Similar associations between markers of antitumor immune response and improved outcomes were also found in several other large neoadjuvant trials involving pertuzumab and trastuzumab, including TRYPHAENA and CALGB 40601.[106,132] A secondary analysis of the NeoALTTO trial found that high numbers of tumor-infiltrating lymphocytes were associated with better prognosis regardless of whether patients received trastuzumab or lapatinib.[133] In the metastatic setting, a secondary analysis of the CLEOPATRA trial of trastuzumab and docetaxel plus pertuzumab or placebo found an association between increased tumor-infiltrating lymphocytes and improved outcomes in the metastatic setting regardless of anti-HER2 antibody regimen.[134] Taken together, these data support a role for immune checkpoint blockade and other immunomodulatory therapies in HER2+ breast cancer.

Clinical Trials with Immunomodulatory Agents

HER2 itself is an obvious antigen for the development of vaccines directed against HER2+ tumors, and there has been considerable interest in tumor vaccine development in HER2+ breast cancer, though without significant clinical success. Phase I trials of a peptide-based vaccine utilizing the E75 peptide derived from the HER2 extracellular domain were able to demonstrate HER2-directed T-cell responses that persisted for up to several years when administered with trastuzumab in metastatic HER2+ breast cancer but did not demonstrate any clinical benefit, perhaps due to the advanced disease setting.[135] Subsequent trials focused on use in the adjuvant setting, but the largest phase III adjuvant trial of this vaccine (Table 12.5) was halted early due to futility by the independent data monitoring committee. Additional ongoing trials are evaluating this vaccine in combination with trastuzumab and in the setting of ductal carcinoma in situ (Table 12.5). Additional vaccine approaches in early-phase trials include the combination of peptide vaccines with chemotherapy in addition to trastuzumab, peptide-based vaccines derived from the HER2 intracellular or transmembrane domains, DNA-based vaccines, dendritic cell vaccines, whole tumor cell vaccines, and the *ex vivo* expansion and re-infusion of autologous HER2-specific T-cells after vaccination.[136]

Given the success of immune checkpoint blockade in other solid tumor settings, a number of exciting trials are expanding the study of these agents to HER2+ breast cancer. Available agents include the anti-PD1 antibodies pembrolizumab and nivolumab, anti—PD-L1 antibodies atezolizumab, avelumab, and durvalumab, and the anti-CTLA4 antibodies ipilimumab and tremelimumab. Of these, pembrolizumab, atezolizumab, and durvalumab are in clinical trials in HER2+ breast cancer (Table 12.5), primarily in the metastatic setting and in combination with anti-HER2 antibodies, including a planned (but not yet recruiting) phase III trial of pembrolizumab versus placebo in combination with standard-of-care trastuzumab, pertuzumab, and paclitaxel as first-line therapy for metastatic disease (NCT03199885).

Taken together, the immunogenicity of HER2 makes HER2+ breast cancer an appealing candidate for both active immunization therapies and immune checkpoint blockade. While many different vaccine strategies are currently being pursued in this setting, none has yet demonstrated promising clinical activity. Meanwhile, the results of the first trials utilizing immune checkpoint blockade in combination with anti-HER2 antibodies in HER2+ breast cancer are eagerly awaited, though it remains to be seen whether their activity in other settings is replicated here.

Side Effect Profile

AEs associated with the anti-PD-1, anti-PD-L1, and anti-CTLA4 antibodies are autoimmune in nature, including rashes, diarrhea/colitis, and thyroiditis, as well as pneumonitis with PD-1 and PD-L1 inhibitors. It remains to

TABLE 12.5
Selected Trials With Immunomodulatory Therapies

Identifier	Phase	Setting	Design	Outcomes
PEMBROLIZUMAB				
NCT03032107	Ib	Advanced H-refractory	Pembrolizumab with T-DM1 in H-refractory advanced HER2+ breast cancer; recruiting	AEs, ORR, PFS
NCT03272334	I/II	Metastatic H-refractory	Pembrolizumab with anti-CD3/ Anti-HER2 armed activated autologous T cells in H-refractory metastatic HER2+ breast cancer; recruiting	AEs/DLTs, serum immune response, ORR
NCT02318901	Ib/II	Metastatic	Pembrolizumab with H or T-DM1 in metastatic HER2+ breast cancer; recruiting	MTD, AEs, ORR, PFS
NCT02129556 (PANACEA)	Ib/II	Advanced H-refractory	Pembrolizumab with trastuzumab in H-refractory advanced HER2+ breast cancer; ongoing	MTD, ORR
NCT03199885	III	Metastatic first-line	H, Pt, and paclitaxel with pembrolizumab or placebo as first-line therapy in metastatic HER2+ breast cancer; not yet recruiting	PFS, CNS mets, AEs including late immune-related
ATEZOLIZUMAB				
NCT02605915	Ib	Metastatic and neoadjuvant	Metastatic disease: H and Pt with atezolizumab with or without docetaxel, or T-DM1 dose escalation with atezolizumab Neoadjuvant: H and Pt with atezolizumab or T-DM1 with atezolizumab in HER2+ breast cancer; recruiting	DLTs, AEs
NCT02924883	II	Advanced H-refractory	T-DM1 with atezolizumab or placebo in H-refractory advanced/metastatic HER2+ breast cancer; ongoing	AEs, PFS, ORR, OS
NCT03125928	II	Advanced first-line	H, Pt, and paclitaxel with atezolizumab as first-line therapy in advanced/metastatic HER2+ breast cancer; recruiting	AEs, ORR,
DURVALUMAB				
NCT02649686	Ib	Metastatic H-refractory	H with durvalumab in H-refractory metastatic HER2+ breast cancer; ongoing	AEs, ORR, CBR
VACCINES				
NCT01570036	II	Early node-positive or high-risk node negative	H and GM-CSF with or without E75 HER2 vaccine in node-positive or high-risk node-negative HER2 1 + or 2 + breast cancer after treatment; recruiting	DFS

TABLE 12.5
Selected Trials With Immunomodulatory Therapies—cont'd

Identifier	Phase	Setting	Design	Outcomes
NCT02297698	II	Early high risk	H and E75 HER2 vaccine with GM-CSF in patients with early-stage HER2+ breast cancer high risk by study definition; recruiting	Invasive DFS, AEs
NCT01479244	III	Early node positive	E75 HER2 vaccine with GM-CSF or placebo in node-positive HER2 1+ or 2+ breast cancer after treatment; terminated because of futility	DFS, OS
NCT02636582	II	DCIS	E75 HER2 vaccine with GM-CSF or placebo in patients with DCIS; recruiting	E75-specific T cell response, AEs.

AE, adverse event; CBR, clinical benefit rate (complete remission + partial response + stable disease for >6 months); DCIS, ductal carcinoma in situ; DFS, disease-free survival; DLT, dose-limiting toxicity; GM-CSF, granulocyte-macrophage colony-stimulating factor; H, trastuzumab; MBC, advanced/metastatic breast cancer; MTD, maximum tolerated dose; ORR, overall response rate (complete remission + partial response); OS, overall survival; pCR, pathologic complete response; PFS, progression-free survival; Pt, pertuzumab; T-DM1, trastuzumab emtansine.

be seen whether new immune-mediated or other toxicities emerge when used in combination with anti-HER2 antibodies.

PARP INHIBITORS

Poly(ADP-ribose) polymerases (PARPs) are nuclear DNA damage sensors involved in recognition and repair of single-strand DNA breaks. Seminal preclinical work in the early 2000s revealed that homozygous BRCA1/2 mutant cells, which are deficient in homologous recombination repair, are profoundly sensitive to PARP inhibition.[137] Since then, several PARP inhibitors have been approved for use in advanced ovarian cancer and are in phase III trials in the metastatic and adjuvant settings for HER2-negative breast cancer arising in the setting of germline BRCA mutations with encouraging preliminary results.[138] Interestingly, there is some preclinical evidence suggesting that HER2 overexpression may also sensitize breast cancer cells to PARP inhibitors. A panel of HER2+ human breast cancer cell lines was found to be sensitive to PARP inhibitors veliparib and olaparib in vitro, whereas HER2 overexpression in HER2-negative breast cancer cells significantly increased their sensitivity to veliparib in vitro and in xenografts.[139] The mechanism was in fact thought to be unrelated to DNA repair and instead possibly due to inhibition of NF-κB by veliparib, though this remains to be investigated. A subsequent study by the same group demonstrated that PARP1 protein and phospho-p65, a marker of NF-κB

pathway activation, were enriched in HER2+ tumors in a set of 307 breast tumor samples, providing additional support for their initial observation.[140] Although these findings require additional preclinical validation, they raise the intriguing possibility that PARP inhibitors could have clinical activity in HER2+ breast cancer, which has not yet been explored in the clinical setting.

CONCLUSION

With the advent of trastuzumab, and more recently trastuzumab emtansine and pertuzumab, the treatment and prognosis of both early-stage and advanced/metastatic HER2+ breast cancer has been revolutionized. As we have outlined above, a number of additional exciting targeted therapies are emerging, which may particularly be of use in patients with intrinsic or acquired anti-HER2 antibody resistance. Ultimately, it is likely that many of these targeted agents will find success only in a particular molecularly determined subgroup of patients and, indeed, that an individual patient's disease will evolve in its sensitivities over time, such that identification of relevant biomarkers to allow effective clinical utilization of such therapies will be essential. Of the spectrum of targeted agents in development, those with particular promise in the broader population include the CDK4/6 inhibitors, the newer PI3K inhibitors, and the pan-HER inhibitor neratinib. Immune checkpoint inhibitors may also show activity in this setting as they have in many others.

DISCLOSURE STATEMENT

O'Regan: Research support: Pfizer, Novartis, Advisor/
honoraria: Pfizer, Eli Lilly

REFERENCES

1. Loibl S, Gianni L. HER2-positive breast cancer. *Lancet.* 2017;389(10087):2415–2429. https://doi.org/10.1016/S0140-6736(16)32417-5.
2. Perez EA, Romond EH, Suman VJ, et al. Trastuzumab plus adjuvant chemotherapy for human epidermal growth factor receptor 2-positive breast cancer: planned joint analysis of overall survival from NSABP B-31 and NCCTG N9831. *J Clin Oncol.* 2014;32(33):3744–3752. https://doi.org/10.1200/JCO.2014.55.5730.
3. Swain SM, Baselga J, Kim S-B, et al. Pertuzumab, trastuzumab, and docetaxel in HER2-positive metastatic breast cancer. *N Engl J Med.* 2015;372(8):724–734. https://doi.org/10.1056/NEJMoa1413513.
4. Yarden Y, Pines G. The ERBB network: at last, cancer therapy meets systems biology. *Nat Rev Cancer.* 2012;12(8):553–563. https://doi.org/10.1038/nrc3309.
5. Rimawi MF, Schiff R, Osborne CK. Targeting HER2 for the treatment of breast cancer. *Annu Rev Med.* 2015;66(1):111–128. https://doi.org/10.1146/annurev-med-042513-015127.
6. Arteaga CL, Engelman JA. ERBB receptors: from oncogene discovery to basic science to mechanism-based cancer therapeutics. *Cancer Cell.* 2014;25(3):282–303. https://doi.org/10.1016/j.ccr.2014.02.025.
7. Rexer BN, Arteaga CL. Intrinsic and acquired resistance to HER2-targeted therapies in HER2 gene-amplified breast cancer: mechanisms and clinical implications. *Crit Rev Oncog.* 2012;17(1):1–16.
8. Hanahan D, Weinberg RA. Hallmarks of cancer: the next generation. *Cell.* 2011;144(5):646–674. https://doi.org/10.1016/j.cell.2011.02.013.
9. Malumbres M, Barbacid M. Cell cycle, CDKs and cancer: a changing paradigm. *Nat Rev Cancer.* 2009;9(3):153–166. https://doi.org/10.1038/nrc2602.
10. Cancer Genome Atlas Network, Getz G, Chin L, Mills GB, Ingle JN. Comprehensive molecular portraits of human breast tumours. *Nature.* 2012;490(7418):61–70. https://doi.org/10.1038/nature11412.
11. Finn RS, Martin M, Rugo HS, et al. Palbociclib and letrozole in advanced breast cancer. *N Engl J Med.* 2016;375(20):1925–1936. https://doi.org/10.1056/NEJMoa1607303.
12. Hortobagyi GN, Stemmer SM, Burris HA, et al. Ribociclib as first-line therapy for HR-positive, advanced breast cancer. *N Engl J Med.* 2016;375(18):1738–1748. https://doi.org/10.1056/NEJMoa1609709.
13. Sledge GW, Toi M, Neven P, et al. MONARCH 2: abemaciclib in combination with fulvestrant in women with HR+/HER2- advanced breast cancer who had progressed while receiving endocrine therapy. *J Clin Oncol.* 2017;35(25):2875–2884. https://doi.org/10.1200/JCO.2017.73.7585.
14. Goetz MP, Toi M, Campone M, et al. MONARCH 3: abemaciclib as initial therapy for advanced breast cancer. *J Clin Oncol.* 2017;35(32):3638–3646. https://doi.org/10.1200/JCO.2017.75.6155.
15. Landis MW, Pawlyk BS, Li T, Sicinski P, Hinds PW. Cyclin D1-dependent kinase activity in murine development and mammary tumorigenesis. *Cancer Cell.* 2006;9(1):13–22. https://doi.org/10.1016/j.ccr.2005.12.019.
16. Yu Q, Sicinska E, Geng Y, et al. Requirement for CDK4 kinase function in breast cancer. *Cancer Cell.* 2006;9(1):23–32. https://doi.org/10.1016/j.ccr.2005.12.012.
17. Choi YJ, Li X, Hydbring P, et al. The requirement for cyclin D function in tumor maintenance. *Cancer Cell.* 2012;22(4):438–451. https://doi.org/10.1016/j.ccr.2012.09.015.
18. Finn RS, Dering J, Conklin D, et al. PD 0332991, a selective cyclin D kinase 4/6 inhibitor, preferentially inhibits proliferation of luminal estrogen receptor-positive human breast cancer cell lines in vitro. *Breast Cancer Res.* 2009;11(5):R77. https://doi.org/10.1186/bcr2419.
19. Goel S, Wang Q, Watt AC, et al. Overcoming therapeutic resistance in HER2-positive breast cancers with CDK4/6 inhibitors. *Cancer Cell.* 2016;29(3):255–269. https://doi.org/10.1016/j.ccell.2016.02.006.
20. Corona SP, Ravelli A, Cretella D, et al. CDK4/6 inhibitors in HER2-positive breast cancer. *Crit Rev Oncol Hematol.* 2017;112:208–214. https://doi.org/10.1016/j.critrevonc.2017.02.022.
21. Guerrero-Zotano A, Mayer IA, Arteaga CL. PI3K/AKT/mTOR: role in breast cancer progression, drug resistance, and treatment. *Cancer Metastasis Rev.* 2016;35(4):515–524. https://doi.org/10.1007/s10555-016-9637-x.
22. Utermark T, Rao T, Cheng H, et al. The p110α and p110β isoforms of PI3K play divergent roles in mammary gland development and tumorigenesis. *Genes Dev.* 2012;26(14):1573–1586. https://doi.org/10.1101/gad.191973.112.
23. Nagata Y, Lan K-H, Zhou X, et al. PTEN activation contributes to tumor inhibition by trastuzumab, and loss of PTEN predicts trastuzumab resistance in patients. *Cancer Cell.* 2004;6(2):117–127. https://doi.org/10.1016/j.ccr.2004.06.022.
24. Yakes FM, Chinratanalab W, Ritter CA, King W, Seelig S, Arteaga CL. Herceptin-induced inhibition of phosphatidylinositol-3 kinase and Akt Is required for antibody-mediated effects on p27, cyclin D1, and antitumor action. *Cancer Res.* 2002;62(14):4132–4141.
25. Berns K, Horlings HM, Hennessy BT, Madiredjo M. A functional genetic approach identifies the PI3K pathway as a major determinant of trastuzumab resistance in breast cancer. *Cancer Cell.* 2007;12(4):395–402. https://doi.org/10.1016/j.ccr.2007.08.030.
26. Chakrabarty A, Bhola NE, Sutton C, et al. Trastuzumab-resistant cells rely on a HER2-PI3K-FoxO-survivin axis and are sensitive to PI3K inhibitors. *Cancer Res.* 2013;73(3):1190–1200. https://doi.org/10.1158/0008-5472.CAN-12-2440.

27. Weigelt B, Warne PH, Downward J. PIK3CA mutation, but not PTEN loss of function, determines the sensitivity of breast cancer cells to mTOR inhibitory drugs. *Oncogene.* 2011;30(29):3222—3233. https://doi.org/10.1038/onc.2011.42.

28. Miller TW, Forbes JT, Shah C, et al. Inhibition of mammalian target of rapamycin is required for optimal antitumor effect of HER2 inhibitors against HER2-overexpressing cancer cells. *Clin Cancer Res.* 2009; 15(23):7266—7276. https://doi.org/10.1158/1078-0432. CCR-09-1665.

29. O'Reilly KE, Rojo F, She Q-B, et al. mTOR inhibition induces upstream receptor tyrosine kinase signaling and activates Akt. *Cancer Res.* 2006;66(3):1500—1508. https://doi.org/10.1158/0008-5472.CAN-05-2925.

30. García-García C, Ibrahim YH, Serra V, et al. Dual mTORC1/2 and HER2 blockade results in antitumor activity in preclinical models of breast cancer resistant to anti-HER2 therapy. *Clin Cancer Res.* 2012;18(9):2603—2612. https://doi.org/10.1158/1078-0432.CCR-11-2750.

31. O'Brien NA, McDonald K, Tong L, et al. Targeting PI3K/mTOR overcomes resistance to HER2-targeted therapy independent of feedback activation of AKT. *Clin Cancer Res.* 2014;20(13):3507—3520. https://doi.org/10.1158/1078-0432.CCR-13-2769.

32. Peddi PF, Hurvitz SA. PI3K pathway inhibitors for the treatment of brain metastases with a focus on HER2+ breast cancer. *J Neurooncol.* 2014;117(1):7—13. https://doi.org/10.1007/s11060-014-1369-6.

33. Baselga J, Cortés J, Im S-A, et al. Biomarker analyses in CLEOPATRA: a phase III, placebo-controlled study of pertuzumab in human epidermal growth factor receptor 2-positive, first-line metastatic breast cancer. *J Clin Oncol.* 2014;32(33):3753—3761. https://doi.org/10.1200/JCO.2013.54.5384.

34. Baselga J, Lewis Phillips GD, Verma S, et al. Relationship between tumor biomarkers and efficacy in EMILIA, a phase III study of trastuzumab emtansine in HER2-positive metastatic breast cancer. *Clin Cancer Res.* 2016;22(15):3755—3763. https://doi.org/10.1158/1078-0432.CCR-15-2499.

35. Perez EA, Dueck AC, McCullough AE, et al. Impact of PTEN protein expression on benefit from adjuvant trastuzumab in early-stage human epidermal growth factor receptor 2-positive breast cancer in the North Central Cancer Treatment Group N9831 trial. *J Clin Oncol.* 2013;31(17):2115—2122. https://doi.org/10.1200/JCO.2012.42.2642.

36. Pogue-Geile KL, Song N, Jeong J-H, et al. Intrinsic subtypes, PIK3CA mutation, and the degree of benefit from adjuvant trastuzumab in the NSABP B-31 trial. *J Clin Oncol.* 2015;33(12):1340—1347. https://doi.org/10.1200/JCO.2014.56.2439.

37. Yardley DA, Noguchi S, Pritchard KI, et al. Everolimus plus exemestane in postmenopausal patients with HR(+) breast cancer: BOLERO-2 final progression-free

survival analysis. *Adv Ther.* 2013;30(10):870—884. https://doi.org/10.1007/s12325-013-0060-1.

38. Wolff AC, Lazar AA, Bondarenko I, et al. Randomized phase III placebo-controlled trial of letrozole plus oral temsirolimus as first-line endocrine therapy in postmenopausal women with locally advanced or metastatic breast cancer. *J Clin Oncol.* 2013;31(2):195—202. https://doi.org/10.1200/JCO.2011.38.3331.

39. Andre F, O'Regan R, Ozguroglu M, et al. Everolimus for women with trastuzumab-resistant, HER2-positive, advanced breast cancer (BOLERO-3): a randomised, double-blind, placebo-controlled phase 3 trial. *Lancet Oncol.* 2014;15(6):580—591. https://doi.org/10.1016/S1470-2045(14)70138-X.

40. Hurvitz SA, Andre F, Jiang Z, et al. Combination of everolimus with trastuzumab plus paclitaxel as first-line treatment for patients with HER2-positive advanced breast cancer (BOLERO-1): a phase 3, randomised, double-blind, multicentre trial. *Lancet Oncol.* 2015;16(7):816—829. https://doi.org/10.1016/S1470-2045(15)00051-0.

41. Andre F, Hurvitz S, Fasolo A, et al. Molecular alterations and everolimus efficacy in human epidermal growth factor receptor 2-overexpressing metastatic breast cancers: combined exploratory biomarker analysis from BOLERO-1 and BOLERO-3. *J Clin Oncol.* 2016;34(18): 2115—2124. https://doi.org/10.1200/JCO.2015.63.9161.

42. Seiler M, Ray-Coquard I, Melichar B, et al. Oral ridaforolimus plus trastuzumab for patients with HER2+ trastuzumab-refractory metastatic breast cancer. *Clin Breast Cancer.* 2015;15(1):60—65. https://doi.org/10.1016/j.clbc.2014.07.008.

43. Hudis C, Swanton C, Janjigian YY, et al. A phase 1 study evaluating the combination of an allosteric AKT inhibitor (MK-2206) and trastuzumab in patients with HER2-positive solid tumors. *Breast Cancer Res.* 2013;15(6): R110. https://doi.org/10.1186/bcr3577.

44. Loibl S, la Peña de L, Nekljudova V, et al. Neoadjuvant buparlisib plus trastuzumab and paclitaxel for women with HER2+ primary breast cancer: a randomised, double-blind, placebo-controlled phase II trial (NeoPHOEBE). *Eur J Cancer.* 2017;85:133—145. https://doi.org/10.1016/j.ejca.2017.08.020.

45. Guerin M, Rezai K, Isambert N, et al. PIKHER2: a phase IB study evaluating buparlisib in combination with lapatinib in trastuzumab-resistant HER2-positive advanced breast cancer. *Eur J Cancer.* 2017;86:28—36. https://doi.org/10.1016/j.ejca.2017.08.025.

46. Saura C, Bendell J, Jerusalem G, et al. Phase Ib study of Buparlisib plus Trastuzumab in patients with HER2-positive advanced or metastatic breast cancer that has progressed on Trastuzumab-based therapy. *Clin Cancer Res.* 2014;20(7):1935—1945. https://doi.org/10.1158/1078-0432.CCR-13-1070.

47. De Palma M, Biziato D, Petrova TV. Microenvironmental regulation of tumour angiogenesis. *Nat Rev Cancer.* 2017; 17(8):457—474. https://doi.org/10.1038/nrc.2017.51.

48. Wen X-F, Yang G, Mao W, et al. HER2 signaling modulates the equilibrium between pro- and antiangiogenic factors via distinct pathways: implications for HER2-targeted antibody therapy. *Oncogene.* 2006;25(52):6986–6996. https://doi.org/10.1038/sj.onc.1209685.

49. Konecny GE, Meng YG, Untch M, et al. Association between HER-2/*neu* and vascular endothelial growth factor expression predicts clinical outcome in primary breast cancer patients. *Clin Cancer Res.* 2004;10(5):1706–1716. https://doi.org/10.1158/1078-0432.CCR-0951-3.

50. Linderholm B, Andersson J, Lindh B, et al. Overexpression of c-erbB-2 is related to a higher expression of vascular endothelial growth factor (VEGF) and constitutes an independent prognostic factor in primary node-positive breast cancer after adjuvant systemic treatment. *Eur J Cancer.* 2004;40(1):33–42. https://doi.org/10.1016/S0959-8049(03)00673-7.

51. Le X-F, Mao W, Lu C, et al. Specific blockade of VEGF and HER2 pathways results in greater growth inhibition of breast cancer xenografts that overexpress HER2. *Cell Cycle.* 2008;7(23):3747–3758. https://doi.org/10.4161/cc.7.23.7212.

52. Martin M, Makhson A, Gligorov J, et al. Phase II study of bevacizumab in combination with trastuzumab and capecitabine as first-line treatment for HER-2-positive locally recurrent or metastatic breast cancer. *Oncologist.* 2012;17(4):469–475. https://doi.org/10.1634/theoncologist.2011-0344.

53. Schwartzberg LS, Badarinath S, Keaton MR, Childs BH. Phase II multicenter study of docetaxel and bevacizumab with or without trastuzumab as first-line treatment for patients with metastatic breast cancer. *Clin Breast Cancer.* 2014;14(3):161–168. https://doi.org/10.1016/j.clbc.2013.12.003.

54. Zhao M, Pan X, Layman R, et al. A Phase II study of bevacizumab in combination with trastuzumab and docetaxel in HER2 positive metastatic breast cancer. *Invest New Drugs.* 2014;32(6):1285–1294. https://doi.org/10.1007/s10637-014-0122-5.

55. Gianni L, Romieu GH, Lichinitser M, et al. AVEREL: a randomized phase III Trial evaluating bevacizumab in combination with docetaxel and trastuzumab as first-line therapy for HER2-positive locally recurrent/metastatic breast cancer. *J Clin Oncol.* 2013;31(14):1719–1725. https://doi.org/10.1200/JCO.2012.44.7912.

56. Arteaga CL, Mayer IA, O'Neill AM, et al. A randomized phase III double-blinded placebo-controlled trial of first-line chemotherapy and trastuzumab with or without bevacizumab for patients with HER2/neu-overexpressing metastatic breast cancer (HER2+ MBC): a trial of the Eastern Cooperative Oncology Group (E1105). *J Clin Oncol.* 2012;30(suppl 15):605. https://doi.org/10.1200/jco.2012.30.15_suppl.605.

57. Hurvitz SA, Pegram M, Lin L, et al. Final results of a phase II trial evaluating trastuzumab and bevacizumab as first line treatment of HER2-amplified advanced breast cancer. *Cancer Res.* 2009;69(suppl 24):6094. https://doi.org/10.1158/0008-5472.SABCS-09-6094.

58. Drooger JC, van Tinteren H, de Groot SM, et al. A randomized phase 2 study exploring the role of bevacizumab and a chemotherapy-free approach in HER2-positive metastatic breast cancer: the HAT study (BOOG 2008-2003), a Dutch Breast Cancer Research Group trial. *Cancer.* 2016;122(19):2961–2970. https://doi.org/10.1002/cncr.30141.

59. Rugo HS, Chien AJ, Franco SX, et al. A phase II study of lapatinib and bevacizumab as treatment for HER2-overexpressing metastatic breast cancer. *Breast Cancer Res Treat.* 2012;134(1):13–20. https://doi.org/10.1007/s10549-011-1918-z.

60. Sideras K, Dueck AC, Hobday TJ, et al. North central cancer treatment group (NCCTG) N0537: phase II trial of VEGF-trap in patients with metastatic breast cancer previously treated with an anthracycline and/or a taxane. *Clin Breast Cancer.* 2012;12(6):387–391. https://doi.org/10.1016/j.clbc.2012.09.007.

61. Moreno-Aspitia A, Morton RF, Hillman DW, et al. Phase II trial of sorafenib in patients with metastatic breast cancer previously exposed to anthracyclines or taxanes: North Central Cancer Treatment Group and Mayo Clinic Trial N0336. *J Clin Oncol.* 2009;27(1):11–15. https://doi.org/10.1200/JCO.2007.15.5242.

62. Burstein HJ, Elias AD, Rugo HS, et al. Phase II study of sunitinib malate, an oral multitargeted tyrosine kinase inhibitor, in patients with metastatic breast cancer previously treated with an anthracycline and a taxane. *J Clin Oncol.* 2008;26(11):1810–1816. https://doi.org/10.1200/JCO.2007.14.5375.

63. Cardoso F, Canon J-L, Amadori D, et al. An exploratory study of sunitinib in combination with docetaxel and trastuzumab as first-line therapy for HER2-positive metastatic breast cancer. *Breast.* 2012;21(6):716–723. https://doi.org/10.1016/j.breast.2012.09.002.

64. Bachelot T, Garcia-Saenz JA, Verma S, et al. Sunitinib in combination with trastuzumab for the treatment of advanced breast cancer: activity and safety results from a phase II study. *BMC Cancer.* 2014;14(1):166. https://doi.org/10.1186/1471-2407-14-166.

65. Cristofanilli M, Johnston SRD, Manikhas A, et al. A randomized phase II study of lapatinib + pazopanib versus lapatinib in patients with HER2+ inflammatory breast cancer. *Breast Cancer Res Treat.* 2013;137(2):471–482. https://doi.org/10.1007/s10549-012-2369-x.

66. Johnston SRD, Gómez H, Stemmer SM, et al. A randomized and open-label trial evaluating the addition of pazopanib to lapatinib as first-line therapy in patients with HER2-positive advanced breast cancer. *Breast Cancer Res Treat.* 2013;137(3):755–766. https://doi.org/10.1007/s10549-012-2399-4.

67. Smith JW, Buyse ME, Rastogi P, et al. Epirubicin with cyclophosphamide followed by docetaxel with trastuzumab and bevacizumab as neoadjuvant therapy for HER2-positive locally advanced breast cancer or as adjuvant therapy for HER2-positive pathologic stage III breast cancer: a phase II trial of the NSABP Foundation Research Group, FB-5. *Clin Breast Cancer.* 2017;17(1):48–54.e3. https://doi.org/10.1016/j.clbc.2016.07.008.

68. Slamon DJ, Swain SM, Buyse M, et al. Primary Results from BETH, a Phase 3 Controlled Study of Adjuvant Chemotherapy and Trastuzumab ± Bevacizumab in Patients with HER2-positive, Node-positive or High Risk Node-negative Breast Cancer; 2013. http://www.abstracts2view.com/sabcs13/view.php?nu=SABCS13L_875&terms=.

69. Yardley DA, Raefsky E, Castillo R, et al. Phase II study of neoadjuvant weekly nab-paclitaxel and carboplatin, with bevacizumab and trastuzumab, as treatment for women with locally advanced HER2+ breast cancer. *Clin Breast Cancer*. 2011;11(5):297–305. https://doi.org/10.1016/j.clbc.2011.04.002.

70. Coudert B, Pierga J-Y, Mouret-Reynier M-A, et al. Use of [(18)F]-FDG PET to predict response to neoadjuvant trastuzumab and docetaxel in patients with HER2-positive breast cancer, and addition of bevacizumab to neoadjuvant trastuzumab and docetaxel in [(18)F]-FDG PET-predicted non-responders (AVATAXHER): an open-label, randomised phase 2 trial. *Lancet Oncol*. 2014;15(13):1493–1502. https://doi.org/10.1016/S1470-2045(14)70475-9.

71. Ritter CA, Perez-Torres M, Rinehart C, Guix M. Human breast cancer cells selected for resistance to trastuzumab in vivo overexpression epidermal growth factor receptor and ErbB ligands and remain dependent on the ErbB receptor network. *Clin Cancer Res*. 2007;13(16):4909–4919. https://doi.org/10.1158/1078-0432.CCR-07-0701.

72. Dua R, Zhang J, Nhonthachit P, Penuel E, Petropoulos C, Parry G. EGFR over-expression and activation in high HER2, ER negative breast cancer cell line induces trastuzumab resistance. *Breast Cancer Res Treat*. 2010;122(3):685–697. https://doi.org/10.1007/s10549-009-0592-x.

73. Arpino G, Gutierrez C, Weiss H, et al. Treatment of human epidermal growth factor receptor 2-overexpressing breast cancer xenografts with multiagent HER-targeted therapy. *JNCI J Natl Cancer Inst*. 2007;99(9):694–705. https://doi.org/10.1093/jnci/djk151.

74. Cheng H, Ballman K, Vassilakopoulou M, et al. EGFR expression is associated with decreased benefit from trastuzumab in the NCCTG N9831 (Alliance) trial. *Br J Cancer*. 2014;111(6):1065–1071. https://doi.org/10.1038/bjc.2014.442.

75. Cameron D, Casey M, Oliva C, Newstat B, Imwalle B, Geyer CE. Lapatinib plus capecitabine in women with HER-2-positive advanced breast cancer: final survival analysis of a phase III randomized trial. *Oncologist*. 2010;15(9):924–934. https://doi.org/10.1634/theoncologist.2009-0181.

76. Diéras V, Miles D, Verma S, et al. Trastuzumab emtansine versus capecitabine plus lapatinib in patients with previously treated HER2-positive advanced breast cancer (EMILIA): a descriptive analysis of final overall survival results from a randomised, open-label, phase 3 trial. *Lancet Oncol*. 2017;18(6):732–742. https://doi.org/10.1016/S1470-2045(17)30312-1.

77. Gelmon KA, Boyle FM, Kaufman B, et al. Lapatinib or trastuzumab plus taxane therapy for human epidermal growth factor receptor 2-positive advanced breast cancer: final results of NCIC CTG MA.31. *J Clin Oncol*. 2015;33(14):1574–1583. https://doi.org/10.1200/JCO.2014.56.9590.

78. Crown J, Kennedy MJ, Tresca P, et al. Optimally tolerated dose of lapatinib in combination with docetaxel plus trastuzumab in first-line treatment of HER2-positive metastatic breast cancer. *Ann Oncol*. 2013;24(8):2005–2011. https://doi.org/10.1093/annonc/mdt222.

79. Esteva FJ, Franco SX, Hagan MK, et al. An open-label safety study of lapatinib plus trastuzumab plus paclitaxel in first-line HER2-positive metastatic breast cancer. *Oncologist*. 2013;18(6):661–666. https://doi.org/10.1634/theoncologist.2012-0129.

80. Blackwell KL, Burstein HJ, Storniolo AM, et al. Overall survival benefit with lapatinib in combination with trastuzumab for patients with human epidermal growth factor receptor 2-positive metastatic breast cancer: final results from the EGF104900 Study. *J Clin Oncol*. 2012;30(21):2585–2592. https://doi.org/10.1200/JCO.2011.35.6725.

81. Lin NU, Guo H, Yap JT, et al. Phase II study of lapatinib in combination with trastuzumab in patients with human epidermal growth factor receptor 2-positive metastatic breast cancer: clinical outcomes and predictive value of early [18F]Fluorodeoxyglucose positron emission tomography imaging (TBCRC 003). *J Clin Oncol*. 2015;33(24):2623–2631. https://doi.org/10.1200/JCO.2014.60.0353.

82. Vogel CL, Cobleigh MA, Tripathy D, et al. Efficacy and safety of trastuzumab as a single agent in first-line treatment of HER2-overexpressing metastatic breast cancer. *J Clin Oncol*. 2002;20(3):719–726. https://doi.org/10.1200/JCO.2002.20.3.719.

83. Bachelot T, Romieu G, Campone M, et al. Lapatinib plus capecitabine in patients with previously untreated brain metastases from HER2-positive metastatic breast cancer (LANDSCAPE): a single-group phase 2 study. *Lancet Oncol*. 2013;14(1):64–71. https://doi.org/10.1016/S1470-2045(12)70432-1.

84. Lin NU, Diéras V, Paul D, et al. Multicenter phase II study of lapatinib in patients with brain metastases from HER2-positive breast cancer. *Clin Cancer Res*. 2009;15(4):1452–1459. https://doi.org/10.1158/1078-0432.CCR-08-1080.

85. Burstein HJ, Sun Y, Dirix LY, et al. Neratinib, an irreversible ErbB receptor tyrosine kinase inhibitor, in patients with advanced ErbB2-positive breast cancer. *J Clin Oncol*. 2010;28(8):1301–1307. https://doi.org/10.1200/JCO.2009.25.8707.

86. Martin M, Bonneterre J, Geyer CE, et al. A phase two randomised trial of neratinib monotherapy versus lapatinib plus capecitabine combination therapy in patients with HER2+ advanced breast cancer. *Eur J Cancer*. 2013;49(18):3763–3772. https://doi.org/10.1016/j.ejca.2013.07.142.

87. Swaby R, Blackwell K, Jiang Z, et al. Neratinib in combination with trastuzumab for the treatment of advanced breast cancer: a phase I/II study. *J Clin Oncol.* 2009;27(15S):1004. https://doi.org/10.1200/jco.2009.27.15s.1004.

88. Jankowitz RC, Abraham J, Tan AR, et al. Safety and efficacy of neratinib in combination with weekly paclitaxel and trastuzumab in women with metastatic HER2-positive breast cancer: an NSABP Foundation Research Program phase I study. *Cancer Chemother Pharmacol.* 2013;72(6):1205–1212. https://doi.org/10.1007/s00280-013-2262-2.

89. Awada A, Dirix L, Manso Sanchez L, et al. Safety and efficacy of neratinib (HKI-272) plus vinorelbine in the treatment of patients with ErbB2-positive metastatic breast cancer pretreated with anti-HER2 therapy. *Ann Oncol.* 2012;24(1):109–116. https://doi.org/10.1093/annonc/mds284.

90. Saura C, Garcia-Saenz JA, Xu B, et al. Safety and efficacy of neratinib in combination with capecitabine in patients with metastatic human epidermal growth factor receptor 2-positive breast cancer. *J Clin Oncol.* 2014;32(32):3626–3633. https://doi.org/10.1200/JCO.2014.56.3809.

91. Awada A, Colomer R, Inoue K, et al. Neratinib plus paclitaxel vs trastuzumab plus paclitaxel in previously untreated metastatic ERBB2-positive breast cancer: the NEfERT-T randomized clinical trial. *JAMA Oncol.* 2016;2(12):1557–1564. https://doi.org/10.1001/jamaoncol.2016.0237.

92. Freedman RA, Gelman RS, Wefel JS, et al. Translational Breast Cancer Research Consortium (TBCRC) 022: a phase II trial of neratinib for patients with human epidermal growth factor receptor 2-positive breast cancer and brain metastases. *J Clin Oncol.* 2016;34(9):945–952. https://doi.org/10.1200/JCO.2015.63.0343.

93. Freedman RA, Gelman RS, Melisko ME, et al. TBCRC 022: phase II trial of neratinib + capecitabine for patients (Pts) with human epidermal growth factor receptor 2 (HER2+) breast cancer brain metastases (BCBM). *J Clin Oncol.* 2017;35(suppl 15):1005. https://doi.org/10.1200/JCO.2017.35.15_suppl.1005.

94. Lin NU, Winer EP, Wheatley D, et al. A phase II study of afatinib (BIBW 2992), an irreversible ErbB family blocker, in patients with HER2-positive metastatic breast cancer progressing after trastuzumab. *Breast Cancer Res Treat.* 2012;133(3):1057–1065. https://doi.org/10.1007/s10549-012-2003-y.

95. Harbeck N, Huang C-S, Hurvitz S, et al. Afatinib plus vinorelbine versus trastuzumab plus vinorelbine in patients with HER2-overexpressing metastatic breast cancer who had progressed on one previous trastuzumab treatment (LUX-Breast 1): an open-label, randomised, phase 3 trial. *Lancet Oncol.* 2016;17(3):357–366. https://doi.org/10.1016/S1470-2045(15)00540-9.

96. Cortés J, Diéras V, Ro J, et al. Afatinib alone or afatinib plus vinorelbine versus investigator's choice of treatment for HER2-positive breast cancer with progressive brain metastases after trastuzumab, lapatinib, or both (LUX-Breast 3): a randomised, open-label, multicentre, phase 2 trial. *Lancet Oncol.* 2015;16(16):1700–1710. https://doi.org/10.1016/S1470-2045(15)00373-3.

97. Piccart-Gebhart M, Holmes E, Baselga J, et al. Adjuvant lapatinib and trastuzumab for early human epidermal growth factor receptor 2-positive breast cancer: results from the randomized phase III adjuvant lapatinib and/or trastuzumab treatment optimization trial. *J Clin Oncol.* 2016;34(10):1034–1042. https://doi.org/10.1200/JCO.2015.62.1797.

98. Untch M, Loibl S, Bischoff J, et al. Lapatinib versus trastuzumab in combination with neoadjuvant anthracycline-taxane-based chemotherapy (GeparQuinto, GBG 44): a randomised phase 3 trial. *Lancet Oncol.* 2012;13(2):135–144. https://doi.org/10.1016/S1470-2045(11)70397-7.

99. Guarneri V, Frassoldati A, Bottini A, et al. Preoperative chemotherapy plus trastuzumab, lapatinib, or both in human epidermal growth factor receptor 2-positive operable breast cancer: results of the randomized phase II CHER-LOB study. *J Clin Oncol.* 2012;30(16):1989–1995. https://doi.org/10.1200/JCO.2011.39.0823.

100. Hurvitz SA, Miller JM, Dichmann R, et al. Abstract S1-02: final analysis of a phase II 3-arm randomized trial of neoadjuvant trastuzumab or lapatinib or the combination of trastuzumab and lapatinib, followed by six cycles of docetaxel and carboplatin with trastuzumab and/or lapatinib in patients with HER2+ breast cancer (TRIO-US B07). *Cancer Res.* 2014;73(suppl 24):S1–S02–S1–02. https://doi.org/10.1158/0008-5472.SABCS13-S1-02.

101. Holmes FA, Nagarwala YM, Espina VA, et al. Correlation of molecular effects and pathologic complete response to preoperative lapatinib and trastuzumab, separately and combined prior to neoadjuvant breast cancer chemotherapy. *J Clin Oncol.* 2011;29(suppl 15):506. https://doi.org/10.1200/jco.2011.29.15_suppl.506.

102. Rimawi MF, Mayer IA, Forero A, et al. Multicenter phase II study of neoadjuvant lapatinib and trastuzumab with hormonal therapy and without chemotherapy in patients with human epidermal growth factor receptor 2-overexpressing breast cancer: TBCRC 006. *J Clin Oncol.* 2013;31(14):1726–1731. https://doi.org/10.1200/JCO.2012.44.8027.

103. Rimawi MF, Niravath PA, Wang T, et al. Abstract S6-02: TBCRC023: a randomized multicenter phase II neoadjuvant trial of lapatinib plus trastuzumab, with endcorine therapy and without chemotherapy, for 12 vs. 24 weeks in patients with HER2 overexpressing breast cancer. *Cancer Res.* 2015;75(suppl 9):S6–S02–S6–02. https://doi.org/10.1158/1538-7445.SABCS14-S6-02.

104. Baselga J, Bradbury I, Eidtmann H, et al. Lapatinib with trastuzumab for HER2-positive early breast cancer (Neo-ALTTO): a randomised, open-label, multicentre, phase 3 trial. *Lancet.* 2012;379(9816):633–640. https://doi.org/10.1016/S0140-6736(11)61847-3.

105. Robidoux A, Tang G, Rastogi P, et al. Lapatinib as a component of neoadjuvant therapy for HER2-positive operable breast cancer (NSABP protocol B-41): an open-label, randomised phase 3 trial. *Lancet Oncol.* 2013;14(12): 1183—1192. https://doi.org/10.1016/S1470-2045(13) 70411-X.

106. Carey LA, Berry DA, Cirrincione CT, et al. Molecular heterogeneity and response to neoadjuvant human epidermal growth factor receptor 2 targeting in CALGB 40601, a randomized phase III trial of paclitaxel plus trastuzumab with or without lapatinib. *J Clin Oncol.* 2016;34(6):542—549. https://doi.org/10.1200/ JCO.2015.62.1268.

107. Chan A, Delaloge S, Holmes FA, et al. Neratinib after trastuzumab-based adjuvant therapy in patients with HER2-positive breast cancer (ExteNET): a multicentre, randomised, double-blind, placebo-controlled, phase 3 trial. *Lancet Oncol.* 2016;17(3):367—377. https://doi.org/ 10.1016/S1470-2045(15)00551-3.

108. Jacobs SA, Robidoux A, Garcia J, et al. Abstract PD5-04: NSABP FB-7: a phase II randomized trial evaluating neoadjuvant therapy with weekly paclitaxel (P) plus neratinib (N) or trastuzumab (T) or neratinib and trastuzumab (N+T) followed by doxorubicin and cyclophosphamide (AC) with postoperative T in women with locally advanced HER2-positive breast cancer. *Cancer Res.* 2016;76(suppl 4):PD5—04—PD5—04. https://doi.org/ 10.1158/1538-7445.SABCS15-PD5-04.

109. Park JW, Liu MC, Yee D, et al. Adaptive randomization of neratinib in early breast cancer. *N Engl J Med.* 2016;375(1): 11—22. https://doi.org/10.1056/NEJMoa1513750.

110. Hanusch C, Schneeweiss A, Loibl S, et al. Dual blockade with AFatinib and trastuzumab as NEoadjuvant treatment for patients with locally advanced or operable breast cancer receiving taxane-anthracycline containing chemotherapy-DAFNE (GBG-70). *Clin Cancer Res.* 2015;21(13): 2924—2931. https://doi.org/10.1158/1078-0432.CCR-14-2774.

111. Geyer CE, Forster J, Lindquist D, et al. Lapatinib plus capecitabine for HER2-positive advanced breast cancer. *N Engl J Med.* 2006;355(26):2733—2743. https:// doi.org/10.1056/NEJMoa064320.

112. Wong K-K, Fracasso PM, Bukowski RM, et al. A phase I study with neratinib (HKI-272), an irreversible pan ErbB receptor tyrosine kinase inhibitor, in patients with solid tumors. *Clin Cancer Res.* 2009;15(7):2552—2558. https://doi.org/10.1158/1078-0432.CCR-08-1978.

113. Lu Y, Zi X, Zhao Y, Mascarenhas D, Pollak M. Insulin-like growth factor-I receptor signaling and resistance to trastuzumab (Herceptin). *J Natl Cancer Inst.* 2001;93(24): 1852—1857.

114. Nahta R, Yuan LXH, Zhang B, Kobayashi R, Esteva FJ. Insulin-like growth factor-I receptor/human epidermal growth factor receptor 2 heterodimerization contributes to trastuzumab resistance of breast cancer cells. *Cancer Res.* 2005;65(23):11118—11128. https://doi.org/10.1158/ 0008-5472.CAN-04-3841.

115. Yerushalmi R, Gelmon KA, Leung S, et al. Insulin-like growth factor receptor (IGF-1R) in breast cancer subtypes. *Breast Cancer Res Treat.* 2012;132(1): 131—142. https://doi.org/10.1007/s10549-011-1529-8.

116. Harris LN, You F, Schnitt SJ, et al. Predictors of resistance to preoperative trastuzumab and vinorelbine for HER2-positive early breast cancer. *Clin Cancer Res.* 2007;13(4): 1198—1207. https://doi.org/10.1158/1078-0432.CCR-06-1304.

117. Shattuck DL, Miller JK, Carraway KL, Sweeney C. Met receptor contributes to trastuzumab resistance of Her2-overexpressing breast cancer cells. *Cancer Res.* 2008;39(7): 720—727. https://doi.org/10.1016/j.ctrv.2013.01.006.

118. Liu L, Shi H, Liu Y, et al. Synergistic effects of foretinib with HER-targeted agents in MET and HER1- or HER2-coactivated tumor cells. *Mol Cancer Ther.* 2011;10(3): 518—530. https://doi.org/10.1158/1535-7163.MCT-10-0698.

119. Minuti G, Cappuzzo F, Duchnowska R, et al. Increased MET and HGF gene copy numbers are associated with trastuzumab failure in HER2-positive metastatic breast cancer. *Br J Cancer.* 2012;107(5):793—799. https:// doi.org/10.1038/bjc.2012.335.

120. Hanker AB, Garrett JT, Estrada MV, et al. HER2-Overexpressing Breast Cancers Amplify FGFR Signaling upon Acquisition of Resistance to Dual Therapeutic Blockade of HER2. *Clin Cancer Res.* 2017;23(15): 4323—4334. https://doi.org/10.1158/1078-0432.CCR-16-2287.

121. Qu X, Wu Z, Dong W, et al. Update of IGF-1 receptor inhibitor (ganitumab, dalotuzumab, cixutumumab, teprotumumab and figitumumab) effects on cancer therapy. *Oncotarget.* 2017;8(17):29501—29518. https://doi.org/ 10.18632/oncotarget.15704.

122. Scagliotti GV, Novello S, Pawel von J. The emerging role of MET/HGF inhibitors in oncology. *Cancer Treat Rev.* 2013;39(7):793—801. https://doi.org/10.1016/ j.ctrv.2013.02.001.

123. Mo H-N, Liu P. Targeting MET in cancer therapy. *Chronic Dis Transl Med.* 2017;3(3):148—153. https://doi.org/ 10.1016/j.cdtm.2017.06.002.

124. Babina IS, Turner NC. Advances and challenges in targeting FGFR signalling in cancer. *Nat Rev Cancer.* 2017; 17(5):318—332. https://doi.org/10.1038/nrc.2017.8.

125. Musolino A, Campone M, Neven P, et al. Phase II, randomized, placebo-controlled study of dovitinib in combination with fulvestrant in postmenopausal patients with HR(+), HER2(-) breast cancer that had progressed during or after prior endocrine therapy. *Breast Cancer Res.* 2017;19(1):18. https://doi.org/10.1186/ s13058-017-0807-8.

126. Seckl M, Badman PD, Liu X, et al. RADICAL trial: a phase Ib/ IIa study to assess the safety and efficacy of AZD4547 in combination with either anastrozole or letrozole in ER positive breast cancer patients progressing on these aromatase inhibitors (AIs). *J Clin Oncol.* 2017;35(suppl 15):1059. https://doi.org/10.1200/JCO.2017.35.15_suppl.1059.

127. Andre F, Cortés J. Rationale for targeting fibroblast growth factor receptor signaling in breast cancer. *Breast Cancer Res Treat.* 2015;150(1):1–8. https://doi.org/10.1007/s10549-015-3301-y.

128. Ma H, Zhang T, Shen H, Cao H, Du J. The adverse events profile of anti-IGF-1R monoclonal antibodies in cancer therapy. *Br J Clin Pharmacol.* 2014;77(6):917–928. https://doi.org/10.1111/bcp.12228.

129. Dieras V, Campone M, Yardley DA, et al. Randomized, phase II, placebo-controlled trial of onartuzumab and/or bevacizumab in combination with weekly paclitaxel in patients with metastatic triple-negative breast cancer. *Ann Oncol.* 2015;26(9):1904–1910. https://doi.org/10.1093/annonc/mdv263.

130. Tolaney SM, Nechushtan H, Ron I-G, et al. Cabozantinib for metastatic breast carcinoma: results of a phase II placebo-controlled randomized discontinuation study. *Breast Cancer Res Treat.* 2016;160(2):305–312. https://doi.org/10.1007/s10549-016-4001-y.

131. Bianchini G, Gianni L. The immune system and response to HER2-targeted treatment in breast cancer. *Lancet Oncol.* 2014;15(2):e58–e68. https://doi.org/10.1016/S1470-2045(13)70477-7.

132. Ignatiadis M, Van den Eynden GG, Salgado R, et al. Tumor infiltrating lymphocytes before and after dual HER2 blockade in HER2-amplified early breast cancer: a TRYPHAENA substudy. *J Clin Oncol.* 2016;34(suppl 15):11507–11507. https://doi.org/10.1200/JCO.2016.34.15_suppl.11507.

133. Salgado R, Denkert C, Campbell C, et al. Tumor-infiltrating lymphocytes and associations with pathological complete response and event-free survival in HER2-positive early-stage breast cancer treated with lapatinib and trastuzumab: a secondary analysis of the NeoALTTO trial. *JAMA Oncol.* 2015;1(4):448–454. https://doi.org/10.1001/jamaoncol.2015.0830.

134. Luen SJ, Salgado R, Fox S, et al. Tumour-infiltrating lymphocytes in advanced HER2-positive breast cancer treated with pertuzumab or placebo in addition to trastuzumab and docetaxel: a retrospective analysis of the CLEOPATRA study. *Lancet Oncol.* 2017;18(1):52–62. https://doi.org/10.1016/S1470-2045(16)30631-3.

135. Disis ML, Wallace DR, Gooley TA, et al. Concurrent trastuzumab and HER2/neu-specific vaccination in patients with metastatic breast cancer. *J Clin Oncol.* 2009;27(28):4685–4692. https://doi.org/10.1200/JCO.2008.20.6789.

136. Milani A, Sangiolo D, Montemurro F, Aglietta M, Valabrega G. Active immunotherapy in HER2 overexpressing breast cancer: current status and future perspectives. *Ann Oncol.* 2013;24(7):1740–1748. https://doi.org/10.1093/annonc/mdt133.

137. Farmer H, McCabe N, Lord CJ, et al. Targeting the DNA repair defect in BRCA mutant cells as a therapeutic strategy. *Nature.* 2005;434(7035):917–921. https://doi.org/10.1038/nature03445.

138. Robson ME, Im S-A, Senkus E, et al. OlympiAD: phase III trial of olaparib monotherapy versus chemotherapy for patients (pts) with HER2-negative metastatic breast cancer (mBC) and a germline BRCAmutation (gBRCAm). *J Clin Oncol.* 2017;35(suppl 18):LBA4-LBA4. https://doi.org/10.1200/JCO.2017.35.18_suppl.LBA4.

139. Nowsheen S, Cooper T, Bonner JA, LoBuglio AF, Yang ES. HER2 overexpression renders human breast cancers sensitive to PARP inhibition independently of any defect in homologous recombination DNA repair. *Cancer Res.* 2012;72(18):4796–4806. https://doi.org/10.1158/0008-5472.CAN-12-1287.

140. Stanley J, Klepczyk L, Keene K, et al. PARP1 and phospho-p65 protein expression is increased in human HER2-positive breast cancers. *Breast Cancer Res Treat.* 2015;150(3):569–579. https://doi.org/10.1007/s10549-015-3359-6.

141. Chow LW-C, Xu B, Gupta S, et al. Combination neratinib (HKI-272) and paclitaxel therapy in patients with HER2-positive metastatic breast cancer. *Br J Cancer.* 2013;108(10):1985–1993. https://doi.org/10.1038/bjc.2013.178.

142. Gajria D, King T, Pannu H, et al. Abstract P5-18-04: tolerability and efficacy of targeting both mTOR and HER2 signaling in trastuzumab-refractory HER2+ metastatic breast cancer. *Cancer Res.* 2014;72(suppl 24):P5-P18-04-P5-18-04. https://doi.org/10.1158/0008-5472.SABCS12-P5-18-04.

CHAPTER 13

Harnessing the Immune System in HER2+ Disease

WILLIAM R. GWIN, III, MD • MARY L. (NORA) DISIS, MD

INTRODUCTION

The recognition of HER2 receptor overexpression in a subset of breast cancer patients and its persistence in disease that is refractory to HER2-directed therapy have driven an extensive effort by multiple investigators to induce immunity against the HER2 receptor itself. These efforts have principally focused on inducing HER2-specific immunity through vaccination using multiple vaccine platforms as well as cellular therapy. Unfortunately for our patients, there is evidence that during HER2+ oncogenesis, there is a significant stepwise loss of HER2-specific immune system activation. The highest levels of HER2-specific immunogenicity are reported in healthy individuals, decreased levels are noted in HER2+ ductal carcinoma in situ (DCIS), and the lowest levels are found in HER2+ invasive breast carcinoma.[1] The HER2-specific monoclonal antibody trastuzumab can partially restore this immunogenicity, which perhaps could be further augmented with HER2 vaccination.[2] Beyond directing the immune system to target HER2, additional therapeutic approaches are also being pursued to augment anticancer immunity. Th1 immunity is a critical component of antitumor immunity, as it represents an adaptive immune response that mediates a direct cytotoxic effect on tumor cells.[3] Approaches that have been investigated to stimulate Th1 immunity include augmenting natural killer (NK) cell function, suppressing Treg populations, vaccination against tumor-associated antigens (TAA), and targeting immune checkpoint molecules. In this chapter, we will describe the HER2+ tumor microenvironment and discuss immunomodulatory therapies for HER2+ breast cancer in a review of the prior, ongoing, and future immune therapeutic approaches in HER2+ breast cancer.

THE IMMUNE MILIEU OF HER2+ TUMORS

Interactions between the immune system and the tumor microenvironment are a relatively new and active area of research. To fully harness the immune system to combat cancer, it is necessary to consider the tumor microenvironment. In and around HER2+ breast cancer cells are tumor-infiltrating lymphocytes (TILs), HER2-specific CD4 T cells, NK cells, and immunosuppressive regulatory T cells (Treg) (Fig. 13.1). Some aspects of the tumor immune microenvironment are specific to HER2+ breast cancer, whereas other alterations are reported across multiple tumor types. Herein, we describe our current understanding of the adaptive immune system (i.e., T and B lymphocytes) in HER2+ breast tumors, followed by studies into the nature of the innate immune system (i.e., dendritic cells [DCs], NK cells, and macrophages).

The Adaptive Immune System: T Lymphocytes and B Lymphocytes

The adaptive immune system is composed of lymphocytes that create immunologic memory after an initial response to a specific pathogen, which leads to an enhanced, highly specific response to subsequent encounters with that pathogen. The immediate interaction of immune cells and malignant cells occurs both at the interface of normal and tumor tissue as well as within the tumor microenvironment itself. The role of TILs in disease prognosis has been the subject of significant debate, spurring recent analyses of TILs in large phase III studies with HER2+ breast cancer patients.[4,5] Investigations have continued to further define TILs, particularly the overall TIL content, TIL anatomic location, and TIL subtypes and their roles in prognosis (Table 13.1). In addition, more comprehensive approaches to TIL evaluation are being pursued in multiple tumor types. For example, the "Immunoscore" is a prognostic immune biomarker that quantitates the immune cell composition of the tumor microenvironment, specifically CD8+ and CD45RO+ T cells, and associates the resulting score with clinical survival endpoints in colorectal cancer.[6,7]

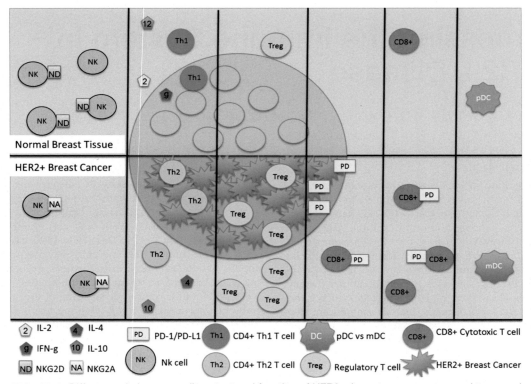

FIG. 13.1 Differences in immune cell content and function of HER2+ breast cancers compared to normal breast tissue. (1) Natural Killer cell (NK) function, in HER2+ breast cancer NK cells are inhibited through the upregulation of the NK cell inhibitory factor NKG2A and the down regulation of the activating factor NKG2D. (2) Th1 vs Th2 immune environment. In the HER2+ breast cancer microenvironment, CD4+Th2 T cells secrete IL-4 and IL-10 that suppress local anti-cancer immune responses. While normal breast tissue also contain CD4+Th1 T cells that secrete IL-2, INF-γ, among other cytokines capable of driving destructive immune responses. (3) Regulatory T cells (Tregs) are increased in HER2+ breast cancers. (4). Immune check point molecules, in some HER2+ breast cancers there is an upregulation of PD-1 and PD-L1 on both malignant and immune cells. (5) Dendritic cells, the presence of intratumoral monocytic dendritic cells (mDCs) are associated with HER2 over-expression while circulating plasmacytoid dendritic cells (pDCs) have been associated with improved survival.

In HER2+ breast cancer, we are working to understand how to incorporate immune biomarkers into a comprehensive assessment of the HER2+ breast cancer immune microenvironment.

Tumor-infiltrating lymphocytes predict response to chemotherapy and HER2-targeted therapy in HER2+ disease

In HER2+ breast cancer, the TIL content of the tumor microenvironment and its relationship with prognosis has been extensively studied. A recent review of 15 TIL studies in breast cancer (n = 13,914) revealed that most HER2+ breast cancers (n = 929) contain some degree of infiltrating lymphocytes (76%–89%), with lymphocyte-predominate disease (defined as >50%–60% TIL) noted in a minority of cases (11%–24%).[8] Clinically, a pathologic analysis of HER2+ breast cancers in the phase III studies GeparDuo and GeparTrio revealed a significant relationship between increasing TIL levels and pathologic complete response (pCR) to neoadjuvant chemotherapy.[4] Patients with lymphocyte-predominant HER2+ breast cancer (defined as tumors with >60% infiltrating lymphocytes in those studies) had a significantly higher rate of pCR than tumors with no TILs (31% vs. 4.3%, $P = .016$).[4] A retrospective analysis of the randomized, adjuvant trastuzumab FinHER study revealed a significant association between an increase in TILs and decreased distant metastasis-free

TABLE 13.1
Immune Biomarkers in HER2+ Breast Cancer

Immune Biomarker	Levels Associated With HER2+ Breast Cancer Cases	Association With Clinical Outcomes	References
ADAPTIVE IMMUNE RESPONSES			
CD8+ T cells (CTLs)	• Present in >60% • 52% with high CTL infiltrate • Associated with HER2 expression ($P < .001$)	• Improved survival ($P = .009$)	• Bailur et al.[26] • Mohammed et al.[97]
CD4+ helper T cells (Th1)	• Decreased levels through HER2 oncogenesis	• Increased levels associated with improved survival ($P = .002$)	• Datta et al.[1,92]
CD4+ helper T cells (Th2)	• Increased through HER2 oncogenesis	• Increased levels associated with decreased survival ($P = .002$)	• Datta et al.[1,92]
Regulatory T Cells (Tregs)	• Present in 70% • 65% classified as Treg high	• Shorter DFS (HR 3.13), OS (HR = 7.69), decreased pCR (OR = 0.15)	• Bense et al.[11]
PD-1/PD-L1	• 33% of HER2+/HR− • 28% of HER2+/HR+ Luminal B	• Worse OS (HR 3.68)	• Muenst et al.[16] • Qin et al.[21]
Dendritic cells (DCs)	• No evidence of decreased number of DCs	• Intratumoral pCD123+ DC associated with worse OS (58% vs. 93%) and shorter RFS (37% vs. 90%)	• Bailur et al.[26]
Natural killer cells (NK cells)	• Lower number of NK cells ($P < .05$)	• Activating factors associated with improved DMFS (89% vs. 42% ($P = .01$)	• Muraro et al.[31] • Mamessier et al.[32,33]
Macrophages and tumor-associated macrophages (TAMs)	• Increased CD163+ TAM ($P < .001$)	• CD68+ macrophages associated with worse BCa-specific survival ($P < .001$) and DFS ($P = .004$)	• Mahmoud et al.[40]
Mast cells	• No evidence of lower levels	• Presence associated with shorter DFS (HR = 5.85) and shorter OS (HR = 5.33)	• Bense et al.[11]
γδ T cells	• No evidence of lower levels	• Presence associated with prolonged OS (HR = 0.27) and higher pCR (OR = 1.55)	• Bense et al.[11]

survival (DMFS) in patients randomized to receive trastuzumab (2mg/kg, weekly) with each 10% increase in TIL being significantly[9] associated with an improvement in DMFS (P = .025). In a retrospective pathologic evaluation of the BIG 02-98 adjuvant chemotherapy trial, the relationship between quantity and location of stromal lymphocytic infiltration versus intratumoral lymphocytic infiltration was investigated. Analysis of HER2+ breast cancer cases from this trial revealed a significant relationship between increasing stromal lymphocytic infiltration (by 10% increments) and disease-free survival (DFS) and overall survival (OS) with anthracycline-based chemotherapy (DFS P = .042; OS P = .018).[5]

A type 1 (antitumor) immune environment is progressively lost during HER2 oncogenesis and replaced with a type 2 (tumor-tolerant) immune environment

In addition to the level and location of TIL infiltration, the content and functional nature of TILs and their relationship with disease progression has been investigated, specifically evaluating for Type 1 versus Type 2 immunity. Type 1 immunity involves the activation and propagation of CD4+ T-helper-1 (Th1) cells that create an antitumor immune response through the secretion of Type 1 cytokines, such as INF-γ. These cytokines, along with the presence of tumor antigens, activate antigen-presenting cells (APCs) (e.g., DCs), that in turn present the TAA to CD8+ cytotoxic T cells (CTLs), leading to the activation and propagation of the CTL to kill the tumor cells. In a systemic review of TILs in breast cancer by Stanton et al., 61% of HER2+ tumors contained at least one CD8+ T cell per high powered field (range 40%–83%) and 52% of HER2+ tumors were classified as having a high CD8+ T cell infiltrate.[8]

In HER2+ breast cancer, there is evidence of progressive loss of HER2-specific Th1 antitumor activity through the process of HER2 oncogenesis. HER2-negative breast cancer patients maintain anti-HER2 immune activation, whereas HER2+ DCIS demonstrates a statistically significant decrease in HER2-targeted CD4+ T cells (P < .0001), and there is an even lower level of HER2-specific T cells in invasive HER2+ breast cancer (P ≤ .001).[1] This loss of HER2-specific Th1 immunity was not due to defects in immune competence, T cell anergy, or increase in immunosuppressive phenotypes (i.e., Tregs) but rather due to a shift in antitumor Th1 activity to tumor-tolerant Th2 phenotypes.[1]

In contrast to the anticancer Th1 CD4+ T cells and CD8+ T cells involved in Type 1 antitumor immunity, a Type 2 immune environment contains CD4+ T-helper-2 (Th2) cells that secrete cytokines, such as IL-4, IL-6, and IL-10, which limit the acute inflammatory response and prevent the activation of CTL. This immune environment also involves the presence of other cell types that represent an immunosuppressive immune element within the tumor microenvironment, including CD4+CD25+FOXP3+ regulatory T cells (Treg) and myeloid-derived suppressor cells (MDSCs). Although only small numbers of HER2+ breast cancers have been evaluated for Tregs in clinical studies, 70% of evaluated HER2+ breast cancer cases contained a FOXP3+ infiltrate, with the majority of these cases (67%) classified as FOXP3+ high in Stanton et al.'s review.[8] A study in the adjuvant setting revealed that HER2+ breast cancers can be associated with the presence of FOXP3+ Tregs (P = .002) outside of the tumor beds in stromal lymphoid aggregates, and the presence of FOXP3+ Tregs in these lymphoid aggregates was associated with a shorter relapse-free survival (P = .025).[10] In another study of HER2+ breast cancer patients treated with neoadjuvant or adjuvant therapy, increased Tregs were associated with a lower pCR rate in response to neoadjuvant therapy (odds ratio [OR] = 0.15, 95% confidence interval [CI] 0.03–0.69), shorter DFS (hazard ratio [HR] = 3.13, 95% CI = 1.23–7.89), and shorter OS (HR = 7.69, 95% CI = 3.43–17.23).[11] Finally, the clinical relevance of circulating levels of Tregs in HER2+ breast cancer patients receiving trastuzumab (6mg/kg, 3 week cycles) reveals that progression-free survival (PFS) in metastatic patients was inversely related to the number of peripheral blood Tregs (area under the curve = 0.970, P = .004).[12]

Several studies have sought to define the relationship between clinical outcome in HER2+ breast cancer and comprehensive assessment of the immune environment through analysis of Th1- versus Th2-linked gene signatures as well as through evaluation of markers related to immune activation and immunosuppression. A study of gene expression data grouped into recognized Th1 and Th2 signaling pathways revealed that HER2+ tumors with low TGF-β (Th2) and high IL-12 (Th1) pathways had significantly better clinical outcome than with either activated pathway alone (HR = 0.19, CI 0.06–0.62, P = .002).[13] The mRNA analysis of tumor samples from the GeparSixto neoadjuvant study with taxane (Paclitaxel 80mg/m^{2}weekly) + anthracycline (Liposomal doxorubicin 30mg/m^2 weekly) ± platinum (Carboplatinum AUC 1.5 weekly) therapy revealed that an increased rate of pCR to neoadjuvant chemotherapy in HER2+ tumors was associated with an increase in immune activation markers CCL5 (P = .00,008), CXCL9 (P = .0001), CD8A (P = .002), IGKC

($P = .002$), and CD21 ($P = .001$), as well as an increase in immunosuppression markers PD-1 ($P = 0,003$), PDL-1 ($P = .00,002$), CTLA4 ($P = .001$), and FOXP3 ($P = .005$) by univariate analysis.[14] Prior studies have also reported positive clinical correlations of immunosuppressive markers,[15] and it is increasingly felt that immune factors (whether immune-activating or immunosuppressive) represent an "inflamed" tumor environment.

In regards to the role of the immunosuppressive PD-1/PD-L1 checkpoint expression in HER2+ breast cancers, a tissue microarray study evaluating the association between PD-L1 expression and intrinsic breast cancer subtype revealed PD-L1 expression in 28.8% of Luminal B HER2+ cases and 33.9% of HER2+ subtype cases compared with 30.7% of triple negative breast cancer (TNBC) cases with PD-L1 expression.[16] Another study of PD-L1 expression across all breast cancer subtypes (n = 465) revealed that high PD-L1 expression was significantly associated with HER2+ disease ($P = .003$) as well as high levels of TILs ($P < .001$).[17] A smaller analysis of 44 breast cancers revealed that expression of PD-L1 in TILs was also associated with HER2+ status ($P = .019$) and tumor lymphocyte infiltration ($P = .001$), among other parameters.[18] In this study, PD-L1 expression was present both on TILs as well as on tumor cells.

In addition to activated T cells, the expression of PD-L1 and PD-L2 has been reported on other immune cells, including monocytes and DCs.[19] In a study of 600+ breast cancer cases, the presence of PD-1+ TILs was associated with significantly worse OS in the Luminal B HER2+ subtype (HR = 3.689, $P < .001$).[16] In a tissue array analysis of >1000 breast cancers, PD-L1 was an independent indicator of poor prognosis in HER2+ breast cancers and was associated with shorter DFS (HR = 1.866, $P = .001$) and OS (HR = 1.517, $P = .036$). This is an area of ongoing investigation, as the prognostic significance of PD-L1 in HER2+ breast cancer is conflicting. Some reports suggest an association with improved survival,[17,20] whereas other reports suggest an association with worse clinical prognosis.[16,21] Interestingly, PD-L1 was detected in 60% of breast cancer patients treated with neoadjuvant chemotherapy but in only 37% of patients who had not received neoadjuvant chemotherapy,[22] suggesting that systemic therapy may upregulate this inhibitory signaling pathway.

As there has been extensive variation in the immune cell subtypes analyzed in HER2+ breast cancers, there is a need for the development and standardization of a comprehensive immune analysis program in HER2+ breast cancers.[23] As noted above, the "Immunoscore" was developed in colorectal cancer and is an example of a prognostic immune biomarker that quantitates the immune cell composition of the tumor microenvironment, specifically CD8+ and CD45RO+ T cells, and associates the resulting immune score with clinical survival endpoints.[6,7] A recent study has evaluated PD-L1 expression in HER2+ breast cancer patients (n = 167) using a similar concept and revealed that 53.3% of cases had either PD-L1 positivity in tumor cells or high levels of PD-L1 in TILs. A high PD-L1 Immunoscore in TILs and high total PD-L1 Immunoscore in tumor cells plus TILs was significantly associated with high histologic grade ($P < .001$), high TIL level ($P < .001$), an increased number of tertiary lymphoid structures around the invasive carcinoma ($P = .002$), and a better DFS rate in patients with hormone receptor-negative (HR−), HER2+ breast cancer ($P = .039$).[24] This being said, in HER2+ breast cancer, investigations are ongoing regarding how to incorporate immune biomarkers such as PD-L1, Tbet+ CD4+ T cells, and Tregs into a comprehensive assessment of the immune contexture of the HER2+ breast cancer immune microenvironment and how changes in this immune content may affect clinical endpoints.

The Innate Immune System in HER2+ Breast Cancer; Dendritic Cells, Natural Killer Cells, and Macrophages

The innate immune system evolutionarily developed as the first line of defense against infectious agents (e.g., bacteria and viruses) as well as for the removal of damaged and dead cells.[25] In contrast to the adaptive immune system, the innate immune system does not provide long-lasting immunity.

Dendritic cells in HER2+ breast cancer

DCs are APCs that act as messengers between the innate and adaptive immune system. Immature DCs sample the surrounding environment for pathogens such as viruses and bacteria. This is done through pattern recognition receptors such as the Toll-like receptors (TLRs). DCs transition from immature to active mature forms with antigen uptake, leading to their migration to activate T cells in local lymph nodes. DCs are typically either classified as monocytic dendritic cells (mDCs) (CD11c+) that produce IL-12 and TLR1-8 or classified as plasmacytoid dendritic cells (pDCs) (CD123+) that produce TNF-a and TLR-7/9.[26] A study evaluating the DC and T cell content of breast cancer tissues revealed that the intratumoral presence of CD3+ T cells and CD208 (DC-LAMP+) mDCs significantly correlated with HER2 overexpression ($P = .009$), although the presence of mDCs had no correlation with recurrence-free survival or OS.[27] This study also suggested that intratumoral CD123+ pDCs were associated with shorter OS (93% vs. 58% at 60 months) and relapse-free survival (90% vs. 37% at 60 months) across all breast cancer subtypes. In contradiction to this, another study demonstrated that a high level of circulating pDCs, along with low levels of immunosuppressive cells (Treg and MDSCs) and the presence of circulating HER2-specific CD8+ T cells, was associated with a significant improvement in survival across all breast cancer subtypes ($P = .009$).[26] The discrepancy between the level of pDC within the tumor and in the circulation may also reflect functional differences between pDCs found in the tumor microenvironment compared to those found systemically and warrants further investigation.

Natural killer cells are decreased and their function altered in HER2+ breast cancer

NK cells are innate immune cells that have the ability to distinguish normal from malignant cells.[28] In the context of cancer, NK cells become activated and subsequently target and eliminate malignant cells directly through the release of cytotoxic enzymes (e.g., granzymes) while simultaneously recruiting and activating other effector immune cells through the release of soluble factors such as cytokines.[29] NK cells have activating receptors (e.g., NKG2D, DNAM-1) and inhibitory receptors (e.g., NKG2A). NK cells also express the Fc immunoglobulin receptor CD16 (FcγRIII) that mediates antibody-dependent cellular cytotoxicity (ADCC), which is particularly relevant to the antitumor activity of the HER2-targeted monoclonal antibodies trastuzumab and pertuzumab.

In a study of the circulating immune cells in patients with various subtypes of locally advanced breast cancer, it was reported that among the CD3-cell populations, higher numbers of CD16+CD56+ NK cells were detected in HER2-negative cases compared with HER2+ patients ($P = .049$) and healthy donors ($P = .025$).[30] In a second study by the same research team, HER2+ cases showed lower percentages of NK cells at baseline ($P < .05$) and during neoadjuvant chemotherapy ($P < .05$) when compared to the HER2-negative group.[31] Interestingly, HER2+ patients were noted to have an increased percentage of NK cells with the NF-κB nuclear translocation, a marker of NK cell activation, during neoadjuvant chemotherapy with paclitaxel ($80mg/m^2$ weekly) and trastuzumab (2mg/kg, weekly) when compared with prechemotherapy levels ($P < .05$).[31] This is discussed further in the next section of this chapter.

A study that evaluated peripheral blood from patients with breast cancer of various subtypes (including HER2+) and at different stages of disease demonstrated changes in the NK cell phenotype with decreased mean fluorescence index (MFI) for NK cell-activating factors NKG2D ($P \leq .005$), DNAM-1 ($P < .05$), and CD16 ($P < .05$) and increased MFI for NK cell-inhibitory factors including NKG2A ($P \leq .005$). These changes were correlated with a decrease in NK cell degranulation ($P < .05$) and cytotoxicity ($P < .05$).[32] In another study of the level of NK cell activity across stages of HER2+ breast cancer, CD56+ NK cells exhibited a decrease in FcγRIII (CD16) expression in the adjuvant ($P = .006$) and metastatic ($P = .013$) settings. In this same study, peripheral blood NK cells from HER2+ breast cancer patients had decreased levels of activating receptors NKG2D ($P \leq .0005$), DNAM expression ($P \leq .0005$), and cytotoxicity receptor NKp30 ($P \leq .0005$) compared with controls.[33] Although the above evidence suggests that the activating factors are decreased on NK cells, an mRNA expression analysis has revealed that NK cell-activating ligands, specifically MICB (ligand for the activating factor NKG2D) ($P = .02$) and B7-H6 (ligand for the NKp46 receptor) ($P = .01$), were upregulated in the majority of HER2+ breast cancers.[33]

Preclinical models of HER2+ breast cancer (MMTV-Neu) have been evaluated to determine if altered NK cell function is tumor-specific or systemic. At the time of initial tumor development, the levels of NK cell activation receptors NKG2D and DNAM-1 were decreased in the tumor-infiltrating NK cells and peripheral blood NK cells within the same mice. Functional analysis of these tumor-derived NK cells and circulating NK cells in HER2+ tumor-bearing FVB-Neu mice also demonstrated decreased cytotoxicity when compared with controls ($P < .05$).[33]

Genomic analysis of NK-associated factors has demonstrated that HER2+ breast cancer cases associated with increased levels of NKG7 (NK Cell Granule Protein 7), among other lymphocyte-associated genes, had a long-term DMFS of 89% versus 42% ($P = .01$) when compared with HER2+ cases without this associated increase in lymphocyte-related genes.[34] Per Mamessier et al., the alterations found in NK cell receptors in breast cancer could be induced by the breast tumor microenvironment and have suggested that TGF-β1 is a potential causative agent, as it is a powerful inhibitor and has been found to be elevated in advanced breast tumors.[32] Accordingly, blocking TGF-β1 in mice suppresses the occurrence of metastases and restores NK cell activity.[35]

Macrophages and mast cells are immunosuppressive and associated with worse clinical outcome, whereas γδ T cells are associated with improved clinical outcome in HER2+ breast cancer

In evaluating other members of the innate immune system, several studies have evaluated the presence of tumor-associated macrophages, mast cells, and γδ T cells and their relationship to prognosis. Macrophages are phagocytes that engulf and digest cellular debris, foreign substances, microbes, cancer cells, and anything recognized as foreign or abnormal. M1 macrophages are proinflammatory and suppress tumor cells, unlike M2 macrophages, which are immunosuppressive and promote tumor growth[36,37] M2 macrophages express high levels of CD163, and this marker has been used to discriminate between M1 and M2 macrophages.[38] Tumor-associated macrophages resemble M2 macrophages in established tumors, contributing to tumor progression.[39] In a study of >250 breast cancer cases, high CD163 counts were strongly associated with Ki67-high tumors (upper quartile) (OR 5.4, $P < .001$) and positive HER2 status (OR 4.5, $P < .001$). In a study of >1000 breast cancer cases evaluated for the density of CD68+ macrophages (but without differentiating between M1 and M2), a higher total number of macrophages was associated with higher tumor grade (r(s) = 0.39, $P < .001$) and HER-2 positivity ($P < .001$). In addition, by univariate analysis, higher numbers of CD68+ macrophages were significantly associated with worse breast cancer–specific survival ($P < .001$) and shorter disease-free interval ($P = .004$).[40]

Mast cells are recognized to play a role in allergic reactions, but they are also involved in wound healing, defense against pathogens, and immune tolerance.[41] In nonmetastatic HER2+ breast cancer, a higher fraction of mast cells was associated with shorter DFS (HR = 5.85, 95% CI 2.20–15.54) and worse OS (HR = 5.33, 95% CI 2.04–13.91).[11] γδ T cells have been observed to accumulate in breast cancer TILs, have strong suppressive activities on responding T cells, and block the maturation and activities of DCs.[42] In this same study by Bense et al., an increased fraction of γδ T cells was associated with a higher pCR rate (OR = 1.55, 95% CI 1.01–2.38), prolonged DFS (HR = 0.68, 95% CI 0.48–0.98), and a prolonged OS (HR = 0.27, 95% CI 0.10–0.73).[11]

IMMUNOMODULATING EFFECTS OF HER2-TARGETED ANTIBODIES

A number of commonly used systemic therapies for HER2+ breast cancer are now recognized to have immunomodulatory properties, including trastuzumab, pertuzumab, taxane chemotherapies, and cyclophosphamide (Table 13.2).

TABLE 13.2
Systemic Therapies and Immune Effects in HER2+ Breast Cancer

Systemic Therapy	Immune Effects	References
Trastuzumab	• Antibody-dependent cellular cytotoxicity (ADCC) • Antibody-dependent cell-mediated phagocytosis • Increase HER2-specific Th1 immunity and decreases HER2-specific Th2 immunity	Arnould et al.[47], Lazar et al.[48] Petricevic et al.[12] Taylor et al.[51]
Pertuzumab	• ADCC	Scheuer et al.[65], Diessner et al.[66]
T-DM1	• ADCC	Juntilla et al.[98]
Taxanes	• Increase in serum Th1 cytokines levels • Increases NK cells • Depletes myeloid-derived suppressor cells • Promotes maturation of DCs	Tsavaris et al.[74] Miura et al.[77] Sevko et al.[72] Machiels et al.[76]
Cyclophosphamide	Low-dose cyclophosphamide: • Induces selective apoptosis of CD4+ Tregs • Enhances HER-2-specific antibody response Standard dose cyclophosphamide • Does not augment HER-2–specific antibody responses	Chen et al.[80]

HER2-Specific Monoclonal Antibody Therapy: Trastuzumab

The first major advance in the systemic clinical management of targeted therapy for HER2+ breast cancer was the development of the anti-HER2 monoclonal antibody trastuzumab.[43] Trastuzumab is a humanized IgG1 kappa monoclonal antibody that binds to domain IV of the HER2 receptor.[44] Trastuzumab was originally discovered through the screening of anti-HER2 monoclonal antibodies,[45] and development led to a humanized version of the murine antibody 4D5, now known as trastuzumab.[46] Although originally thought to function through passive immunization, the mechanisms behind trastuzumab's efficacy are now recognized to be much more complex. A key mechanism of anticancer activity of trastuzumab is ADCC,[47] in which the Fc portion of the monoclonal antibody trastuzumab engages with the FcγR on immune effector cells such as NK cells, stimulating the immune system to kill the tumor cells.[48]

Trastuzumab response and TILs

As was described previously, the pathologic analysis from the FinHER study of adjuvant chemotherapy ± trastuzumab (2mg/kg, weekly)[9] revealed a significant association between the increase in TILs and decreased distant disease-free survival (DDFS) in patients randomized to receive trastuzumab.[9] This study also noted that each 10% increase in TIL was significantly associated with an improvement in DDFS ($P = .025$). As the tumor microenvironment is critical to trastuzumab ADCC anticancer activity, investigators have evaluated whether the mere presence of TILs is sufficient or if a certain number of TILs predicts response to trastuzumab. In an analysis of the N9831 trial of adjuvant anthracycline (doxorubicin 60 mg/m^2 and cyclophosphamide 600 mg/m^2 every 3 weeks)/taxane (paclitaxel 80 mg/m^2 weekly) chemotherapy alone or this same chemotherapy with trastuzumab (2mg/kg, weekly), there was a significant interaction between treatment arm and lymphocyte-predominant breast cancer (LPBC) status ($P = .03$) as evaluated by stromal TILs (STILs). Interestingly, patients with LPBC tumors did not appear to derive any additional benefit from the addition of trastuzumab therapy (HR 2.43, 95% CI 0.58–10.22, $P = .22$). This is in contrast to patients with non-LPBC tumors, who appeared to derive benefit from the addition of trastuzumab (HR 0.49, 95% CI 0.35–0.69, $P < .001$) to chemotherapy.[49] This study suggests that patients with high levels of STILs found in LPBC did not benefit from the addition of trastuzumab, but this observation was limited by the small number of patients with LPBC in this study and thus warrants further investigation.

Trastuzumab may induce a stimulatory environment for TILs. Genomic biomarker analysis for pCR was performed on historical tumor tissue for 45 patients who had received neoadjuvant taxane (paclitaxel 80 mg/m^2 weekly)/anthracycline (FEC - 5-fluorouracil 500 mg/m^2, cyclophosphamide 500 mg/m^2, and epirubicin 75 mg/m^2) chemotherapy with or without trastuzumab. This investigation revealed that only one pathway, the CD40 signaling pathway (involving 64 genes out of 1275 distinct gene sets), revealed significant enrichment in patients who had received trastuzumab and had achieved a pCR compared with those receiving chemotherapy alone. The false discovery rate associated for this observation was 0.0022.[50]

Trastuzumab therapy increases HER2-specific Th1 immunity in HER2+ breast cancer

There is increasing evidence that trastuzumab may function to partially immunize against the HER2 receptor. In a small study of HER2+ breast cancer patients treated with trastuzumab based therapy, baseline anti-HER2 antibody immunity was detected in 29% of study patients. This percentage significantly increased to 56% ($P < .001$) after trastuzumab therapy. When evaluating HER2-specific T cell responses in this study, it was reported that 60% of trastuzumab-treated patients had an increase in their HER2-specific Th1 T cell responses after trastuzumab treatment. Interestingly, this HER2-specific T cell immunity persisted beyond the completion of trastuzumab therapy.[51]

In a retrospective evaluation of patients who had received neoadjuvant chemotherapy ± trastuzumab for their HER2+ breast cancer, the presence of T-bet+ lymphocytes (Th1) after neoadjuvant therapy was significantly increased in patients who received trastuzumab (2mg/kg weekly)-taxane (docetaxel 100 mg m^2 or docetaxel 75 mg m^2 + carboplatin AUC 6) chemotherapy compared with chemotherapy alone ($P = .0008$). In addition, the presence of T-bet+ lymphocytes in peritumoral lymphoid structures after neoadjuvant trastuzumab-containing therapy was independently associated with improved recurrence-free survival ($P = .04$).[52]

Trastuzumab mediates anticancer activity principally through antibody-dependent cellular cytotoxicity involving NK cells

Activation of ADCC has been described as a major mechanism of action mediating the anticancer activity of trastuzumab,[53–55] but there is a wide range of ADCC activity among HER2+ breast cancer patients.[56] Because NK cells are thought to mediate the highest level of ADCC in HER2+ breast cancers, alterations in

NK cell function have been the most widely reported mechanism to explain this variability.[56] In patients receiving neoadjuvant trastuzumab, for example, the efficiency of trastuzumab-dependent ADCC is mainly due to NK lytic efficiency.[57] In one neoadjuvant study, the level of ADCC at diagnosis (baseline) was slightly higher in patients who achieved a pCR (mean ± standard deviation [minimum − maximum value], 20.83 ± 18.00 [$4.33 - 72.54$]) compared with partial responders (16.63 ± 14.98 [$0.00 - 46.70$]), although this was not statistically significant. Interestingly, patients in this study who achieved a pCR also demonstrated a slight recovery of ADCC lysis, whereas partial responders demonstrated the opposite trend.[31]

There have been some conflicting data in the literature regarding the level of ADCC in HER2+ metastatic breast cancer treated with trastuzumab compared with the activity found in earlier stages of disease.[56] Petricevic et al. evaluated ADCC activity and antibody-dependent cell-mediated phagocytosis secondary to trastuzumab in patients undergoing trastuzumab-based treatment in the adjuvant and metastatic settings as well as from trastuzumab treatment–naïve patients. In comparison with healthy controls, ADCC activity was significantly depressed in the metastatic ($P = .002$), adjuvant ($P = .02$), and trastuzumab-naïve ($P < .001$) patient cohorts. In the adjuvant trastuzumab population, markers of this reduced ADCC activity were found to be inversely correlated with the expression of CD107a ($P = .034$), a degranulation marker indicating cytotoxic activation, on CD56+ NK cells. Of note, ADCC activity in these patient cohorts were similar, regardless of treatment duration or additional chemotherapy,[12] suggesting that trastuzumab stimulates ADCC in the metastatic setting as effectively as in the adjuvant setting.[12]

A small neoadjuvant clinical trial in HER2+ patients of chemotherapy (docetaxel 100 mg m² every three weeks) ± trastuzumab (2mg/kg weekly) demonstrated a significant increase in the number of NK cells ($P = .043$) and T cells expressing the activation marker Granzyme B (associated with cell lytic capability) ($P = .032$) in the tumors of patients treated with trastuzumab compared with tumors from patients receiving similar chemotherapy without trastuzumab.[47] Indeed, this has been supported by other studies that have reported a higher efficiency of ADCC and NK-mediated cell lysis in clinical responders to trastuzumab when compared with nonresponders.[57,58] Interestingly, neoadjuvant paclitaxel (80 mg/m² weekly)/trastuzumab (2mg/kg, weekly) treatment induced a significant increase in the number of NK cells independently of pathologic response (pCR or pathologic partial response [PR]) ($P < .05$).[31]

The interaction between trastuzumab and immune effector cells is mediated through the Fc domain on trastuzumab and the Fc γ receptor (FcγR) on effector cells. FcγRs are divided into activating and inhibitory groups. Some common single-nucleotide polymorphisms in the coding regions of the FcγR genes have been associated with differential antibody-binding affinities and functional outcomes.[54] Associations of FcγR gene polymorphisms with clinical response among trastuzumab-treated patients have been equivocal, some finding positive associations[54,59] with others finding no associations.[60] In a study by Musolino et al., patients who were prospectively treated with taxane + trastuzumab were evaluated for any association between FcγR polymorphisms and ADCC activity and clinical survival. The ADCC analysis showed that human peripheral blood mononuclear cells (PBMCs) with the FcγRIIIa-158 V/V genotype and/or FcγRIIa-131 H/H genotype had a significantly higher trastuzumab-mediated cytotoxicity than PBMCs harboring other genotypes (71% vs. 38%, $P = .04$). This study also demonstrated that the V/V and/or H/H genotypes were significantly correlated with objective response rate (ORR) (OR 8.7, 95% CI 1.4−53.8, $P = .02$) and PFS (HR 5.3, 95% CI 1.6−16.9, $P = .005$).[54] One of the larger retrospective trials to evaluate the role of Fcγ polymorphisms and clinical outcome after trastuzumab treatment in the N9831 trial found patients with genotypes *FCB3A-158V/V* or *FCB3A-158V/F* received greater clinical benefits from trastuzumab (HR 0.31, 95% CI 0.22−0.43; $P < .001$) than patients who were homozygous for the low-affinity allele (HR 0.71, 95% CI 0.51−1.01, $P = .05$).[61]

To explore if alterations of the Fc domain on trastuzumab might increase ADCC, Fc variant trastuzumab antibodies (Abs) have been tested in cell lines expressing low to amplified levels of HER2. Two specific variants, S239D_I332E and S239D_I332E_A330L, provided substantial ADCC enhancements over nonvariant trastuzumab across a broad range of antigen expression levels. In addition, at barely observable HER2 antigen expression (e.g., the MCF7 cell line), ADCC was improved using the variant Abs above the detectable threshold,[48] supporting the testing of such antibodies in HER2 low-expressing breast cancers.

Optimizing the Fc domain of a HER2 monoclonal antibody has now been translated into the clinical development of the monoclonal Ab margetuximab (MGAH22). Margetuximab was originally derived from the parent antibody of trastuzumab. Margetuximab and trastuzumab bind the same HER2 epitope with similar affinity and exhibit similar tumor-directed, effector cell-independent, antiproliferative activity in breast cancer cells in vitro in the absence of immune effectors.[62] However, the Fc domain of margetuximab was designed to increase binding to both isoforms of FcγRIIIA stimulatory receptors on NK cells and macrophages relative to trastuzumab.[62] In the phase I study of margetuximab in patients with treatment-refractory HER2-overexpressing malignancies, margetuximab mediated greater ex vivo ADCC activity compared with trastuzumab as indicated by lower EC_{50} and greater maximum cytotoxicity ($P < .0001$) in patient PBMCs. In addition, tumor reductions were observed in over half (18/23, 78%) of the response-evaluable patients with breast cancer, including durable (>30 weeks) responders.[63]

HER2-Specific Monoclonal Antibody Therapy: Pertuzumab

With the intent of developing additional anti-HER2 monoclonal antibodies, preclinical antibody screening found that the 2C4 monoclonal antibody bound to the dimerization domain of HER2 (domain II), providing the potential to prevent HER2-mediated cellular signaling by preventing homo- and heterodimerization. The variable region of 2C4 was cloned into a vector containing human κ and CH1 domains to construct a mouse-human chimeric antigen-binding fragment (Fab) and creating pertuzumab, a recombinant, humanized monoclonal IgG1 anti-HER2 antibody targeting the extracellular dimerization domain of the HER2 receptor.[64] Pertuzumab was developed clinically and is now FDA approved in HER2+ breast cancer. Similar to trastuzumab, preclinical studies have shown that pertuzumab induces ADCC against HER2-expressing cells and induces cell death.[65–67]

Pertuzumab mediates ADCC similar to trastuzumab and may augment ADCC when used in combination with trastuzumab

In preclinical models, both trastuzumab and pertuzumab effectively induce ADCC in HER2-overexpressing preclinical models,[65,66] although some data suggest that pertuzumab may be slightly less efficient at inducing ADCC.[67] Preclinical data are conflicting on whether there is an additive effect on the level of ADCC activity with trastuzumab/pertuzumab combination therapy. In one preclinical study, there was no increased ADCC activity with the combination of the two agents.[65] A separate preclinical study reported that the combined application of trastuzumab and pertuzumab antibodies in ADCC killing assays significantly improved target cell lysis through ADCC compared with the application of only one antibody ($P < .05$).[66] A study by Toth et al. offers a possible explanation for

this discrepancy: antibody dose-response curves of in vitro ADCC show that antibody-mediated killing can be saturated. Thus, the combination of trastuzumab and pertuzumab exerts an additive effect only at subsaturation doses. The additive effect in vivo indicates that therapeutic tissue levels likely do not saturate ADCC,[67] but there is a threshold at which raising the dose of antibody will yield no improvement in ADCC.

IMMUNE MODULATION WITH CYTOTOXIC THERAPY

Historically, chemotherapeutic agents were felt to be purely immunosuppressive. Recent evidence challenges this perception and supports that a number of chemotherapeutic agents have immunomodulating properties, most commonly through the induction of immunogenic cell death (ICD). Common chemotherapies used in HER2+ breast cancer management, including cyclophosphamide and the taxanes docetaxel and paclitaxel, are now recognized to possess immunomodulatory abilities as outlined below.

Taxanes and Immune Modulation in HER2+ Breast Cancer

Microtubule inhibitors such as taxane chemotherapies induce ICD through endoplasmic reticulum stress, leading to translocation of calreticulin to the plasma membrane, inducing immunomediated phagocytosis.[68] Subsequently, tumor antigens are presented by DCs,[69] leading to the augmentation of Type I immunity through increasing cytotoxic T cell infiltration.[70,71] The taxane paclitaxel also depletes MDSCs,[72] this is achieved through active metabolite accumulation in MDSCs.[73] A small clinical study in breast cancer patients evaluated the immune effects of taxanes and revealed that paclitaxel (200 mg/m^2 every three weeks) and docetaxel (100 mg m^2 every three weeks) therapies lead to an increase in serum Th1 cytokine levels when compared with control patients. Significant increases were noted in IFN-γ ($P < .0001$), IL-2 ($P < .0001$), IL-6 ($P = .007$), and granulocyte-macrophage colony-stimulating factor (GM-CSF) ($P = .001$) cytokines. In addition, enhanced activity was noted in NK and lymphocyte-activated killer cells. Both taxanes led to a decrease in the serum levels of IL-1 and TNF-α cytokines.[74] In preclinical studies, low-dose paclitaxel also promotes TLR4-dependent maturation of DCs in mice.[75] This DC maturation stimulates the CD4+ T-helper phenotype by increasing the type 1 (Th1) response while not affecting the Th2 response as measured by IFN-γ versus IL-4 enzyme-linked immunospot (ELISpot) and results in the secretion of proinflammatory cytokines, which enhances the priming and lytic activity of CD8+ T cells.[76]

In a small clinical study (n = 20) looking at the effects of paclitaxel on ADCC when given in combination with trastuzumab, patients were given either trastuzumab (2mg/kg, weekly) + paclitaxel (80 mg/m^2 weekly) or trastuzumab (2mg/kg, weekly) alone. The mean ADCC level increased 20% after trastuzumab monotherapy and 126% ($P < .05$) after combination therapy with trastuzumab and paclitaxel. All patients receiving combination therapy had increased ADCC levels. The number of NK cells increased by 51% after trastuzumab monotherapy and 112% ($P < .05$) after combination therapy.[77]

Cyclophosphamide

Cyclophosphamide is an option for systemic therapy in the adjuvant and neoadjuvant management of HER2+ breast cancers in combination with either a taxane or an anthracycline (e.g., doxorubicin, epirubicin). Cyclophosphamide has been extensively studied in regard to its ability to modulate the tumor immune environment, particularly at doses lower than those given clinically. Breast cancer patients receiving dose-dense therapy with doxorubicin (60 mg/m2) and cyclophosphamide (600 mg/m2) followed by Paclitaxel (175mg/m2 every three weeks) were noted to have a significant increase in circulating MDSCs when compared with baseline ($P < .00001$).[78] It has also been recognized that alternate dosing schedules of cyclophosphamide may have significantly different effects on the immune system. Clinical metronomic dosing of cyclophosphamide (50 mg orally, twice a day for one week on and one week off) has been reported to induce a significant decrease in circulating CD4+CD25+ Tregs ($P < .0001$), an effect which appeared to be selective for Tregs, as other T cell subtypes were not decreased. Interestingly, NK cell function (as measured by cytotoxicity) in these metronomically treated patients was significantly increased from baseline ($P = .01$) and to a level not significantly different from noncancer patients.[79] Low-dose cyclophosphamide given 1–3 days before antigen exposure overcomes systemic immune tolerance to enhance both antibody and T cell responses, whereas the same treatment given after or at the same time as antigen exposure induces antigen-specific tolerance.[80] In preclinical models, low-dose cyclophosphamide depletes Tregs, promotes DC maturation, shifts the CD4+ T-helper phenotype from Th2 to Th1, induces the differentiation of T-helper type 17 cells, and promotes the evolution of a durable CD44^{hi} T cell memory response through IFNα secretion. In addition, cyclophosphamide

doses of 200–300 mg/m^2 given 1 day prior to vaccination or 600 mg/m^2 given 7 days prior to vaccination can decrease Tregs.[79,81]

HER2 VACCINES

Cancer vaccines have been and continue to be developed to elicit Th1 tumor antigen-specific immune responses to augment existing immunity.[1] In breast cancer, the most common target for vaccination has been the HER2 receptor. The early development of HER2 cancer vaccines principally used peptide constructs that elicited primarily CD8+ cytotoxic T lymphocyte (CTL) immunity. The cancer vaccine approach to HER2+ breast cancer has evolved to include immune adjuvants such as GM-CSF and POLY-ICLC (an immune stimulant composed of carboxymethylcellulose, polyinosinic-polycytidylic acid, and poly-L-lysin double-stranded RNA), DNA-based vaccine strategies, and novel delivery platforms, including plasmid and viral vectors. HER2 vaccine strategies have been evaluated in the in situ, neoadjuvant, adjuvant, and metastatic settings.

Early HER2-targeted vaccines used HER2 peptide epitopes that activated CTLs. These approaches have been reported to induce HER2-specific CD8 T cell responses, yet these responses were short lived.[82] The desire to induce a long-lasting HER2-specific immunity led to the development of HER2 peptide vaccines that were able to activate both CD4+ and CD8+ T cells and induce a delayed-type hypersensitivity (CD4-mediated) as well as prolonged HER2-specific CD8+ T cell responses.[83,84] Of the peptide approaches, the E75 (NeuVax, nelipepimut-S) peptide vaccine, derived from the extracellular domain of HER2 and given with GM-CSF, is the most advanced in clinical testing. In the clinical testing of this vaccine as adjuvant therapy in breast cancer patients with any level of HER2 expression (immunohistochemistry [IHC] grade 1 to 3+), 5-year disease-free survival was increased in vaccinated patients versus unvaccinated patients (89.7% vs. 80.2%, $P = .08$).[85] There was a trend toward benefit in patients with low levels of HER2 expression (IHC 1 to 2+, FISH negative) with 5-year disease-free survival of 88.1% in the vaccinated patients and 77.5% in the unvaccinated ($P = .16$). This study also revealed that the NeuVax vaccine–induced epitope spreading to other epitopes within the HER2 molecule (intraantigen spreading) and to other TAA (interantigen spreading) decreased the levels of Tregs and the TGF-B cytokine, and increased the level of memory T cells.[85] Unfortunately, the phase III PRESENT trial of NeuVax in women with early-stage node-positive breast cancer with low-to-intermediate HER2 expression (HER2 1+ by IHC or HER2 2+ by IHC) was halted because of futility.

As noted above, there is evidence that trastuzumab functions to immunize a minority of patients against the HER2 protein, but induction of HER2-specific T cell immunity is variable.[2] Accordingly, vaccination against HER2 has been combined with trastuzumab as well as other systemic therapies with the intent of augmenting HER2-specific immunity and clinical responses. A trastuzumab plus vaccine strategy designed to elicit HER2-specific T-helper (Th) immunity was used in a small trial of HER2+ breast cancer patients with minimal residual disease after neoadjuvant therapy. In this study, HER2 vaccination combined with trastuzumab augmented HER2-specific CTL immunity in the majority of patients (84%) and induced epitope spreading in the majority of patients (74%). Interestingly, the greater the HER2 intramolecular epitope spreading T cell response, the greater the decrease in serum TGF-β ($r = 0.614$; $P = 0.0003$).[2] Another study combining HER2 vaccination with the VRP-HER2 vaccine with HER2-directed therapy also highlights the use of viral vectors to deliver DNA sequences of HER2 using alphavirus-like replicon particles (VRP).[86] This construct is based on the attenuated Venezuelan equine encephalitis virus, which highly expresses heterologous proteins, targets expression to DCs, and induces robust humoral and cellular immune responses against the vectored gene products.[87,88] Analysis to date of this study demonstrates that this combination is well tolerated and that combination of trastuzumab and VRP-HER2 augmented HER2-specific immunity. Clinical follow-up to date is greater than 26 months in this heavily pretreated metastatic population and has not met median OS.[89]

Cell-based vaccine therapies include those containing autologous APCs that are pulsed with a tumor antigen ex vivo. Lapuleucel-T is a cell-based therapeutic derived from autologous APCs loaded with extensive recombinant HER2 sequences (HER500) linked to a GM-CSF domain. Treatment with lapuleucel-T was associated with a significant increase in IFN-γ ELISPOT response to HER2 antigens at week 8 (median 16 spots/ 3×10^5 PBMC; $P = .0010$) compared with baseline (median 0.0 spots/3×10^5 PBMC). In this study, clinical response was limited with one patient having a partial response and three patients having stable disease (SD) for >1 year.[90]

Another phase I study evaluated the feasibility of expanding HER2 vaccine-primed peripheral blood T cells ex vivo and the safety of infusing these primed T cells. HER2-specific T cells significantly increased in vivo compared with preinfusion levels ($P = .010$) and persisted in 4/6 patients (66%) over 70 days after the first infusion. Partial clinical responses were observed in 43% of patients.[91]

In a pilot study in the adjuvant setting, patients who did not achieve a pCR to neoadjuvant chemotherapy + trastuzumab received adjuvant HER2-pulsed type 1-polarized dendritic cell (DC1) vaccination. The DC1 vaccine platform has been developed to be rapidly activated from peripheral blood monocytes using INF-γ and lipopolysaccharide (LPS, a TLR 4 agonist) to induce mature DCs that express high levels of costimulatory molecules and substantial amounts of IL-12. Immunogenicity against HER2 was improved in DC1-treated patients following HER2-pulsed DC1 vaccination.[92]

IMMUNE CHECKPOINT BLOCKADE

An area of increased investigation in all breast cancer subtypes is the immunomodulatory and therapeutic role of the immune checkpoint molecules CTLA-4, PD-1, and PD-L1. CTLA-4 functions by downregulating immune responses. It is constitutively expressed in Tregs but only upregulated on conventional T cells after activation. PD-1 and its ligand PD-L1 are members of the CD28/CTL-4 signaling family and function as a negative regulatory pathway on T cell function after their activation by antigen.[16] Monoclonal Abs targeting these checkpoints have demonstrated clinical benefits and have received FDA approval in melanoma, non–small cell lung cancer, renal cell carcinoma, and bladder cancer, among others.

PD-1 and PD-L1 are expressed in a significant number of HER2+ breast cancers, supporting the clinical testing of PD-1 and PD-L1 monoclonal antibodies in HER2+ breast cancer. The challenge has been in predicting which patients will respond to these therapies, as the use of PD-L1 IHC as a predictive biomarker has not been reliable because of multiple issues, including variability among the available detection antibodies, no consensus regarding the IHC cut off for PD-L1 positivity, and variability in tissue preparation and processing. In the JAVELIN study of the anti-PD-L1 monoclonal antibody avelumab (10 mg/kg intravenously every 2 weeks), there were no partial or complete responses in HER2+ patients (n = 26), two responses among the hormone-receptor positive HER2-negative cohort (n = 72), and three among the TNBC patients (n = 58). The preliminary correlative studies from this clinical trial suggested that PD-L1 expression of 10% or greater by tumor-associated immune cells was uncommon (8.8% of the

136 patients) but was associated with a higher response rate (16.7% vs. 1.6%).[93]

Combining trastuzumab with anti-PD-1 antibodies showed greater tumor regression in mouse models of HER2+ mammary tumors compared with either antibody alone ($P = .0097$).[94] It has also recently been demonstrated in breast cancer–bearing mice that a combination regimen of an anti-PD-1 antibody and a multipeptide vaccine derived from breast cancer antigens, including HER2, prolonged the vaccine-induced PFS period and increased the median survival by nearly threefold when compared with vaccine alone ($P = .0002$). This research also demonstrated that PD-1 blockade enhances breast cancer vaccine efficacy by altering both CD8 T cell and DC components of the tumor microenvironment.[95]

Interestingly, the addition of trastuzumab has been reported to upregulate PD-1/PD-L1 on the cell surface. The ongoing phase Ib/II PANACEA clinical trial of pembrolizumab (200mg) + trastuzumab (6mg/kg) every three weeks in HER2+ breast cancer patients who have progressed on prior trastuzumab was reported at the San Antonio Breast Cancer Symposium in 2017. In the PD-L1-positive intention-to-treat population, the trial met its primary endpoint with an ORR of 15% and disease control rate of 25%. In PD-L1-positive patients with 5% or more TILs present in the metastatic lesion, the ORR was 39% and the disease control rate was 47%, suggesting that quantification of TILs may help identify patients who will most benefit from this treatment. No clinical responses were observed in the PD-L1–negative cohort.[96]

CONCLUSION

HER2+ breast cancer is immunogenic and possesses a unique immune phenotype. The progressive loss of HER2-specific Th1 immunity noted through each step of HER2 oncogenesis highlights an immune escape mechanism used by HER2+ breast cancers. Countering this, trastuzumab seems to partially restore this HER2-specific immunity, and ongoing vaccine studies have illustrated a potential to further augment this HER2-specific immunity. In addition, the stromal TIL, and particularly its content of immunostimulatory and immunosuppressive cells, is predictive of response to both systemic chemotherapy and HER2-directed therapy and holds the potential to predict response to additional immunomodulatory therapies currently under development.

REFERENCES

1. Datta J, Rosemblit C, Berk E, et al. Progressive loss of anti-HER2 CD4(+) T-helper type 1 response in breast tumorigenesis and the potential for immune restoration. *Oncoimmunology.* 2015;4(10):e1022301. https://doi.org/10.1080/2162402x.2015.1022301. Epub 2015/10/10. PubMed PMID: 26451293; PMCID: PMC4589053.
2. Disis ML, Wallace DR, Gooley TA, et al. Concurrent trastuzumab and HER2/neu-specific vaccination in patients with metastatic breast cancer. *J Clin Oncol.* 2009;27(28): 4685–4692. https://doi.org/10.1200/jco.2008.20.6789. Epub 2009/09/02. PubMed PMID: 19720923; PMCID: PMC2754913.
3. Sica A, Larghi P, Mancino A, et al. Macrophage polarization in tumour progression. *Semin Cancer Biol.* 2008;18(5): 349–355. https://doi.org/10.1016/j.semcancer.2008.03.004. Epub 2008/05/10. PubMed PMID: 18467122.
4. Denkert C, Loibl S, Noske A, et al. Tumor-associated lymphocytes as an independent predictor of response to neoadjuvant chemotherapy in breast cancer. *J Clin Oncol.* 2010; 28(1):105–113. https://doi.org/10.1200/jco.2009.23.7370. Epub 2009/11/18. PubMed PMID: 19917869.
5. Loi S, Sirtaine N, Piette F, et al. Prognostic and predictive value of tumor-infiltrating lymphocytes in a phase III randomized adjuvant breast cancer trial in node-positive breast cancer comparing the addition of docetaxel to doxorubicin with doxorubicin-based chemotherapy: BIG 02-98. *J Clin Oncol.* 2013;31(7):860–867. https://doi.org/10.1200/jco.2011.41.0902. Epub 2013/01/24. PubMed PMID: 23341518.
6. Galon J, Costes A, Sanchez-Cabo F, et al. Type, density, and location of immune cells within human colorectal tumors predict clinical outcome. *Science (New York, NY).* 2006;313(5795):1960–1964. https://doi.org/10.1126/science.1129139. Epub 2006/09/30. PubMed PMID: 17008531.
7. Pages F, Berger A, Camus M, et al. Effector memory T cells, early metastasis, and survival in colorectal cancer. *N Engl J Med.* 2005;353(25):2654–2666. https://doi.org/10.1056/NEJMoa051424. Epub 2005/12/24. PubMed PMID: 16371631.
8. Stanton SE, Adams S, Disis ML. Variation in the incidence and magnitude of tumor-infiltrating lymphocytes in breast cancer subtypes: a systematic review. *JAMA Oncol.* 2016; 2(10):1354–1360. https://doi.org/10.1001/jamaoncol.2016.1061. Epub 2016/06/30. PubMed PMID: 27355489.
9. Loi S, Michiels S, Salgado R, et al. Tumor infiltrating lymphocytes are prognostic in triple negative breast cancer and predictive for trastuzumab benefit in early breast cancer: results from the FinHER trial. *Ann Oncol.* 2014;25(8):1544–1550. https://doi.org/10.1093/annonc/mdu112. Epub 2014/03/13. PubMed PMID: 24608200.
10. Gobert M, Treilleux I, Bendriss-Vermare N, et al. Regulatory T cells recruited through CCL22/CCR4 are selectively

activated in lymphoid infiltrates surrounding primary breast tumors and lead to an adverse clinical outcome. *Cancer Res.* 2009;69(5):2000–2009. https://doi.org/10.1158/0008-5472.can-08-2360. Epub 2009/02/27. PubMed PMID: 19244125.

11. Bense RD, Sotiriou C, Piccart-Gebhart MJ, et al. Relevance of tumor-infiltrating immune cell composition and functionality for disease outcome in breast cancer. *J Natl Cancer Inst.* 2017;109(1). https://doi.org/10.1093/jnci/djw192. Epub 2016/10/16. PubMed PMID: 27737921.

12. Petricevic B, Laengle J, Singer J, et al. Trastuzumab mediates antibody-dependent cell-mediated cytotoxicity and phagocytosis to the same extent in both adjuvant and metastatic HER2/neu breast cancer patients. *J Transl Med.* 2013;11:307. https://doi.org/10.1186/1479-5876-11-307. Epub 2013/12/18. PubMed PMID: 24330813; PMCID: PMC4029549.

13. Teschendorff AE, Gomez S, Arenas A, et al. Improved prognostic classification of breast cancer defined by antagonistic activation patterns of immune response pathway modules. *BMC Cancer.* 2010;10:604. https://doi.org/10.1186/1471-2407-10-604. Epub 2010/11/06. PubMed PMID: 21050467; PMCID: PMC2991308.

14. Denkert C, von Minckwitz G, Brase JC, et al. Tumor-infiltrating lymphocytes and response to neoadjuvant chemotherapy with or without carboplatin in human epidermal growth factor receptor 2-positive and triple-negative primary breast cancers. *J Clin Oncol.* 2015;33(9):983–991. https://doi.org/10.1200/jco.2014.58.1967. Epub 2014/12/24. PubMed PMID: 25534375.

15. Jacquemier J, Bertucci F, Finetti P, et al. High expression of indoleamine 2,3-dioxygenase in the tumour is associated with medullary features and favourable outcome in basal-like breast carcinoma. *Int J Cancer.* 2012;130(1):96–104. https://doi.org/10.1002/ijc.25979. Epub 2011/02/18. PubMed PMID: 21328335.

16. Muenst S, Soysal SD, Gao F, Obermann EC, Oertli D, Gillanders WE. The presence of programmed death 1 (PD-1)-positive tumor-infiltrating lymphocytes is associated with poor prognosis in human breast cancer. *Breast Cancer Res Treat.* 2013;139(3):667–676. https://doi.org/10.1007/s10549-013-2581-3. Epub 2013/06/13. PubMed PMID: 23756627; PMCID: PMC3885332.

17. Bae SB, Cho HD, Oh MH, et al. Expression of programmed death receptor ligand 1 with high tumor-infiltrating lymphocytes is associated with better prognosis in breast cancer. *J Breast Cancer.* 2016;19(3):242–251. https://doi.org/10.4048/jbc.2016.19.3.242. Epub 2016/10/11. PubMed PMID: 27721873; PMCID: PMC5053308.

18. Ghebeh H, Mohammed S, Al-Omair A, et al. The B7-H1 (PD-L1) T lymphocyte-inhibitory molecule is expressed in breast cancer patients with infiltrating ductal carcinoma: correlation with important high-risk prognostic factors. *Neoplasia (New York, NY).* 2006;8(3):190–198. https://doi.org/10.1593/neo.05733. Epub 2006/04/14. PubMed PMID: 16611412; PMCID: PMC1578520.

19. Brown JA, Dorfman DM, Ma FR, et al. Blockade of programmed death-1 ligands on dendritic cells enhances T cell activation and cytokine production. *J Immunol (Baltim, Md: 1950).* 2003;170(3):1257–1266. Epub 2003/01/23. PubMed PMID: 12538684.

20. Schalper KA, Velcheti V, Carvajal D, et al. In situ tumor PD-L1 mRNA expression is associated with increased TILs and better outcome in breast carcinomas. *Clin Cancer Res.* 2014;20(10):2773–2782. https://doi.org/10.1158/1078-0432.ccr-13-2702. Epub 2014/03/22. PubMed PMID: 24647569.

21. Qin T, Zeng YD, Qin G, et al. High PD-L1 expression was associated with poor prognosis in 870 Chinese patients with breast cancer. *Oncotarget.* 2015;6(32):33972–33981. https://doi.org/10.18632/oncotarget.5583. Epub 2015/09/18. PubMed PMID: 26378017; PMCID: PMC4741818.

22. Ghebeh H, Lehe C, Barhoush E, et al. Doxorubicin downregulates cell surface B7-H1 expression and upregulates its nuclear expression in breast cancer cells: role of B7-H1 as an anti-apoptotic molecule. *Breast Cancer Res.* 2010;12(4):R48. https://doi.org/10.1186/bcr2605. Epub 2010/07/16. PubMed PMID: 20626886; PMCID: PMC2949635.

23. Fridman WH, Zitvogel L, Sautes-Fridman C, Kroemer G. The immune contexture in cancer prognosis and treatment. *Nat Rev Clin Oncol.* 2017;14(12):717–734. https://doi.org/10.1038/nrclinonc.2017.101. Epub 2017/07/26. PubMed PMID: 28741618.

24. Kim A, Lee SJ, Kim YK, et al. Programmed death-ligand 1 (PD-L1) expression in tumour cell and tumour infiltrating lymphocytes of HER2-positive breast cancer and its prognostic value. *Sci Rep.* 2017;7(1):11671. https://doi.org/10.1038/s41598-017-11905-7. Epub 2017/09/17. PubMed PMID: 28916815; PMCID: PMC5601941.

25. Elliott MR, Ravichandran KS. The dynamics of apoptotic cell clearance. *Dev Cell.* 2016;38(2):147–160. https://doi.org/10.1016/j.devcel.2016.06.029. Epub 2016/07/28. PubMed PMID: 27459067; PMCID: PMC4966906.

26. Kini Bailur J, Gueckel B, Pawelec G. Prognostic impact of high levels of circulating plasmacytoid dendritic cells in breast cancer. *J Transl Med.* 2016;14(1):151. https://doi.org/10.1186/s12967-016-0905-x. Epub 2016/05/29. PubMed PMID: 27234566; PMCID: PMC4884426.

27. Treilleux I, Blay JY, Bendriss-Vermare N, et al. Dendritic cell infiltration and prognosis of early stage breast cancer. *Clin Cancer Res.* 2004;10(22):7466–7474. https://doi.org/10.1158/1078-0432.ccr-04-0684. Epub 2004/12/01. PubMed PMID: 15569976.

28. Trinchieri G. Biology of natural killer cells. *Adv Immunol.* 1989;47:187–376. Epub 1989/01/01. PubMed PMID: 2683611.

29. Vivier E, Tomasello E, Baratin M, Walzer T, Ugolini S. Functions of natural killer cells. *Nat Immunol.* 2008;9(5):503–510. https://doi.org/10.1038/ni1582. Epub 2008/04/22. PubMed PMID: 18425107.

30. Muraro E, Martorelli D, Turchet E, et al. A different immunologic profile characterizes patients with HER-2-

overexpressing and HER-2-negative locally advanced breast cancer: implications for immune-based therapies. *Breast Cancer Res.* 2011;13(6):R117. https://doi.org/10.1186/bcr3060. Epub 2011/11/25. PubMed PMID: 22112244; PMCID: PMC3326559.

31. Muraro E, Comaro E, Talamini R, et al. Improved natural killer cell activity and retained anti-tumor CD8(+) T cell responses contribute to the induction of a pathological complete response in HER2-positive breast cancer patients undergoing neoadjuvant chemotherapy. *J Transl Med.* 2015;13:204. https://doi.org/10.1186/s12967-015-0567-0. Epub 2015/06/28. PubMed PMID: 26116238; PMCID: PMC4483222.

32. Mamessier E, Sylvain A, Thibult ML, et al. Human breast cancer cells enhance self tolerance by promoting evasion from NK cell antitumor immunity. *J Clin Investig.* 2011;121(9):3609−3622. https://doi.org/10.1172/jci45816. Epub 2011/08/16. PubMed PMID: 21841316; PMCID: PMC3171102.

33. Mamessier E, Sylvain A, Bertucci F, et al. Human breast tumor cells induce self-tolerance mechanisms to avoid NKG2D-mediated and DNAM-mediated NK cell recognition. *Cancer Res.* 2011;71(21):6621−6632. https://doi.org/10.1158/0008-5472.can-11-0792. Epub 2011/09/23. PubMed PMID: 21937679.

34. Alexe G, Dalgin GS, Scanfeld D, et al. High expression of lymphocyte-associated genes in node-negative HER2+ breast cancers correlates with lower recurrence rates. *Cancer Res.* 2007;67(22):10669−10676. https://doi.org/10.1158/0008-5472.can-07-0539. Epub 2007/11/17. PubMed PMID: 18006808.

35. Thiery JP, Sleeman JP. Complex networks orchestrate epithelial-mesenchymal transitions. *Nat Rev Mol Cell Biol.* 2006;7(2):131−142. https://doi.org/10.1038/nrm1835. Epub 2006/02/24. PubMed PMID: 16493418.

36. Liguori M, Solinas G, Germano G, Mantovani A, Allavena P. Tumor-associated macrophages as incessant builders and destroyers of the cancer stroma. *Cancers.* 2011;3(4):3740−3761. https://doi.org/10.3390/cancers3043740. Epub 2011/01/01. PubMed PMID: 24213109; PMCID: PMC3763394.

37. Quatromoni JG, Eruslanov E. Tumor-associated macrophages: function, phenotype, and link to prognosis in human lung cancer. *Am J Transl Res.* 2012;4(4):376−389. Epub 2012/11/13. PubMed PMID: 23145206; PMCID: PMC3493031.

38. Heusinkveld M, van der Burg SH. Identification and manipulation of tumor associated macrophages in human cancers. *J Transl Med.* 2011;9:216. https://doi.org/10.1186/1479-5876-9-216. Epub 2011/12/20. PubMed PMID: 22176642; PMCID: PMC3286485.

39. Klingen TA, Chen Y, Aas H, Wik E, Akslen LA. Tumor-associated macrophages are strongly related to vascular invasion, non-luminal subtypes, and interval breast cancer. *Hum Pathol.* 2017;69:72−80. https://doi.org/10.1016/j.humpath.2017.09.001. Epub 2017/09/20. PubMed PMID: 28923419.

40. Mahmoud SM, Lee AH, Paish EC, Macmillan RD, Ellis IO, Green AR. Tumour-infiltrating macrophages and clinical outcome in breast cancer. *J Clin Pathol.* 2012;65(2):159−163. https://doi.org/10.1136/jclinpath-2011-200355. Epub 2011/11/04. PubMed PMID: 22049225.

41. Theoharides TC, Valent P, Akin C. Mast cells, mastocytosis, and related disorders. *N Engl J Med.* 2015;373(19):1885−1886. https://doi.org/10.1056/NEJMc1510021. Epub 2015/11/05. PubMed PMID: 26535528.

42. Peng G, Wang HY, Peng W, Kiniwa Y, Seo KH, Wang RF. Tumor-infiltrating gammadelta T cells suppress T and dendritic cell function via mechanisms controlled by a unique toll-like receptor signaling pathway. *Immunity.* 2007;27(2):334−348. https://doi.org/10.1016/j.immuni.2007.05.020. Epub 2007/07/28. PubMed PMID: 17656116.

43. Slamon DJ, Leyland-Jones B, Shak S, et al. Use of chemotherapy plus a monoclonal antibody against HER2 for metastatic breast cancer that overexpresses HER2. *N Engl J Med.* 2001;344(11):783−792. https://doi.org/10.1056/nejm200103153441101. Epub 2001/03/15. PubMed PMID: 11248153.

44. Cho HS, Mason K, Ramyar KX, et al. Structure of the extracellular region of HER2 alone and in complex with the Herceptin Fab. *Nature.* 2003;421(6924):756−760. https://doi.org/10.1038/nature01392. Epub 2003/03/01. PubMed PMID: 12610629.

45. Lewis GD, Figari I, Fendly B, et al. Differential responses of human tumor cell lines to anti-p185HER2 monoclonal antibodies. *Cancer Immunol Immunother.* 1993;37(4):255−263. Epub 1993/09/01. PubMed PMID: 8102322.

46. Carter P, Presta L, Gorman CM, et al. Humanization of an anti-p185HER2 antibody for human cancer therapy. *Proc Natl Acad Sci USA.* 1992;89(10):4285−4289. Epub 1992/05/15. PubMed PMID: 1350088; PMCID: PMC49066.

47. Arnould L, Gelly M, Penault-Llorca F, et al. Trastuzumab-based treatment of HER2-positive breast cancer: an antibody-dependent cellular cytotoxicity mechanism? *Br J Cancer.* 2006;94(2):259−267. https://doi.org/10.1038/sj.bjc.6602930. Epub 2006/01/13. PubMed PMID: 16404427; PMCID: PMC2361112.

48. Lazar GA, Dang W, Karki S, et al. Engineered antibody Fc variants with enhanced effector function. *Proc Natl Acad Sci USA.* 2006;103(11):4005−4010. https://doi.org/10.1073/pnas.0508123103. Epub 2006/03/16. PubMed PMID: 16537476; PMCID: PMC1389705.

49. Perez EA, Ballman KV, Tenner KS, et al. Association of stromal tumor-infiltrating lymphocytes with recurrence-free survival in the N9831 adjuvant trial in patients with early-stage HER2-positive breast cancer. *JAMA Oncol.* 2016;2(1):56−64. https://doi.org/10.1001/jamaoncol.2015.3239. Epub 2015/10/16. PubMed PMID: 26469139; PMCID: PMC4713247.

50. Esteva FJ, Wang J, Lin F, et al. CD40 signaling predicts response to preoperative trastuzumab and concomitant paclitaxel followed by 5-fluorouracil, epirubicin, and cyclophosphamide in HER-2-overexpressing breast cancer. *Breast Cancer Res.* 2007;9(6):R87. https://doi.org/

10.1186/bcr1836. Epub 2007/12/19. PubMed PMID: 18086299; PMCID: PMC2246190.

51. Taylor C, Hershman D, Shah N, et al. Augmented HER-2 specific immunity during treatment with trastuzumab and chemotherapy. *Clin Cancer Res.* 2007;13(17): 5133–5143. https://doi.org/10.1158/1078-0432.ccr-07-0507. Epub 2007/09/06. PubMed PMID: 17785568.

52. Ladoire S, Arnould L, Mignot G, et al. T-bet expression in intratumoral lymphoid structures after neoadjuvant trastuzumab plus docetaxel for HER2-overexpressing breast carcinoma predicts survival. *Br J Cancer.* 2011;105(3): 366–371. https://doi.org/10.1038/bjc.2011.261. Epub 2011/07/14. PubMed PMID: 21750556; PMCID: PMC3172914.

53. Barok M, Isola J, Palyi-Krekk Z, et al. Trastuzumab causes antibody-dependent cellular cytotoxicity-mediated growth inhibition of submacroscopic JIMT-1 breast cancer xenografts despite intrinsic drug resistance. *Mol Cancer Ther.* 2007;6(7):2065–2072. https://doi.org/10.1158/1535-7163.mct-06-0766. Epub 2007/07/11. PubMed PMID: 17620435.

54. Musolino A, Naldi N, Bortesi B, et al. Immunoglobulin G fragment C receptor polymorphisms and clinical efficacy of trastuzumab-based therapy in patients with HER-2/neu-positive metastatic breast cancer. *J Clin Oncol.* 2008;26(11): 1789–1796. https://doi.org/10.1200/jco.2007.14.8957. Epub 2008/03/19. PubMed PMID: 18347005.

55. Clynes RA, Towers TL, Presta LG, Ravetch JV. Inhibitory Fc receptors modulate in vivo cytotoxicity against tumor targets. *Nat Med.* 2000;6(4):443–446. https://doi.org/10.1038/74704. Epub 2000/03/31. PubMed PMID: 10742152.

56. Kute T, Stehle Jr JR, Ornelles D, Walker N, Delbono O, Vaughn JP. Understanding key assay parameters that affect measurements of trastuzumab-mediated ADCC against Her2 positive breast cancer cells. *Oncoimmunology.* 2012; 1(6):810–821. https://doi.org/10.4161/onci.20447. Epub 2012/11/20. PubMed PMID: 23162748; PMCID: PMC3489736.

57. Varchetta S, Gibelli N, Oliviero B, et al. Elements related to heterogeneity of antibody-dependent cell cytotoxicity in patients under trastuzumab therapy for primary operable breast cancer overexpressing Her2. *Cancer Res.* 2007; 67(24):11991–11999. https://doi.org/10.1158/0008-5472.can-07-2068. Epub 2007/12/20. PubMed PMID: 18089830.

58. Beano A, Signorino E, Evangelista A, et al. Correlation between NK function and response to trastuzumab in metastatic breast cancer patients. *J Transl Med.* 2008;6:25. https://doi.org/10.1186/1479-5876-6-25. Epub 2008/05/20. PubMed PMID: 18485193; PMCID: PMC2415031.

59. Tamura K, Shimizu C, Hojo T, et al. FcgammaR2A and 3A polymorphisms predict clinical outcome of trastuzumab in both neoadjuvant and metastatic settings in patients with HER2-positive breast cancer. *Ann Oncol.* 2011; 22(6):1302–1307. https://doi.org/10.1093/annonc/mdq585. Epub 2010/11/27. PubMed PMID: 21109570.

60. Hurvitz SA, Betting DJ, Stern HM, et al. Analysis of Fcgamma receptor IIIa and IIa polymorphisms: lack of correlation with outcome in trastuzumab-treated breast cancer patients. *Clin Cancer Res.* 2012;18(12):3478–3486. https://doi.org/10.1158/1078-0432.ccr-11-2294. Epub 2012/04/17. PubMed PMID: 22504044; PMCID: PMC3821872.

61. Gavin PG, Song N, Kim SR, et al. Association of polymorphisms in FCGR2A and FCGR3A with degree of trastuzumab benefit in the adjuvant treatment of ERBB2/HER2-positive breast cancer: analysis of the NSABP B-31 trial. *JAMA Oncol.* 2017;3(3):335–341. https://doi.org/10.1001/jamaoncol.2016.4884. Epub 2016/11/05. PubMed PMID: 27812689; PMCID: PMC5344747.

62. Nordstrom JL, Gorlatov S, Zhang W, et al. Anti-tumor activity and toxicokinetics analysis of MGAH22, an anti-HER2 monoclonal antibody with enhanced Fcgamma receptor binding properties. *Breast Cancer Res.* 2011;13(6): R123. https://doi.org/10.1186/bcr3069. Epub 2011/12/02. PubMed PMID: 22129105; PMCID: PMC3326565.

63. Bang YJ, Giaccone G, Im SA, et al. First-in-human phase 1 study of margetuximab (MGAH22), an Fc-modified chimeric monoclonal antibody, in patients with HER2-positive advanced solid tumors. *Ann Oncol.* 2017;28(4): 855–861. https://doi.org/10.1093/annonc/mdx002. Epub 2017/01/26. PubMed PMID: 28119295.

64. Adams CW, Allison DE, Flagella K, et al. Humanization of a recombinant monoclonal antibody to produce a therapeutic HER dimerization inhibitor, pertuzumab. *Cancer Immunol Immunother.* 2006;55(6):717–727. https://doi.org/10.1007/s00262-005-0058-x. Epub 2005/09/10. PubMed PMID: 16151804.

65. Scheuer W, Friess T, Burtscher H, Bossenmaier B, Endl J, Hasmann M. Strongly enhanced antitumor activity of trastuzumab and pertuzumab combination treatment on HER2-positive human xenograft tumor models. *Cancer Res.* 2009;69(24):9330–9336. https://doi.org/10.1158/0008-5472.can-08-4597. Epub 2009/11/26. PubMed PMID: 19934333.

66. Diessner J, Bruttel V, Becker K, et al. Targeting breast cancer stem cells with HER2-specific antibodies and natural killer cells. *Am J Cancer Res.* 2013;3(2):211–220. Epub 2013/04/18. PubMed PMID: 23593542; PMCID: PMC3623839.

67. Toth G, Szoor A, Simon L, Yarden Y, Szollosi J, Vereb G. The combination of trastuzumab and pertuzumab administered at approved doses may delay development of trastuzumab resistance by additively enhancing antibody-dependent cell-mediated cytotoxicity. *mAbs.* 2016;8(7):1361–1370. https://doi.org/10.1080/19420862.2016.1204503. Epub 2016/07/06. PubMed PMID: 27380003; PMCID: PMC5058622.

68. Chao MP, Jaiswal S, Weissman-Tsukamoto R, et al. Calreticulin is the dominant pro-phagocytic signal on multiple human cancers and is counterbalanced by CD47. *Sci Transl Med.* 2010;2(63):63ra94. https://doi.org/10.1126/scitranslmed.3001375. Epub 2010/12/24. PubMed PMID: 21178137; PMCID: PMC4126904.

69. Senovilla L, Vitale I, Martins I, et al. An immunosurveil-lance mechanism controls cancer cell ploidy. *Sci (New York, NY)*. 2012;337(6102):1678−1684. https://doi.org/10.1126/science.1224922. Epub 2012/09/29. PubMed PMID: 23019653.

70. Galluzzi L, Buque A, Kepp O, Zitvogel L, Kroemer G. Immunological effects of conventional chemotherapy and targeted anticancer agents. *Cancer Cell*. 2015;28(6):690−714. https://doi.org/10.1016/j.ccell.2015.10.012. Epub 2015/12/19. PubMed PMID: 26678337.

71. Lo CS, Sanii S, Kroeger DR, et al. Neoadjuvant chemo-therapy of ovarian cancer results in three patterns of tumor-infiltrating lymphocyte response with distinct im-plications for immunotherapy. *Clin Cancer Res*. 2017;23(4):925−934. https://doi.org/10.1158/1078-0432.ccr-16-1433. Epub 2016/09/08. PubMed PMID: 27601594.

72. Sevko A, Michels T, Vrohlings M, et al. Antitumor effect of paclitaxel is mediated by inhibition of myeloid-derived suppressor cells and chronic inflammation in the sponta-neous melanoma model. *J Immunol (Baltim Md 1950)*. 2013;190(5):2464−2471. https://doi.org/10.4049/jim-munol.1202781. Epub 2013/01/30. PubMed PMID: 23359505; PMCID: PMC3578135.

73. Liechtenstein T, Perez-Janices N, Gato M, et al. A highly efficient tumor-infiltrating MDSC differentiation system for discovery of anti-neoplastic targets, which circumvents the need for tumor establishment in mice. *Oncotarget*. 2014;5(17):7843−7857. https://doi.org/10.18632/onco-target. 2279. Epub 2014/08/26. PubMed PMID: 25151659; PMCID: PMC4202165.

74. Tsavaris N, Kosmas C, Vadiaka M, Kanelopoulos P, Boulamatsis D. Immune changes in patients with advanced breast cancer undergoing chemotherapy with taxanes. *Br J Cancer*. 2002;87(1):21−27. https://doi.org/10.1038/sj.bjc.6600347. Epub 2002/06/27. PubMed PMID: 12085250; PMCID: PMC2364288.

75. Pfannenstiel LW, Lam SS, Emens LA, Jaffee EM, Armstrong TD. Paclitaxel enhances early dendritic cell maturation and function through TLR4 signaling in mice. *Cell Immunol*. 2010;263(1):79−87. https://doi.org/10.1016/j.cellimm.2010.03.001. Epub 2010/03/30. PubMed PMID: 20346445; PMCID: PMC2862830.

76. Machiels JP, Reilly RT, Emens LA, et al. Cyclophosphamide, doxorubicin, and paclitaxel enhance the antitumor im-mune response of granulocyte/macrophage-colony stimu-lating factor-secreting whole-cell vaccines in HER-2/neu tolerized mice. *Cancer Res*. 2001;61(9):3689−3697. Epub 2001/04/28. PubMed PMID: 11325840.

77. Miura D, Yoneyama K, Furuhata Y, Shimizu K. Paclitaxel enhances antibody-dependent cell-mediated cytotoxicity of trastuzumab by rapid recruitment of natural killer cells in HER2-positive breast cancer. *J Nippon Med Sch (Nippon Ika Daigaku zasshi)*. 2014;81(4):211−220. Epub 2014/09/05. PubMed PMID: 25186575.

78. Diaz-Montero CM, Salem ML, Nishimura MI, Garrett-Mayer E, Cole DJ, Montero AJ. Increased circulating myeloid-derived suppressor cells correlate with clinical cancer stage, metastatic tumor burden, and doxorubicin-cyclophosphamide chemotherapy. *Cancer Immunol Immunother*. 2009;58(1):49−59. https://doi.org/10.1007/s00262-008-0523-4. Epub 2008/05/01. PubMed PMID: 18446337; PMCID: PMC3401888.

79. Ghiringhelli F, Menard C, Puig PE, et al. Metronomic cyclophosphamide regimen selectively depletes CD4+CD25+ regulatory T cells and restores T and NK effector functions in end stage cancer patients. *Cancer Immunol Immunother*. 2007;56(5):641−648. https://doi.org/10.1007/s00262-006-0225-8. Epub 2006/09/09. PubMed PMID: 16960692.

80. Chen G, Emens LA. Chemoimmunotherapy: reengineering tumor immunity. *Cancer Immunol Immunother*. 2013;62(2):203−216. https://doi.org/10.1007/s00262-012-1388-0. Epub 2013/02/08. PubMed PMID: 23389507; PMCID: PMC3608094.

81. Nizar S, Copier J, Meyer B, et al. T-regulatory cell modula-tion: the future of cancer immunotherapy? *Br J Cancer*. 2009;100(11):1697−1703. https://doi.org/10.1038/sj.bjc.6605040. Epub 2009/04/23. PubMed PMID: 19384299; PMCID: PMC2695683.

82. Knutson KL, Schiffman K, Cheever MA, Disis ML. Immuni-zation of cancer patients with a HER-2/neu, HLA-A2 pep-tide, p369-377, results in short-lived peptide-specific immunity. *Clin Cancer Res*. 2002;8(5):1014−1018. Epub 2002/05/15. PubMed PMID: 12006513.

83. Disis ML, Schiffman K, Gooley TA, McNeel DG, Rinn K, Knutson KL. Delayed-type hypersensitivity response is a pre-dictor of peripheral blood T-cell immunity after HER-2/neu peptide immunization. *Clin Cancer Res*. 2000;6(4):1347−1350. Epub 2000/04/25. PubMed PMID: 10778962.

84. Knutson KL, Schiffman K, Disis ML. Immunization with a HER-2/neu helper peptide vaccine generates HER-2/neu CD8 T-cell immunity in cancer patients. *J Clin Investig*. 2001;107(4):477−484. https://doi.org/10.1172/jci11752. Epub 2001/02/22. PubMed PMID: 11181647; PMCID: PMC199268.

85. Mittendorf EA, Clifton GT, Holmes JP, et al. Final report of the phase I/II clinical trial of the E75 (nelipepimut-S) vac-cine with booster inoculations to prevent disease recur-rence in high-risk breast cancer patients. *Ann Oncol*. 2014;25(9):1735−1742. https://doi.org/10.1093/annonc/mdu211. Epub 2014/06/08. PubMed PMID: 24907636; PMCID: PMC4143091.

86. Rayner JO, Dryga SA, Kamrud KI. Alphavirus vectors and vaccination. *Rev Med Virol*. 2002;12(5):279−296. https://doi.org/10.1002/rmv.360. Epub 2002/09/05. PubMed PMID: 12211042.

87. Pushko P, Parker M, Ludwig GV, Davis NL, Johnston RE, Smith JF. Replicon-helper systems from attenuated Vene-zuelan equine encephalitis virus: expression of heterolo-gous genes in vitro and immunization against heterologous pathogens in vivo. *Virology*. 1997;239(2):389−401. https://doi.org/10.1006/viro.1997.8878. Epub 1998/01/22. PubMed PMID: 9434729.

88. Pushko P, Bray M, Ludwig GV, et al. Recombinant RNA replicons derived from attenuated Venezuelan equine

encephalitis virus protect guinea pigs and mice from Ebola hemorrhagic fever virus. *Vaccine.* 2000;19(1):142−153. Epub 2000/08/05. PubMed PMID: 10924796.

89. Gwin WR, et al. Effect of alphavirus vaccine encoding HER2 during concurrent anti-HER2 therapies on induction of oligoclonal T cell and antibody responses against HER2. *J Clin Oncol.* 2015;33:3081.

90. Park JW, Melisko ME, Esserman LJ, Jones LA, Wollan JB, Sims R. Treatment with autologous antigen-presenting cells activated with the HER-2 based antigen Lapuleucel-T: results of a phase I study in immunologic and clinical activity in HER-2 overexpressing breast cancer. *J Clin Oncol.* 2007;25(24):3680−3687. https://doi.org/10.1200/jco.2006.10.5718. Epub 2007/08/21. PubMed PMID: 17704416.

91. Disis ML, Dang Y, Coveler AL, et al. HER-2/neu vaccine-primed autologous T-cell infusions for the treatment of advanced stage HER-2/neu expressing cancers. *Cancer Immunol Immunother.* 2014;63(2):101−109. https://doi.org/10.1007/s00262-013-1489-4. Epub 2013/10/29. PubMed PMID: 24162107; PMCID: PMC3945106.

92. Datta J, Berk E, Xu S, et al. Anti-HER2 CD4(+) T-helper type 1 response is a novel immune correlate to pathologic response following neoadjuvant therapy in HER2-positive breast cancer. *Breast Cancer Res.* 2015;17:71. https://doi.org/10.1186/s13058-015-0584-1. Epub 2015/05/23. PubMed PMID: 25997452; PMCID: PMC4488128.

93. Dirix LY, Takacs I, Jerusalem G, et al. Avelumab, an anti-PD-L1 antibody, in patients with locally advanced or metastatic breast cancer: a phase 1b JAVELIN Solid Tumor study. *Breast Cancer Res Treat.* 2017. https://doi.org/10.1007/s10549-017-4537-5. Epub 2017/10/25. PubMed PMID: 29063313.

94. Stagg J, Loi S, Divisekera U, et al. Anti-ErbB-2 mAb therapy requires type I and II interferons and synergizes with anti-PD-1 or anti-CD137 mAb therapy. *Proc Natl Acad Sci USA.* 2011;108(17):7142−7147. https://doi.org/10.1073/pnas.1016569108. Epub 2011/04/13. PubMed PMID: 21482773; PMCID: PMC3084100.

95. Karyampudi L, Lamichhane P, Scheid AD, et al. Accumulation of memory precursor CD8 T cells in regressing tumors following combination therapy with vaccine and anti-PD-1 antibody. *Cancer Res.* 2014;74(11):2974−2985. https://doi.org/10.1158/0008-5472.can-13-2564. Epub 2014/04/15. PubMed PMID: 24728077; PMCID: PMC4313351.

96. Loi S, et al. *Abstract GS2-06: Phase Ib/II Study Evaluating Safety and Efficacy of Pembrolizumab and Trastuzumab in Patients with Trastuzumab-Resistant HER2-Positive Metastatic Breast Cancer: Results from the PANACEA (IBCSG 45-13/BIG 4-13/KEYNOTE-014) Study.* 2018.

97. Mohammed ZM, Going JJ, Edwards J, Elsberger B, McMillan DC. The relationship between lymphocyte subsets and clinico-pathological determinants of survival in patients with primary operable invasive ductal breast cancer. *Br J Cancer.* 2013;109:1676−1684.

98. Junttila TT, Li G, Parsons K, Phillips GL, Sliwkowski MX. Trastuzumab-DM1 (T-DM1) retains all the mechanisms of action of trastuzumab and efficiently inhibits growth of lapatinib insensitive breast cancer. *Breast Cancer Res Treat.* 2011;128:347−356.

CHAPTER 14

Biosimilars for HER2-Positive Breast Cancer

HOPE S. RUGO, MD

INTRODUCTION

The use of trastuzumab, combined with the ability to identify breast cancers overexpressing HER2 or with *HER2* gene amplification, has dramatically changed the outcome of both early- and late-stage HER2 positive (HER2+) breast cancers, with improved response, duration of response, progression-free survival (PFS), and overall survival (OS).[1] The success of trastuzumab is due to the ability to identify a subset of tumors that almost all appear to respond to this targeted biologic agent, as well as the synergy of trastuzumab with chemotherapy and continued response to antibody following progression. One of the challenges of success, and for biologics in general, is the significant cost associated with treatment, which limits access in many parts of the world.

What is a biosimilar (Table 14.1)[2]? The concept of generic medications is familiar, whereby simple, small molecule chemicals are recreated, requiring only that the chemical structure and pharmacokinetics are similar to the original product. In contrast, biologics are large, complex molecules made in living cells, and due to variations in production and posttranslational modifications, even the current branded or reference product may be slightly different from the original agent depending on when and where it was produced.[3] Biosimilars are "similar" to these originator biologic compounds, and due to their complexity, the European Medicines Agency (EMA), Food and Drug Administration (FDA), and World Health Organization have developed guidelines for their development.[4] As the patent life ends or is close to ending on a number of novel biologic therapies for cancer therapy, the number of biosimilars in development has exploded, creating a new playing field important to providers, payers, and patients.[5] The primary patent for trastuzumab expired in the European Union (E.U.) in July of 2014 and will expire in the United States (U.S.) in June of 2019.

A number of biosimilars are already in clinical use; in the U.S., the first oncology biosimilar to be approved was for the myeloid growth factor filgrastim, and several agents are in clinical use in Europe. As of early 2018, one trastuzumab biosimilar is approved in the U.S. and two are approved in the E.U.; none is yet in the clinic, and numerous applications are pending.

Two other terms are used in reference to biologics: intended copies of biologic products ("me-too biologics") and biobetters. Intended copies are copies of already licensed biologic products that have not met the regulatory criteria for biosimilars, and biobetters are biologic agents that have been structurally and/or functionally altered to improve or change clinical performance. Biobetters must go through the full biologic agent development and approval process.

REQUIREMENTS FOR BIOSIMILARITY

The evaluation process of a proposed biosimilar is heavily weighted on proving similarity of structure, function, and biologic activity to the reference product[6] (Fig. 14.1). Indeed, there should be "no clinically meaningful differences between the biologic product and the reference product in terms of the safety, purity and potency of the product."[7] Unlike the reference product, which must show improved outcome compared with accepted standard treatment and where both clinical efficacy and safety have already been confirmed, the biosimilar must demonstrate similarity in analytical and preclinical testing, as well as in pharmacodynamics and pharmacokinetics. The final step in proving biosimilarity is to confirm safety and efficacy in the appropriate target population, along with evaluation of immunogenicity. One of the major challenges is defining the optimal population to detect any clinically meaningful differences between the biosimilar and the reference product. The basis for the clinical guidelines

TABLE 14.1
Difference Between Biologics and Generics

	Small Molecule Generics	Biologics
Produced by	Chemical synthesis	Living systems (cultured cells)
Characterization	Characterized with limited physicochemical methods	Comprehensive physicochemical analysis and bioassays
Manufacturing	Easy to reproduce	Manufacturing conditions are difficult and complicated by posttranslational modification
Safety considerations	Target-specific and off-target toxicity	Target-specific toxicity, off-target toxicity, characterization of immunogenicity (e.g., antidrug antibodies)

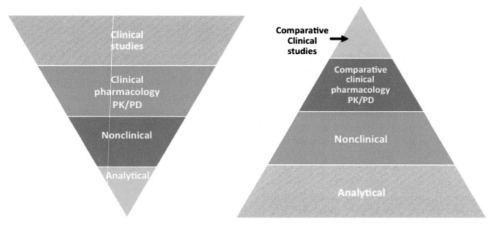

FIG. 14.1 Biosimilar development pathway. *PD*, pharmacodynamics; *PK*, pharmacokinetics.

for biosimilars is in demonstrating equivalence between short-term endpoints within a narrow margin to avoid the costly and larger trials required for approval of the reference product. It is important to ensure that a proposed biosimilarity has met strict regulatory guidelines, as some biologic biosimilars are in use in various countries around the world where the guidelines are much less strict and only a small trial assessing safety is required for approval.

ANALYTIC ASSESSMENT OF BIOSIMILARS

Extensive analytic assessment of proposed biosimilars is required.[8] This includes evaluation of primary (amino acid sequence), secondary, and tertiary structures, as well as posttranslational modifications (e.g., glycoforms, sialylation) and assessment of impurities. Similarity is required, as biologic products cannot be

identical, with drift seen even in the originator biologic.[3] Next, analytic testing must demonstrate similar biologic activity by functional characterization; for trastuzumab biosimilars, this includes assessment of HER2 by cellular and Fcγ receptor binding assays, antibody-dependent cellular cytotoxicity, and inhibition of proliferation, among others. Safety studies are also conducted in cardiomyocytes, and pharmacokinetic and toxicology studies are performed in nonhuman primates.

CLINICAL STUDIES

Assessment of biosimilarity starts with a comparison of pharmacokinetics between the proposed biosimilar and the originator biologic in a small number of patients. In the case of trastuzumab, U.S.- and E.U.-sourced trastuzumab is compared with the proposed biosimilar in healthy adults.[9,10] The final assessment of biosimilarity is a phase III trial comparing the proposed biosimilar with the originator product in a highly sensitive setting in which the primary endpoint is a marker of short-term efficacy. These trials must also include short- and long-term safety, evaluation of pharmacokinetics and immunogenicity with antidrug antibodies, and long-term measures of efficacy.[11]

There has been ongoing discussion about whether it is possible to define the optimal setting in which to evaluate a short-term efficacy endpoint with trastuzumab biosimilars. Centrally determined response rate is a generally acceptable end point that allows a smaller sample size and is a faster method of assessing drug activity. One concern has been the correlation of response with longer-term efficacy endpoints such as event-free survival (EFS) or PFS and OS. Two clinical settings are most relevant, either treatment of metastatic disease in the first-line setting with a primary endpoint of overall response rate (ORR) or as treatment in the neoadjuvant setting with a primary endpoint of pathologic complete response (pCR). For HER2+ disease, improvements in response in the first-line metastatic setting have generally correlated with both improved PFS and OS, and in the neoadjuvant setting, pCR correlates with disease-free survival and OS.[12-14]

Advantages can be found with evaluation of biosimilarity in both the neoadjuvant and metastatic settings. Patients treated in the neoadjuvant setting are naïve to prior therapy, whereas patients in the metastatic setting may have seen adjuvant or neoadjuvant trastuzumab. One metaanalysis of data from a number of clinical trials suggested smaller loss in long-term efficacy using pCR rather than ORR and concluded that the neoadjuvant setting could be the more optimal setting for the evaluation of biosimilars.[15] However, treatment following surgery may vary significantly, which could impact the secondary endpoint of EFS for neoadjuvant biosimilar studies, and exposure to therapy is limited to 1 year. Biosimilar trastuzumab trials in the first-line metastatic setting include a population of patients with limited access to trastuzumab or even HER2 testing, quite similar to the patients enrolled in the original pivotal trials that led to approval of trastuzumab. In addition, patients with stable or responding metastatic disease stay on antibody therapy until progression, providing long-term safety and immunogenicity data. Response rates are a short-term, sensitive measure of the clinical activity of proposed trastuzumab biosimilars; regulatory guidelines support these endpoints. Indeed, both the neoadjuvant and first-line metastatic setting provide the data needed to assess trastuzumab biosimilarity and to support extrapolation of use.

CLINICAL TRIALS

Five phase III trials have reported comparable efficacy using the regulatory guidelines defined by the FDA and EMA, two in the first-line metastatic setting (Table 14.2A) and three in the neoadjuvant setting (Table 14.2B).

The first published trial evaluated the pharmaceutical company Mylan's proposed biosimilar MYL0401O (trastuzumab-dkst, Ogivri) as first-line therapy for metastatic HER2+ breast cancer in a multicenter, double-blind, randomized, parallel group, phase III equivalence study.[16] Eligible patients were randomized to receive a taxane (84% received docetaxel) in combination with either the biosimilar or originator trastuzumab. Chemotherapy was administered for at least 24 weeks,

TABLE 14.2A
Biosimilar Phase III Trials With Primary Efficacy End Points. First-Line Therapy for Metastatic Breast Cancer

Biosimilar	N	Treatment	Primary Endpoint	Results	
				Risk Difference	Risk Ratio
[a]MYL-1401O[16] Trastuzmab-dkst	500	Taxane plus trastuzumab or MYL-1410lO	ORR (24 wk)	5.53 [95% CI −3.08% to 14.04%]	1.09 [90% CI 0.974 to 1.211]
[b]PF-05280014[18]	707	Paclitaxel plus trastuzumab or PF-05280014	ORR (25 wk)	N/A	0.94 [95% CI 0.842 to 1.049]

ORR, overall response rate; *wk*, week.
[a]Equivalence margins: risk difference [−15%, 15%]; risk ratio [0.81, 1.24].
[b]Equivalence margin: risk ratio [0.8, 1.25].

TABLE 14.2B
Biosimilar Phase III Trials With Primary Efficacy End Points. Neoadjuvant Therapy for Early-Stage Breast Cancer

Biosimilar	N	Treatment	Primary Endpoint	Results Risk Difference	Risk Ratio
[a]CT-P6[19]	549	D/FEC plus CT-P6 or trastuzumab × 1 year	Total pCR	−0.04% [95% CI −0.12% to 0.05%]	0.93 [95% CI 0.78, 1.11]
[b]SB-3[20]	800	D/FEC plus SB-3 or trastuzumab × 1 year	Breast pCR	10.70% [95% CI 4.13% to 17.26%]	1.259 [95% CI 1.08 to 1.460]
ABP 980[23]	725	EC followed by paclitaxel with ABP-90 or trastuzumab × 1 year	Total pCR	7.3% [90% CI 1.2% to 13.4%]	1.19 [90% CI 1.03 to 1.37]
[c]PF-05280014[22]	226	D/Ca plus PF-05280014 or trastuzumab × 6 cycles	PK at cycle 6, total pCR	NR	NR

D/Ca, docetaxel 75 mg/m^2 plus carboplatin with area under the curve 6 IV every 3 weeks × 6 cycles; D/FEC, docetaxel 75 mg/m^2 IV every 3 weeks × 4 cycles followed by 5-FU/epirubicin/cyclophosphamide (500 mg/m^2/75 mg/m^2/500 mg/m^2) IV every 3 weeks × 4 cycles with continuation of antibodies for 1 year; EC/paclitaxel, epirubicin 90 mg/m^2 IV every 3 weeks × 4 cycles followed by paclitaxel (weekly or every 3 weeks) × 12 weeks combined with antibodies, followed with antibodies for 1 year with an additional randomization between antibodies in the trastuzumab arm (see text); NR, not reported; pCR, pathologic complete response; PK, pharmacokinetics; total pCR, pCR in breast and lymph nodes.
[a]Equivalence margin: risk difference [−15%, 15%]; risk ratio [0·74, 1·35].
[b]Equivalence margin: risk difference [−13%, 13%]; risk ratio [0.785, 1.546].
[c]Equivalence margin: risk difference [−13%, 13%]; risk ratio [0.76, 1.32].

followed by antibody alone in patients with responding or stable disease until evidence of disease progression or toxicity mandated treatment discontinuation. Of the 458 eligible patients, less than 10% had received adjuvant trastuzumab. The primary outcome was ORR at week 24, and secondary endpoints included time to tumor progression (TTP), PFS, and OS at week 48, as well as development of anti–antibody drug antibodies (ADA) and safety. The ORR at 24 weeks was 69.6% (95% CI 63.62%–75.51%) and 64% (95% CI 57.81%–70.26%) for trastuzumab-dkst and trastuzumab, respectively. The ORR ratio and difference were within the predefined equivalence margins (Table 14.2A). At 48 weeks, there was no statistically significant difference between the biosimilar and trastuzumab in TTP (41.3% vs. 43.0%; −1.7%; 95% CI −11.1% to 6.9%), PFS (44.3% vs. 44.7%; −0.4%; 95% CI −9.4% to 8.7%), or OS (89.1% vs. 85.1%; 4.0%; 95% CI −2.1% to 10.3%). Of note, due to the low number of events, survival data are still immature. There was no clinically significant difference in toxicity, including cardiac events, and ADA were detected in a small number of patients in each arm.

Based on this data, Mylan's proposed biosimilar was approved in the U.S. using "comparisons of extensive structural and functional product characterization, animal data, human pharmacokinetic and pharmacodynamic data, and clinical studies including clinical immunogenicity between Ogivri and U.S.-licensed Herceptin."[17] Furthermore, the FDA approval states that "these data demonstrate that Ogivri is highly similar to U.S.-licensed Herceptin and that there are no clinically meaningful differences between the products." Approval was granted for all indications currently held for trastuzumab, including HER2+ gastric cancer and early- and late-stage breast cancer, although it will not be available in the clinic until the U.S. patent expires in mid-2019.

Another randomized, double-blind, phase III trial has been conducted in the first-line metastatic setting comparing the proposed trastuzumab biosimilar PF-05280014 with trastuzumab given in combination with weekly paclitaxel for at least 33 weeks, followed by antibody therapy alone until progression or toxicity.[18] About 10% of the 707 randomized patients had previous exposure to adjuvant trastuzumab. The primary endpoint of ORR was similar between the two arms at 62.5% (95% CI 57.2%–67.6%) and 66.5% (95% CI 61.3%–71.4%) for the biosimilar and originator, respectively. The risk ratio for response was within the equivalence margin (Table 14.2A), and secondary endpoints, including 1 year PFS (56% vs.

52%) and OS (88.84% vs. 87.96%), were also similar. There was no difference in safety or immunogenicity, and applications for approval are pending.

Three trastuzumab biosimilars have been tested in the neoadjuvant setting, and two are now approved for use in the E.U. The first study to be published, and the first biosimilar to trastuzumab to be approved in the E.U., is CT-P6.[19] In a randomized, double-blind, active-controlled, phase III equivalence trial, patients with stage I–III HER2+ breast cancer were treated with docetaxel 75 mg/m^2 IV every 3 weeks for 4 cycles followed by 5-FU 500 mg/m,^{2} epirubicin 75 mg/m^2 and cyclophosphamide 500 mg/m^2 IV every 3 weeks × 4 cycles (D/FEC) and were randomized to receive either concurrent CT-P6 or trastuzumab. Following chemotherapy, patients underwent surgery followed by infusions of the originally assigned antibody every 3 weeks to complete 1 year of therapy. The primary endpoint was pCR in breast and axillary nodes with secondary endpoints including long-term safety and efficacy 3 years after the last patient started therapy. Efficacy met the predetermined equivalence margin for both risk difference and risk ratio (Table 14.2B) with pCR rates of 46% (95% CI 40.4–53.2) and 50.4% (95% CI 44.1–56.7) for CT-P6 and trastuzumab, respectively. There were no differences in safety or immunogenicity (negative ADAs). Long-term follow-up is ongoing.

The second trastuzumab biosimilar to gain approval in the E.U. is SB-3. In this phase III, randomized, double-blind study, 800 patients with stage II–III HER2+ breast cancer were treated with D/FEC with either SB-3 or trastuzumab followed by surgery and the assigned antibody to complete 1 year.[20] The primary endpoint was breast pCR. Secondary endpoints included pCR in breast and axillary nodes, safety, and EFS and OS at 1 year. Breast pCR was similar between the two arms (51.7% vs. 42.0% in the SB-3 and trastuzumab arms, respectively), and both the risk difference and risk ratio met the equivalence margins (Table 14.2B). pCR in breast and node was also similar (45.8% vs. 35.8%, respectively), and there were no differences in safety endpoints, including cardiac function and immunogenicity. At a median follow-up of just over 1 year, the incidence of treatment-emergent adverse events was comparable between the two arms, and only three patients in each arm had evidence of ADAs. EFS was also similar with a hazard ratio of 0.94 (92.2% and 91.6%, SB-3 vs. trastuzumab; 95% CI 0.59–1.51), as was OS (99.8% and 98.9%).[21]

Two additional neoadjuvant trials have been reported; both agents have applications pending for biosimilar approval. The neoadjuvant PF-0520014 trial randomized 226 patients with early-stage HER2+ disease to receive docetaxel 75 mgm^2 plus carboplatin (area under the curve = 6) IV every 3 weeks × 6 with either the proposed biosimilar or trastuzumab, followed by surgery.[22] The primary endpoint for this trial was noninferiority in the percentage of patients with cycle 5 trough concentration >20 µg/mL, which was achieved in 92.1% and 93.3% of patients receiving PF-0520014 and trastuzumab, respectively, meeting the noninferiority margin for the difference between the two groups of −12.5% (lower limit of 95% CI, −8.02% to 6.49%). Efficacy, measured by pCR in breast and node, was also similar (47.0%, 95% CI 36.9%–57.2% for PF-05280014; and 50.0%, 95% CI 80.2%–93.7% for trastuzumab). Adverse events were similar in number, and ADA rates were very low in both arms.

The ABP-90 phase III neoadjuvant trial has an additional design plan that incorporates switching between the biosimilar and originator antibody.[23] Patients with ≥2 cm HER2+ early-stage breast cancer were treated with epirubicin 90 mg/m^2 plus cyclophosphamide 600 mg/m^2 IV every 3 weeks × 4 cycles, followed by either ABP-90 or trastuzumab with every 3 week or weekly paclitaxel (taxane schedule per investigator choice) for 12 weeks followed by surgery. After surgery, patients initially randomized to ABP-90 continued on this antibody to complete 1 year. Patients initially randomized to trastuzumab were re-randomized to receive either ABP-90 or trastuzumab for their remaining treatment. The primary endpoint was pCR in breast and nodes, which was similar between the two arms at 48% and 40.5% for ABP-90 or trastuzumab, respectively. Both the risk difference and risk ratio fell within the prespecified equivalency margins (Table 14.2B). Patients who switched from trastuzumab to ABP-90 had no difference in safety or efficacy compared with those who stayed on trastuzumab or those who stayed on ABP-90 with short follow-up.[24,25]

All five biosimilars described above have submitted applications for regulatory approval in both the U.S. and E.U. As noted, one biosimilar is approved in the U.S. and two in the E.U. Several other biosimilars have been evaluated in small, randomized trials primarily focusing on safety.

PHARMACOVIGILANCE

Postregulatory approval pharmacovigilance is a critical and required component of the incorporation of biosimilars into clinical practice with guidelines in place in the U.S. and E.U. Pharmacovigilance includes focused monitoring and careful safety reporting with ongoing assessment of the adverse effects to generate postmarketing surveillance data.

EXTRAPOLATION AND INTERCHANGEABILITY

Extrapolation means that the use of an approved biosimilar in one setting could be extrapolated to any setting in which the originator is approved and for which there is sufficient scientific justification for use.[26] Does equivalency in one setting mean that clinicians can be confident in similar effectiveness across indications? Extrapolation is a critical component of biosimilar development and is based on demonstrating comparability of safety, efficacy, and immunogenicity without clinically relevant differences in a sensitive and key clinical indication. It is only with extrapolation that development can be streamlined to reduce the marketed cost of the biosimilar and improve access. Indeed, Mylan's trastuzumab biosimilar was approved for HER2-overexpressing breast cancer and metastatic gastric or gastroesophageal junction adenocarcinoma. Given the efficacy and safety of trastuzumab across indications and with multiple different combinations (including the antibody pertuzumab) without unexpected safety or pharmacokinetic concerns,[14] extrapolation for agents that meet the strict criteria for regulatory approval seems reasonable and safe without additional data.[27]

The FDA has issued draft guidance on biosimilar interchangeability, a designation that would allow pharmacy substitution for biosimilars without concern about safety or efficacy. A biologic product must be tested in a dedicated switching study evaluating pharmacokinetics, pharmacodynamics, immunogenicity, and safety, although demonstration of efficacy is not required for the switch, given that the study designs would not allow this. No product has yet received this designation. A study evaluating the safety of switching from the originator trastuzumab to a biosimilar in the adjuvant setting[24] is the first step in approaching interchangeability. It is not clear which trials or how much data will be required to obtain this designation. In general, physicians as prescribers should be involved in these decisions on an individual patient level.

Naming

The naming of biosimilars follows regulatory guidelines and differs between the U.S. and E.U., as well as other countries. The U.S. FDA has determined that biosimilars will use the generic name followed by a series of four meaningless initials to avoid association with specific companies. For example, Mylan's trastuzumab biosimilar is named trastuzumab-dkst (brand name Ogivri).

FUTURE STEPS

The good news is that there are now approved trastuzumab biosimilars in oncology that are expected to be available for clinical use in the near future. One trastuzumab biosimilar is approved in the U.S. and two are approved in the E.U., with many applications pending. It is encouraging to see similar efficacy and safety at the completion of adjuvant therapy, as well as after maintenance therapy in the metastatic setting. Use of biosimilar trastuzumab with extrapolation was recently endorsed by the St. Gallen International Expert Consensus Conference.[28]

Biosimilars of trastuzumab, a life-saving biologic therapy, are expected to reduce cost and to improve access to biologic therapy worldwide.[29]

It has been estimated that use of biosimilars will result in at least a 20%−30% cost reduction, and this may increase with increasing competition. Given that breast cancer is the most common cancer diagnosis in women worldwide and that HER2+ disease comprises about 20% of those cases, the availability of lower-cost trastuzumab biosimilars also has the potential to significantly improve disease outcomes. In countries where the originator product is readily available, availability of lower-cost alternatives that have been rigorously tested following international regulatory guidelines will help defray the overall increasing costs of oncologic care with an expanding range of biologic therapies.

REFERENCES

1. Jiang H, Rugo HS. Human epidermal growth factor receptor 2 positive (HER2+) metastatic breast cancer: how the latest results are improving therapeutic options. *Ther Adv Med Oncol.* 2015;7(6):321−339.
2. Buske C, Ogura M, Kwon HC, Yoon SW. An introduction to biosimilar cancer therapeutics: definitions, rationale for development and regulatory requirements. *Future Oncol.* 2017;13(15s):5−16.
3. Kim S, Song J, Park S, et al. Drifts in ADCC-related quality attributes of Herceptin(R): impact on development of a trastuzumab biosimilar. *MAbs.* 2017;9(4):704−714.
4. Coiffier B. Preparing for a new generation of biologic therapies: understanding the development and potential of biosimilar cancer therapeutics. *Future Oncol.* 2017; 13(15s):1−3.
5. Reinke T. The biosimilar pipeline seams seem to Be bursting. *Manag Care.* 2017;26(3):24−25.

6. Rugo HS, Linton KM, Cervi P, Rosenberg JA, Jacobs I. A clinician's guide to biosimilars in oncology. *Cancer Treat Rev.* 2016;46:73–79.

7. FDA. *Guidance for Industry: Scientific Considerations in Demonstrating Biosimilarity to a Reference Product*; 2015. http://www.fda.gov/downloads/DrugsGuidanceCompliance RegulatoryInformation/Guidances/UCM291128.pdf.

8. Hurst S, Ryan AM, Ng CK, et al. Comparative nonclinical assessments of the proposed biosimilar PF-05280014 and trastuzumab (Herceptin(R)). *BioDrugs.* 2014;28(5):451–459.

9. Yin D, Barker KB, Li R, et al. A randomized phase 1 pharmacokinetic trial comparing the potential biosimilar PF-05280014 with trastuzumab in healthy volunteers (REFLECTIONS B327-01). *Br J Clin Pharmacol.* 2014;78(6): 1281–1290.

10. Esteva FJ, Stebbing J, Wood-Horrall RN, Winkle PJ, Lee SY, Lee SJ. A randomised trial comparing the pharmacokinetics and safety of the biosimilar CT-P6 with reference trastuzumab. *Cancer Chemother Pharmacol.* 2018.

11. Markus R, Liu J, Ramchandani M, Landa D, Born T, Kaur P. Developing the totality of evidence for biosimilars: regulatory considerations and building confidence for the healthcare community. *BioDrugs.* 2017;31(3):175–187.

12. Cortazar P, Zhang L, Untch M, et al. Pathological complete response and long-term clinical benefit in breast cancer: the CTNeoBC pooled analysis. *Lancet.* 2014;384(9938): 164–172.

13. Slamon D, Eiermann W, Robert N, et al. Adjuvant trastuzumab in HER2-positive breast cancer. *N Engl J Med.* 2011; 365(14):1273–1283.

14. Swain SM, Kim SB, Cortes J, et al. Pertuzumab, trastuzumab, and docetaxel for HER2-positive metastatic breast cancer (CLEOPATRA study): overall survival results from a randomised, double-blind, placebo-controlled, phase 3 study. *Lancet Oncol.* 2013;14(6):461–471.

15. Jackisch C, Scappaticci FA, Heinzmann D, et al. Neoadjuvant breast cancer treatment as a sensitive setting for trastuzumab biosimilar development and extrapolation. *Future Oncol.* 2015;11(1):61–71.

16. Rugo HS, Barve A, Waller CF, et al. Effect of a proposed trastuzumab biosimilar compared with trastuzumab on overall response rate in patients with ERBB2 (HER2)-positive metastatic breast cancer: a randomized clinical trial. *JAMA.* 2017;317(1):37–47.

17. FDA. *FDA Approves Ogivri as a Biosimilar to Herceptin*; 2017. https://www.fda.gov/Drugs/InformationOnDrugs/Approved Drugs/ucm587404.htm.

18. Pegram M, Tan-Chiu E, Freyman A, et al. A randomized, double-blind study of PF-05280014 (a potential trastuzumab biosimilar) vs trastuzumab, both in combination with paclitaxel, as first-line treatment for HER2-positive metastatic breast cancer. *ESMO Conf Proc.* 2017: Abstr #238PD.

19. Stebbing J, Baranau Y, Baryash V, et al. CT-P6 compared with reference trastuzumab for HER2-positive breast cancer: a randomised, double-blind, active-controlled, phase 3 equivalence trial. *Lancet Oncol.* 2017.

20. Pivot X, Bondarenko I, Nowecki Z, et al. Phase III, randomized, double-blind study comparing the efficacy, safety, and immunogenicity of SB3 (trastuzumab biosimilar) and reference trastuzumab in patients treated with neoadjuvant therapy for human epidermal growth factor receptor 2-positive early breast cancer. *J Clin Oncol.* 2018: JCO2017740126.

21. Pivot X, Bondarenko I, Nowecki Z, et al. A phase III study comparing SB3 (a proposed trastuzumab biosimilar) and trastuzumab reference product in HER2-positive early breast cancer treated with neoadjuvant-adjuvant treatment: final safety, immunogenicity and survival results. *Eur J Cancer.* 2018;93:19–27.

22. Lammers PE, Dank M, Masetti R, et al. A randomized, double-blind study of PF-05280014 (a potential biosimilar) vs trastuzumab, both given with docetaxel (D) and carboplatin (C), as neoadjuvant treatment for operable human epidermal growth factor receptor 2-positive (HER21) breast cancer. *ESMO Conf Proc.* 2017: Abstr # 154PD.

23. von Minckwitz G, Ponomarova O, Morales S, Zhang N, Hanes V. Efficacy and safety of biosimilar ABP 980 compared with trastuzumab in HER2 positive early breast cancer. *ESMO Conf Proc.* 2017: Abstr #151PD.

24. von Minckwitz G, Turdean M, Zhang N, Santi P, Hanes V. Biosimilar ABP 980 in patients with early breast cancer: results of single switch from trastuzumab to ABP 980. *SABCS Conf Proc.* 2017: Abstr #P5-20-13.

25. Kolberg H-C, Demetriou GS, Zhang N, Tomasevic Z, Hanes V. Safety results from a randomized, double-blind, phase 3 study of ABP 980 compared with trastuzumab in patients with breast cancer. *SABCS Conf Proc.* 2017: Abstr #PD3–10.

26. Declerck P, Danesi R, Petersel D, Jacobs I. The language of biosimilars: clarification, definitions, and regulatory aspects. *Drugs.* 2017;77(6):671–677.

27. Cohen HP, Blauvelt A, Rifkin RM, Danese S, Gokhale SB, Woollett G. Switching reference Medicines to biosimilars: a systematic literature review of clinical outcomes. *Drugs.* 2018.

28. Curigliano G, Burstein HJ, Winer EP, et al. De-escalating and escalating treatments for early-stage breast cancer: the St. Gallen international Expert Consensus Conference on the primary therapy of early breast cancer 2017. *Ann Oncol.* 2017;28(8):1700–1712.

29. Yu B. Greater potential cost savings with biosimilar use. *Am J Manag Care.* 2016;22(5):378.

Index

Note: Page numbers followed by "f" indicate figures, "t" indicate tables.

Printed in the United States
By Bookmasters